Arts and Health Promotion

J. Hope Corbin • Mariana Sanmartino
Emily Alden Hennessy • Helga Bjørnøy Urke
Editors

Arts and Health Promotion

Tools and Bridges for Practice, Research, and Social Transformation

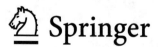 Springer

Editors
J. Hope Corbin ⓘD
Department of Health and
Community Studies
Western Washington University
Bellingham, WA, USA

Emily Alden Hennessy ⓘD
Department of Psychology
Institute for Collaboration on Health
Intervention & Policy
University of Connecticut
Storrs, CT, USA

Mariana Sanmartino ⓘD
Grupo de Didáctica de las Ciencias
IFLYSIB, CONICET - UNLP
Grupo ¿De qué hablamos
cuando hablamos de Chagas?
La Plata, Buenos Aires, Argentina

Helga Bjørnøy Urke ⓘD
Faculty of Psychology, Department of
Health Promotion and Development
University of Bergen
Bergen, Norway

This book is an open access publication.
ISBN 978-3-030-56419-3   ISBN 978-3-030-56417-9   (eBook)
https://doi.org/10.1007/978-3-030-56417-9

Foreword

As a scientific discipline, health promotion has expanded beyond its earlier roots of one-way information dissemination in health education into to a broader, more inclusive approach that considers community perspectives. Since the Ottawa Charter, the field of health promotion has been evolving at a rapid pace, as our understanding of human behavior has deepened; our policy and programs have become more nuanced. The Charter, and subsequent global agreements and frameworks, has further expanded our work and led to the current emphasis on the Social Determinants of Health in designing and developing health-promoting settings, initiatives, and policies.

The potential of the Arts as a powerful force to guide and influence health promotion offers endless possibilities to reach and engage the public in new and creative action around health-related issues and well-being. In its myriad forms (painting, plays, photography, song, etc.), the Arts provide a solid medium through which the fusion of culture as well as equity and human rights concerns can be integrated into health promotion policy and practice. Artistic approaches serve the social justice aims of health promotion by providing tangible means to facilitate the amplification of sidelined "voices" and increasing the visibility of invisible or hidden aspects of health and well-being.

This book, *Arts and Health Promotion: Tools and Bridges for Practice, Research, and Social Transformation,* positions the transformative role of the co-creation of knowledge and illustrates how various creative forms of expression have been applied and can be advanced into an important new dimension of health promotion. Filled with rich examples using different art forms to promote health through practice, research, and social mobilization, this book is a "must read" for policymakers and field practitioners. It is also an excellent resource for students, researchers, and scholars, as preparation for the next generation of health promoters.

The book also illustrates a commitment to shaking up traditional flows of knowledge. The examples of arts-based health promotion presented in the book reflect many homegrown projects from across the globe that demonstrate alternatives to top-down interventions. This volume is a great example of why organizations such as the International Union for Health Promotion and Education (IUHPE) are so important. The IUHPE's bringing together of practitioners, researchers, and policy-makers helps strengthen the field of health promotion by setting the foundation for this exploration of the Arts as a multiway communication channel that can be used and adapted to respond to new and ongoing local problems and global challenges, such as COVID-19, climate change, and systemic racism and resulting inequities. The editorial team's roots as leaders of a network within the IUHPE and the contributions to the volume of many IUHPE members demonstrate how global connections can contribute to equity and diversity of thought.

Erma Manoncourt, PhD
Board Member and Co-Chair, Global Working Group on the Social Determinants of Health, International Union of Health Promotion and Education (IUHPE)
Adjunct Professor, PSIA–Sciences PO
Paris, France

Acknowledgments

The editors would like to thank all the contributors to this volume. We are grateful to have been able to work with you over the past 3 years to bring your important work to publication. We are also grateful to Maurice Mittelmark and Erma Manoncourt for their support before and during this project and to Janet Kim at Springer— who has a wonderful way of working and walked with us every step of the journey. Many thanks to Jenn Cassie, our phenomenal copyeditor, and to the anonymous peer reviewers who made great suggestions to improve the work.

We are incredibly appreciative of the professional network of the International Union for Health Promotion and Education (IUHPE), which served as the birthplace of this work, connected us with many of our authors, and strives to provide space and opportunities for the global learning needed to authentically promote health and social justice.

We would also like to thank our families. Especially our children (Simón, Kell, Roque, Tessa, Sunniva, Saoirse, Ola, and Caoimhe)—two of whom were born over the course of this process and all of whom served as both inspiration and support by demonstrating endless patience with their busy mothers, especially during the final push under COVID-19 shelter-in-place orders.

Lastly, we would like to acknowledge the support of the World Health Organization, Vall d'Hebron Institut de Recerca, Western Washington University, and the University of Bergen who all made the open access publishing of this book possible.

Contents

Part I Introduction

1 **Exploring the Potential for the Arts to Promote Health
  and Social Justice** 3
  Helga Bjørnøy Urke, Emily Alden Hennessy, Mariana Sanmartino,
  and J. Hope Corbin

Part II Arts and Health Promotion: Tools and Bridges for Practice

2 **Drawing as a Salutogenic Therapy Aid for Grieving Adolescents** ... 19
  Masego Katisi, Philip Jefferies, and Mpho Sebako

3 **Promoting Spiritual Health: Using Poetry as a Coping
  Strategy for Iranian Women Post-divorce** 41
  Fatemeh Zarei

4 **Student Creativity and Professional Artwork in a School Food
  Intervention in Denmark** 53
  Dorte Ruge

5 **Creatively Healthy: Art in a Care Home Setting in Scotland** 67
  Gillian C. Barton

6 **CuidarNos: Art and Social Work to Address Trauma
  Among Gender-based Violence Advocates After Hurricane
  María in Puerto Rico** 85
  Heriberto Ramírez-Ayala, Elithet Silva-Martínez,
  and Jenice M. Vázquez-Pagán

7 **Community Theater for Health Promotion in Japan** 103
  Hikari Sandhu, Naoki Hirose, Kazuya Yui, and Masamine Jimba

Part III   Arts and Health Promotion: Tools and Bridges for Research

8   Lights, Camera, (Youth Participatory) Action! Lessons
     from Filming a Documentary with Trans and Gender
     Non-conforming Youth in the USA   123
     Robert A. Marx and Page Valentine Regan

9   From Arts to Action: Project SHINE as a Case Study of Engaging
     Youth in Efforts to Develop Sustainable Water, Sanitation,
     and Hygiene Strategies in Rural Tanzania and India   141
     Anise Gold-Watts, Marte Hovdenak, Aruna Ganesan,
     and Sheri Bastien

10   Photovoice for Health Promotion Research, Empowerment,
     and Advocacy: Young Refugee Stories from Turkey   165
     Ozge Karadag Caman

11   Reframing Health Promotion Research and Practice in Australia
     and the Pacific: The Value of Arts-Based Practices   179
     Wendy Madsen, Michelle Redman-MacLaren, Vicki Saunders,
     Cathy O'Mullan, and Jenni Judd

12   A Kaleidoscope of Words and Senses to (Re)Think the Chagas
     Problem: Experiences in Argentina and Brazil   197
     Carolina Amieva, Carolina Carrillo, Cecilia Mordeglia,
     María Cecilia Gortari, María Soledad Scazzola,
     and Mariana Sanmartino

13   Mapping the Discourse on the Health-Promoting Impacts
     of Community Arts   217
     Charlotte Lombardo

**Part IV   Arts and Health Promotion: Tools and Bridges
            for Social Transformation**

14   Art and Co-creation for the Community Promotion
     of Affective Sexual Health in Catalonia   235
     Jordi Gómez i Prat, Isabel Claveria Guiu, Mario Torrecillas,
     Arturo Solari, and Hakima Ouaarab Esadek

15   ArtScience for Health Awareness in Brazil.   251
     Tania C. de Araújo-Jorge, Roberto Todor,
     Rita C. Machado da Rocha, Sheila S. de Assis,
     Cristina X. A. Borges, Telma T. Santos, Valeria S. Trajano,
     Lucia R. de La Rocque, Anunciata C. M. Braz Sawada,
     and Luciana Ribeiro Garzoni

16 The Western Australian Indigenous Storybook Spins
    Special Yarns 267
    Melissa Stoneham, Christina R. Davies, and Ray Christophers

17 Silent Silhouettes: A Living Reminder of the Urgent Action
    Needed to End Gender-based Violence in Trinidad and Tobago 279
    Stephanie Leitch

18 Movimiento Ventana: An Alternative Proposal to Mental Health
    in Nicaragua 295
    Andrea Deleo, Roberta Romero, and Enmanuelle A. Zelaya

19 Using Art to Bridge Research and Policy: An Initiative
    of the United States National Academy of Medicine 313
    Charlee Alexander, Kyra Cappelucci, and Laura DeStefano

20 Art and Innovation at International Health Promotion
    Conferences 329
    Christa Ayele, J. Hope Corbin, Emily Alden Hennessy,
    Mariana Sanmartino, and Helga Bjørnøy Urke

Part V   Conclusion

21 Arts, Health Promotion, and Social Justice: Synergy in Motion 345
    J. Hope Corbin, Mariana Sanmartino, Helga Bjørnøy Urke,
    and Emily Alden Hennessy

Index 357

About the Editors

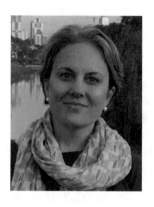

J. Hope Corbin is Associate Professor and Director of the Human Services Program in the Department of Health and Community Studies at Western Washington University in Bellingham. Her scholarship focuses on intersectoral collaboration to reduce inequity in the social determinants of health and on partnership as a mechanism for leveraging diverse ways of knowing, and power, for emancipatory health promotion. She is particularly interested in North-South partnership and promoting equity in global health promotion research. She is also focused on how incorporating the arts in health promotion practice, research, and social mobilization can provide a promising pathway toward transformation, liberation, and healing for individuals, settings, communities, and societies. Hope serves as Vice President for the International Union for Health Promotion and Education's (IUHPE) North American Region, Faculty Mentor to the IUHPE's Student and Early Career Network, and Deputy Editor-in-Chief of *Health Promotion International*.

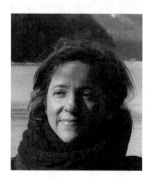

Mariana Sanmartino (PhD in Education Sciences) is a biologist and a specialist in Social Sciences and Health and in Epistemologies of the South. She works as a researcher for the National Board of Scientific and Technical Research (CONICET) in the Grupo de Didáctica de las Ciencias in La Plata, Argentina. She is the founder and coordinator of the group ¿De qué hablamos cuando hablamos de Chagas? (What do we speak about when we speak about Chagas?), whose main objective is to promote an understanding of Chagas disease from an integrated and innovative perspective, linking multiple voices, diverse artistic expressions, and unconventional scenarios. The guiding thread of her career is the search for elements that make it possible to understand the problem of Chagas from an integral perspective, highlighting the role of education and communication as key tools to address this complex and current issue. Mariana is member of the Advisory Board of the International Federation of Associations of People Affected by Chagas Disease (FINDECHAGAS) and serves as part of the Technical Group No.6 on Information, Education and Communication (TG6-IEC Chagas) of the WHO Chagas disease control program.

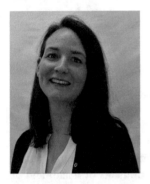

Emily Alden Hennessy (PhD in Community Research and Action) is a Research Assistant Professor at the Institute for Collaboration on Health, Intervention and Policy, University of Connecticut, Storrs, Connecticut. Her scholarship focuses on adolescent and emerging adult health and development, with a focus on problematic substance use and recovery. In this work, she combines developmental and ecological perspectives to address programs and settings for youth health, such as families and schools. Her work also involves various qualitative and quantitative research methodologies and includes developing best practices for evidence syntheses. She is an associate methods editor for the International Coordinating Group of the Campbell Collaboration.

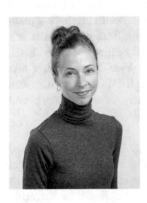

Helga Bjørnøy Urke (PhD in Child Health Promotion) is Associate Professor of Health Promotion and affiliated with the Master's program *Global Development: Theory and Practice,* which includes a specialization in Health Promotion for Development. Her scholarship focuses on early childcare, and child and adolescent mental, physical, and social health and development. The socioecological and resource perspectives dominate in her work, with particular emphasis on the family, school, and community as important health-promoting settings.

Contributors

Charlee Alexander National Academy of Medicine, Washington, DC, USA

Carolina Amieva Grupo de Didáctica de las Ciencias, IFLYSIB, CONICET - UNLP. Grupo ¿De qué hablamos cuando hablamos de Chagas?, La Plata, Buenos Aires, Argentina

Christa Ayele International Union for Health Promotion and Education's Student and Early Career Network, Bergen, Norway

Gillian C. Barton Healthy Workstyles Consultancy, Aberdeen, UK

Sheri Bastien Department of Public Health Science, Faculty of Landscape and Society, Norwegian University of Life Sciences, Ås, Norway
Department of Community Health Sciences, Cumming School of Medicine, University of Calgary, Calgary, AB, Canada

Cristina X. A. Borges Laboratory of Innovations in Therapies, Education and Bioproducts, Oswaldo Cruz Institute (LITEB-IOC/Fiocruz), Oswaldo Cruz Foundation (Fiocruz), Rio de Janeiro, Brazil

Anunciata C. M. Braz Sawada Laboratory of Innovations in Therapies, Education and Bioproducts, Oswaldo Cruz Institute (LITEB-IOC/Fiocruz), Oswaldo Cruz Foundation (Fiocruz), Rio de Janeiro, Brazil

Ozge Karadag Caman Center for Sustainable Development, Earth Institute, Columbia University, New York, NY, USA

Kyra Cappelucci National Academy of Medicine, Washington, DC, USA

Carolina Carrillo Instituto de Ciencias y, Tecnología Dr. César Milstein, CONICET. Grupo ¿De qué hablamos cuando hablamos de Chagas?, Buenos Aires, Argentina

Ray Christophers Nirrumbuk Environmental Health & Services, Nirrumbuk Aboriginal Corporation, Broome, WA, Australia

J. Hope Corbin Department of Health and Community Studies, Western Washington University, Bellingham, WA, USA

Rita C. Machado da Rocha Laboratory of Innovations in Therapies, Education and Bioproducts, Oswaldo Cruz Institute (LITEB-IOC/Fiocruz), Oswaldo Cruz Foundation (Fiocruz), Pavilhão Cardoso Fontes, Rio de Janeiro, Brazil

Christina R. Davies Health Humanities – Division of Health Professions Education, School of Allied Health, The University of Western Australia, Perth, WA, Australia

Public Health Advocacy Institute of WA, Curtin University, Perth, WA, Australia

The West Australian Arts and Health Consortium, Perth, WA, Australia

Lucia R. de La Rocque Laboratory of Innovations in Therapies, Education and Bioproducts, Oswaldo Cruz Institute (LITEB-IOC/Fiocruz), Oswaldo Cruz Foundation (Fiocruz), Rio de Janeiro, Brazil

Tania C. de Araújo-Jorge Laboratory of Innovations in Therapies, Education and Bioproducts, Oswaldo Cruz Institute (LITEB-IOC/Fiocruz), Oswaldo Cruz Foundation (Fiocruz), Rio de Janeiro, Brazil

Sheila S. de Assis Laboratory of Innovations in Therapies, Education and Bioproducts, Oswaldo Cruz Institute (LITEB-IOC/Fiocruz), Oswaldo Cruz Foundation (Fiocruz), Rio de Janeiro, Brazil

Andrea Deleo Movimiento Ventana, Managua, Nicaragua

Laura DeStefano National Academy of Medicine, Washington, DC, USA

Hakima Ouaarab Esadek Hospital Universitari Vall d'Hebron. Unitat de Salut Internacional Drassanes. Equip de Salut Pública i Comunitària. PROSICS Barcelona, Barcelona, Catalunya

Aruna Ganesan Sri Narayani Vidyalaya School, Vellore, India

Luciana Ribeiro Garzoni Laboratory of Innovations in Therapies, Education and Bioproducts, Oswaldo Cruz Institute (LITEB-IOC/Fiocruz), Oswaldo Cruz Foundation (Fiocruz), Rio de Janeiro, Brazil

Anise Gold-Watts Department of Public Health Science, Faculty of Landscape and Society, Norwegian University of Life Sciences, Ås, Norway

Jordi Gómez i Prat Hospital Universitari Vall d'Hebron. Unitat de Salut Internacional Drassanes. Equip de Salut Pública i Comunitària. PROSICS Barcelona, Barcelona, Catalunya

María Cecilia Gortari Epidemiología y Salud Pública Básica, Facultad de Ciencias Veterinarias, UNLP, Grupo ¿De qué hablamos cuando hablamos de Chagas?, La Plata, Buenos Aires, Argentina

Isabel Claveria Guiu Hospital Universitari Vall d'Hebron. Unitat de Salut Internacional Drassanes. Equip de Salut Pública i Comunitària. PROSICS Barcelona, Barcelona, Catalunya

Emily Alden Hennessy Department of Psychology, Institute for Collaboration on Health, Intervention & Policy, University of Connecticut, Storrs, CT, USA

Naoki Hirose Global Health Nursing, Graduate School of Biomedical and Health Sciences, Hiroshima University, Hiroshima, Japan

Marte Hovdenak Department of Health Promotion and Development, University of Bergen, Bergen, Norway

Philip Jefferies Resilience Research Centre, Faculty of Health, Dalhousie University, Halifax, Nova Scotia, Canada

Masamine Jimba Department of Community and Global Health, Graduate School of Medicine, The University of Tokyo, Tokyo, Japan

Jenni Judd Centre for Indigenous Health Equity Research, Centre for Emotional Health and Wellbeing, School of Health, Medical and Applied Sciences, Central Queensland University, Bundaberg, QLD, Australia

Masego Katisi Western Norway University of Applied Sciences, Faculty of Health and Social Sciences, Bergen, Norway

Stephanie Leitch WOMANTRA, St. Ann's, Port of Spain, Trinidad and Tobago

Charlotte Lombardo Faculty of Environmental and Urban Change, York University, Toronto, ON, Canada

Wendy Madsen School of Health, Medical and Applied Sciences CQ University, Norman Gardens, QLD, Australia

Robert A. Marx Department of Child and Adolescent Development, San José State University, San Jose, CA, USA

Cecilia Mordeglia Grupo de Didáctica de las Ciencias, IFLYSIB, CONICET - UNLP. Facultad de Ciencias Naturales y Museo, UNLP. Grupo ¿De qué hablamos cuando hablamos de Chagas?, La Plata, Buenos Aires, Argentina

Catherine O'Mullan School of Health, Medical and Applied Sciences, CQ University Bundaberg, Branyan, QLD, Australia

Heriberto Ramírez-Ayala TIPOS, Toa Alta, Puerto Rico

Michelle Redman-MacLaren College of Medicine and Dentistry, James Cook University, Cairns, QLD, Australia

Page Valentine Regan Educational Foundations, Policy, and Practice, University of Colorado, Boulder, CO, USA

Roberta Romero Movimiento Ventana, Managua, Nicaragua

Dorte Ruge University College Lillebælt, Odense, Denmark

Hikari Sandhu Department of Community and Global Health, Graduate School of Medicine, The University of Tokyo, Tokyo, Japan

Mariana Sanmartino Grupo de Didáctica de las Ciencias, IFLYSIB, CONICET - UNLP. Grupo ¿De qué hablamos cuando hablamos de Chagas?, La Plata, Buenos Aires, Argentina

Telma T. Santos Laboratory of Innovations in Therapies, Education and Bioproducts, Oswaldo Cruz Institute (LITEB-IOC/Fiocruz), Oswaldo Cruz Foundation (Fiocruz), Rio de Janeiro, Brazil

Vicki Saunders First Peoples Health Unit, Queensland Conservatorium Research Centre, Griffith University, Gold Coast Campus, Southport, QLD, Australia

María Soledad Scazzola Museo de La Plata, Facultad de Ciencias Naturales y Museo, UNLP. Grupo ¿De qué hablamos cuando hablamos de Chagas?, La Plata, Buenos Aires, Argentina

Mpho Sebako Ark and Mark Trust, Gaborone, Botswana

Elithet Silva-Martínez Beatriz Lassalle Graduate School of Social Work, University of Puerto Rico, San Juan, Puerto Rico

Arturo Solari Private Practice in Expressive Arts Therapist, Girona, Spain

Collaborator at the Unitat de Salut Internacional Drassanes-Vall d'Hebron, Barcelona, Catalunya

Melissa Stoneham Public Health Advocacy Institute of Western Australia, School of Public Health, Curtin University, Perth, Australia

School of Public Health, Edith Cowan University, Joondalup, Australia

Menzies School of Health Research, Casuarina, Australia

Roberto Todor Laboratory of Innovations in Therapies, Education and Bioproducts, Oswaldo Cruz Institute (LITEB-IOC/Fiocruz), Oswaldo Cruz Foundation (Fiocruz), Rio de Janeiro, Brazil

Mario Torrecillas Pequeños Dibujos Animados (PDA-films), Barcelona, Catalunya

Valeria S. Trajano Laboratory of Innovations in Therapies, Education and Bioproducts, Oswaldo Cruz Institute (LITEB-IOC/Fiocruz), Oswaldo Cruz Foundation (Fiocruz), Pavilhão Cardoso Fontes, Rio de Janeiro, Brazil

Helga Bjørnøy Urke Department of Health Promotion and Development, Faculty of Psychology, University of Bergen, Bergen, Norway

Jenice M. Vázquez-Pagán Department of Social Work, Interamerican University of Puerto Rico, San Juan, Puerto Rico

Kazuya Yui Department of Community Medicine, Saku Central Hospital, Saku, Nagano, Japan

Fatemeh Zarei Department of Health Education and Health Promotion, Faculty of Medical Sciences, Tarbiat Modares University, Tehran, Iran

Enmanuelle A. Zelaya Movimiento Ventana, Managua, Nicaragua

Part I
Introduction

Chapter 1
Exploring the Potential for the Arts to Promote Health and Social Justice

Helga Bjørnøy Urke, Emily Alden Hennessy, Mariana Sanmartino, and J. Hope Corbin

1.1 Health, Health Promotion, and the Arts

Health involves the inclusion and combination of "circumstances / representations / elements related to biological, social, cultural, environmental, economical, political, etc. aspects"; as such, it is a dynamic notion that can only be comprehended and discussed in a contextualized way (Sanmartino 2015, p. 87). Thus, the field of health promotion, a discipline that seeks to enable people to increase control over and ultimately improve their health, is grounded in a complex understanding of health:

> To reach a state of complete physical, mental and social well-being, an individual or group must be able to identify and to realize aspirations, to satisfy needs, and to change or cope with the environment. Health is, therefore, seen as a resource for everyday life, not the objective of living. Health is a positive concept emphasizing social and personal resources, as well as physical capacities. Therefore, health promotion is not just the responsibility of the health sector, but goes beyond healthy life-styles to well-being (WHO 1986).

H. B. Urke (✉)
Department of Health Promotion and Development, Faculty of Psychology,
University of Bergen, Bergen, Norway
e-mail: helga.urke@uib.no

E. A. Hennessy
Department of Psychology, Institute for Collaboration on Health, Intervention & Policy,
University of Connecticut, Storrs, CT, USA
e-mail: ehennessy@mgh.harvard.edu

M. Sanmartino
Grupo de Didáctica de las Ciencias, IFLYSIB, CONICET - UNLP. Grupo ¿De qué hablamos cuando hablamos de Chagas?, La Plata, Buenos Aires, Argentina
e-mail: mariana.sanmartino@conicet.gov.ar

J. H. Corbin
Department of Health and Community Studies, Western Washington University,
Bellingham, WA, USA
e-mail: hope.corbin@wwu.edu

© The Author(s) 2021
J. H. Corbin et al. (eds.), *Arts and Health Promotion*,
https://doi.org/10.1007/978-3-030-56417-9_1

Understanding health while acknowledging context and social determinants, and going beyond the absence of infirmity, is not a simple task. Beyond individual characteristics (personality traits, habits, genetics), people also face significant structural (social, cultural, economic, and political) barriers to health which are not easily solved as they involve multiple domains and ecological layers; i.e., dangerous employment conditions, social exclusion, inequitable distribution of public health programs, marginalization due to gender or race/ethnicity status, globalization and economic policy, and urbanization (CSDH 2008). Thus, the influence of these factors on health must be considered from the lens of intersectionality (Crenshaw 1990), recognizing that individual people and communities might live at the intersection of a variety of these social determinants which lead to compounding marginalization and oppression—especially along the lines of race, class, gender identity, sexual orientation, disability, citizenship, age, and other characteristics—and which may exponentially complicate their experience of health (Bauer 2014; Corbin and Bonde 2012). Similarly, historic experiences also impact health (Czyzewski 2011; Menzies 2008; Chandanabhumma and Narasimhan 2019), whether that be at the individual level of previous personal trauma (van der Kolk 2015), intergenerational trauma (DeGruy 2005), or at the national level with the historic experience of colonialism (Ward 2013; Chandanabhumma and Narasimhan 2019) and/or inequitable economic policy (such as structural adjustment programs) (Spencer et al. 2019). For instance, as we write this COVID-19 ravages the world and because of several overlapping facets of historic, economic, and structural oppression, the US has inequitable distributions of both the illness and access to care: for instance, 73% of the deaths in Milwaukee County, Wisconsin in the first 2 months of the pandemic—were African Americans— despite the fact that African Americans make up only 26% of the population in the county (Thebault et al. 2020).

Given these deeply individualized historically and community-based experiences of health, health promotion must seek to promote not only the physical experience of health but also social justice, agency, and self-determination through empowerment, participation, collaboration, and by reducing inequity (Chandanabhumma and Narasimhan 2019). It is in these efforts that the arts have a promising role. Indeed, Bell and Desai (2011) argue that art should have a central role in all social justice practice. To this end, the present book contributes to the wider social justice art field by introducing the specific role of art in health promotion efforts toward social transformation for health equity.

The Lima Declaration on Art, Health, and Development (PAHO 2009) underscores the inherent power of art in facilitating expression across cultural and social diversity and throughout the life course. The Declaration suggests key connections between art and health promotion, emphasizing art as "a powerful tool for promoting and repairing health, allowing individuals and communities to rework critical, painful or problematic situations and promote better and happier scenarios for their lives" (PAHO 2009, p. 3). The Declaration also points to art as a facilitator for active citizenship and social change through "creativity, imagination, critical thinking and love" (PAHO 2009, p. 3).

The opportunities afforded by incorporating a creative approach have been recognized as key to promoting individual and community health and well-being (Clift and Camic 2016; Craemer 2009; Davies et al. 2015; Jensen and Bonde 2018; Kilroy et al. 2007; Shand 2014; Stuckey and Nobel 2010; White 2006). Indeed, to date, there are numerous examples of how health promotion practice and research can incorporate the arts for health and social benefit in a range of settings (Daykin et al. 2008; Djurichkovic 2011; Fancourt and Finn 2019; Gussak 2007; McKay and McKenzie 2018; Raw et al. 2012).

The social dimension of health is emphasized in the Ottawa Charter for Health Promotion (WHO 1986), which argues that health is created in our everyday life contexts where we "learn, work, play and love" (WHO 1986, p. 4). Similarly, art is created in these same settings and may contribute to the promotion of health, well-being, and social change. We argue that the arts can be transformative for the field of health promotion not only by helping us to do the work that we have traditionally done-- better, but by also providing unique avenues to address and redress issues impacting health disparities that we have neglected or failed to consider. That is, scholars have noted that health promotion might be limited by its positionality and framing, and that it may suffer from being situated in a postcolonial context, origi-nating primarily from a Northern/Western perspective (McPhail-Bell et al. 2013). From a critical standpoint, art not only serves as a tool for health promotion but can also be an important bridge toward equity in both health and knowledge exchange. Again, this aligns with social justice art practice, which considers and uses arts to identify and challenge systems that maintain inequity and injustice. Similar to how we in this book argue for the role of art in critical health promotion, social justice art is concerned with amplifying voice and position to other ways of knowing and facilitate alternatives to the dominant discourse and structures (Bell and Desai 2011, see also Chap. 21, this volume).

This book draws together 19 contributed chapters with examples of arts-based health promotion initiatives in over 17 countries. In this chapter, we begin to describe how these projects serve to promote health through the Ottawa Charter action areas, and suggest how the arts can provide further opportunities for research and practice to work toward social transformation. Through this first chapter we hope to establish the value of art for health promotion in the efforts toward health equity and social justice, and to inspire a wide readership and application of the book: practitioners, researchers, artists, and communities worldwide.

1.2 Arts to Address the Five Health Promotion Action Areas

The Ottawa Charter (WHO 1986) defines the core of the field of health promotion and underlines the need for active engagement by all sectors and at all levels of society to fulfill individual and community potential for health and well-being across five action areas: (1) *strengthening community action, (2) developing personal skills, (3) creating supportive environments, (4) reorienting health services,* and *(5) building healthy public policy.* These action areas require concentrated and intentional efforts, and the arts can be easily adapted in many ways to work toward achieving change in each of them.

1.2.1   Strengthen Community Action

Health promotion encourages a bottom-up approach in which individuals take control of their individual and community health (WHO 1986). The creative arts, specifically those coming from community art initiatives, often hold this same
perspective in the way that they encourage individuals' free expression of experiences. This is exemplified in the critical literature review on community arts for
research presented by Lombardo in Chap. 13. Merging participatory art with health
promotion initiatives can also create synergy when aiming to strengthen community
action. In line with the Ottawa Charter's conceptualization of community development, which involves drawing on "existing human and material resources" (WHO
1986, p. 3), community arts can build capacity to enable health or social transformation while also facilitating "constitutive capacity" as an end in itself, building on
existing community strengths and assets (Carson et al. 2007, p. 367). In Chap. 16,
Stoneham and colleagues discuss how Indigenous community members used the
local custom of storytelling to revise negative stereotypes of their communities in
Western Australian media by telling positive stories and showcasing achievements.
Through this common and culturally appropriate approach, the program aimed to
strengthen community action to improve community well-being.

Indeed, many public health projects including the arts often have explicit goals
of strengthening communities by bringing individuals together to collaboratively
and creatively address specific social or health problems (Carson et al. 2007).
Furthermore, the act of collectively experiencing and witnessing art may also generate a deeper shared understanding among community members of the problems
they face and opportunities for addressing them. For example, in Chap. 11, Madsen
and colleagues explore how several community groups from Australia and the
Pacific created a theater production based on experiences of local women to raise
social consciousness on the issue of domestic and family violence in their
community.

From a social justice perspective, art can also be used to instigate and facilitate
social change by providing communities with opportunities to take action (Boal
1995; Freire 1970). In Paulo Freire's *Pedagogy of the Oppressed* (1970), learners
are viewed and met as co-creators of knowledge. Through this approach, critical
consciousness in individuals and communities can be achieved, which in turn facilitates action for social change. Inspired by Freirian thinking, Augusto Boal's *Theatre
of the Oppressed* uses different forms of participatory theater to allow the contribution of new voices and provide space for change to individuals and communities
(Boal 1995; Österlind 2008). Combining art and education enables the creation of
awareness of individual and community situations, as well as the tools with which
to express them. Through acting out situations of oppression, social injustice, liberation etc., Boal's theory posits that individuals and groups will be equipped to act
out the same situations in real life (Boal 1995; Österlind 2008). In Chap. 6, Ramirez
and colleagues describe how *Encuentro CuidarNos*—a collaboration between the
Puerto Rican Coalition Against Domestic Violence and Sexual Assault and the

University of Puerto Rico—employed a combination of art forms (theater, music, drawing, dance) to process the primary and vicarious trauma experienced by gender-based violence service providers and advocates throughout Puerto Rico in the aftermath of Hurricane Maria. Throughout the different phases of the initiative, the participants were guided through ways of processing the trauma at multiple levels simultaneously to process their own experience of the trauma, and to increase their ability to continue their important work through their organizations and within the broader community.

1.2.2   Develop Personal Skills

Facilitation of life-long development and learning to ensure individual and community agency for health and well-being is a core action area in health promotion. Engagement in creative arts has been connected to the development of a range of personal skills in addition to or besides arts-specific skills at the individual level (Cameron et al. 2013; Chatterjee et al. 2018; Chilcote 2007; Kilroy et al. 2007; White 2006). Kilroy et al. (2007) emphasize the "arts in health" field as a holistic approach that recognizes and responds to the whole person, and as such lays foundations for an active personal development through experiencing flow, gaining new expectations and perspectives, and increasing well-being. Indeed, building personal self-esteem and confidence are among the most cited benefits of community-based arts projects (White 2006), which can further lead to leadership and responsibility taking (Cameron et al. 2013). For example, in Chap. 3, Zarei explores the use of poetry to empower Iranian women experiencing divorce to make meaning from their experiences. Similarly, in Marx and Regan's contribution to this book (Chap. 8), researchers undertook a youth participatory action research project with trans- and gender-non-conforming youth to design, film, and edit a documentary about their experience in the United States. Youth wanted to portray both their unique challenges and their strengths through this work, and they were encouraged to learn new technical and advocacy skills as part of the entire project.

Arts have also been presented as very promising for effective health education, especially when developed in a participatory way (Frishkopf et al. 2016; McDonald et al. 2007). Many arts-based approaches offer alternative (non-language) ways to present knowledge and information; as such, they may mitigate barriers to health knowledge, such as illiteracy. For example, as Caman discusses in Chap. 10, photovoice is used as a social connection tool for Syrian youth displaced in Turkey, as well as to identify and communicate health issues facing this vulnerable population. Furthermore, in the aftermath of a disaster, art can function as a tool for "retrieval and reprocessing of traumatic memories that are often encoded in images rather than in words" (Huss et al. 2016, p. 1), a process which contributes to individual emotional development and healing. In Chap. 2, Katisi and colleagues describe their work with youth in Botswana who had lost caregivers to AIDS, exploring the use of a drawing-narrative approach to facilitate emotional recovery from traumatic experiences in children, who oftentimes may not have the appropriate words they need to talk about their experience.

1.2.3   Create Supportive Environments

A third action area for health promotion as defined in the Ottawa Charter is to ensure environments that are supportive for health—from immediate contexts like family, school, and work environments, to the larger community and across natural and built environments (WHO 1986). Indeed, arts-based activities have been shown to be a viable approach to developing supportive environments for a variety of health-related outcomes in a range of settings, including schools (McKay and McKenzie 2018), prisons (Djurichkovic 2011; Gussak 2007), communities (Shand 2014), and elderly care (Kilroy et al. 2007). For example, in Chap. 4, Ruge describes the use of a variety of art (drawing and graphic design) and cooking activities that engaged children, teachers and kitchen personnel and supported discussion of nutrition and healthful eating in schools in Denmark.

Several arts-driven projects have an explicit objective of creating arenas and safe(r) spaces for physical and mental health promotion among diverse groups including recent immigrants, the elderly, and young people (Clift and Hancox 2010; Cohen et al. 2007; Hallam et al. 2011; Jackson et al. 2010; Kilroy et al. 2007; McKay and McKenzie 2018; Shand 2014). Also, for communities that have experienced a disaster event, the use of art for recovery can help mobilize individuals to take control of their lives again while also creating a group narrative of the disaster experience (Huss et al. 2016), and in this way promote social connection and meaning. Related to this action area, in Chap. 7, Sandhu and colleagues present a historic overview of the use of drama to create supportive environments for health in the Nagano Prefecture of Japan in the 1940s.

Creating supportive environments through art can promote social connection by building new relationships among participants (Shand 2014) or by strengthening bonds between family members, such as by involving parents and children in a project together (Jackson et al. 2010). Gold-Watts and colleagues (Chap. 9) attended to linking the school and community environment in rural Tanzania and India by engaging youth in initial arts-based research (including drawing and mapping), which was later presented to their families and the larger community through a community science fair and a community event day.

When considering the neighborhood as another setting in which close relationships are woven, de Araújo Jorge and colleagues (Chap. 15) describe the development and use of ArtScience-based activities with multiple artistic languages and production of materials for health care communication (including photography, handicraft production, and song composition). The aim was to train community agents living in socio-environmentally vulnerable areas to address health awareness related to social, environmental, and biological determinants involved in the transmission of dengue, Zika, chikungunya, and yellow fever by the *Aedes aegypti* mosquito in urban areas of Rio de Janeiro in Brazil.

1.2.4 Reorient Health Services

In agreement with the argument that health is more than the simple absence of disease, the Ottawa Charter argues that "the role of the health sector must move increasingly in a health promotion direction..." (WHO 1986, p. 3). This means acknowledging the contextualized nature of health, and connecting health services to the broader societal levels in culturally sensitive ways (WHO 1986). Although this is a challenging endeavor, a broader approach to health service provision, treatment, and healing is indeed being taken in health sectors around the world, also incorporating the use of arts (McDonald et al. 2007). Several examples exist of health care settings (hospitals, senior homes, etc.) that take a holistic approach to patient treatment and care through art, both using the more traditional art therapies (Fraser et al. 2014) and also adapting art therapy by moving away from a clinical/expert approach to patient participatory approaches (Kilroy et al. 2007; Preti and Welch 2011). In Chap. 5, Barton describes an initiative within a long-term care facility in Scotland that engaged residents, their families, and its staff in a community art project that aimed to build a sense of community, provide an avenue for self-expression, and beautify the clinical space (using clay tiles). Further, in Chap. 18, Deleo and colleagues, describe the experience of a self-managed social movement to promote mental health and reduce stigma around mental illness through the use of dance (Biodanza) and art therapy in the Psychosocial Hospital of Managua, Nicaragua.

Art can also reorient health services by acting as a bridge between the health care sector and other sectors. For example, the use of live music as therapy for hospitalized children seeks to use art as a "cultural bridge between the hospital and the wider community" by introducing a familiar "outside" into the unfamiliar hospital environment often associated with pain and stress/fear (Preti and Welch 2011). In Chap. 14, written by Gomez i Prat and colleagues, the members of a health team in Barcelona share the way in which they work collaboratively with community stakeholders to co-create innovative resources that allow them to work on affective sexual health issues with migrant populations in international health care services using different art forms, including music, documentary films, videos, and more.

1.2.5 Build Healthy Public Policy

Incorporating arts in health promotion and public health in systematic ways requires attention at the policy level—locally, nationally, and perhaps globally. In this regard, the conclusions of the WHO Regional Office for Europe report point to the need to develop effective strategies for synergized collaboration between health and arts sectors to "realize the potential of the arts for improving global health" (Fancourt and Finn 2019, p. 57).

In this sense, the experience shared in Chap. 12 by Amieva and colleagues is a good example of how such work could inform discourse and lead to changes at the policy level, if appropriate advocacy efforts were undertaken across sectors. In their project, an interdisciplinary team of researchers, practitioners, and artists used workshops and literary productions from those workshops to examine the rhetoric around Chagas disease in Argentina and Brazil, with the ultimate aim of improving advocacy and treatment for this complex condition. The proposal of the National Academy of Medicine (USA), discussed by Alexander and colleagues in Chap. 19, could be considered within the same line of reflection. The Academy has begun to use various forms of art, including images, paintings, and street art, as a way to expand its impact and intentionally include underrepresented voices by asking communities to share their understanding and perceptions of health equity and its role in supporting the well-being of all people. In addition, their recent projects ask artists to explore clinician well-being and its connection to quality patient care and a thriving health system.

Finally, considering the indisputable link that should exist between social mobilization and changes in public policies, "artivism" is an essential tool in health promotion. Understanding "artivism" as activism for social change through art, we agree with the words of Salazar and Olivos when they affirm that:

> ARTIVISM configures a collective action developed predominantly in public spaces. It is confrontational because it challenges and questions directly through the symbolic manifestation; and it is culture as it has to do with the change of meanings and shared representations. However, reflection is important because it constitutes a stop along the way, a moment to think about what assumptions we start from, where we are, what we have achieved and how we continue (Salazar and Olivos 2014, p. 5).

Chapter 17 by Leitch focuses on an eloquent example in this regard: the "Silent Silhouettes" project, a roving installation, in the form of wooden sculptures that aim to visualize—in various public locations—the fatal effects of gender-based violence in Trinidad and Tobago.

1.3   About This Book

Given the many opportunities for using the arts in health promotion efforts to address the five action areas of the Ottawa Charter, this book presents and examines the incorporation of arts in three primary ways: as a dynamic and participatory approach to health promotion practice, as a method to enrich and drive research, and finally as a unique avenue to reflect on and pursue social transformation.

Our intention with this book was to provide a broad overview of the potential for incorporating the arts in health promotion practice and research in a concrete way to enable readers to experiment with these ideas in their own work. As we were inviting contributions to the volume, we established foundational criteria to ensure that the resulting work constituted a diverse, inclusive, and representative contribution in the field of arts and health promotion. We sought to include diverse art forms and initiatives that addressed a broad array of health issues and were implemented in a variety of settings and work contexts. We also strove for gender balance among the invited authors, and geographical diversity in the locations of the projects. As a result, this book has 19 contributed chapters spanning projects from Asia, Africa, Latin America, Australia, Europe, and North America. These projects represent a variety of collaborative arrangements including south-south partnerships, north-south partnerships, and smaller-scale national projects. The chapters also describe programs that support diverse populations, including older adults, young people, professionals, whole communities, schoolchildren, divorcees, transgender and non-binary youth, displaced people/migrants, teachers, and Indigenous peoples. It is this broad relevance of art in so many contexts for so many people—the sheer accessibility and tradition of it—that provides the promise for how art might be a pathway to redressing power structures that influence and cause health disparities and impact the field of health promotion and its means of knowledge production.

There are a variety of models in health promotion that could serve to frame the role of arts in promoting health and equity. In the final chapter (Chap. 21), we employ the Bergen Model of Collaborative Functioning (Corbin et al. 2016) to synthesize and analyze the diverse experiences presented in the volume and propose a way of theorizing how arts-based initiatives might contribute to synergy in health promotion research and practice. We use this model given its flexibility in approaching health promotion projects with multiple stakeholders and its attention to both positive outcomes (synergy) and negative outcomes (antagony). Using examples from across the 19 contributed chapters, we argue that the incorporation of arts can facilitate deeper engagement with one's self and with others, as well as support the process of making sense of context. We also argue that art can promote social justice and contribute to social transformation by amplifying voice, leveraging power, and honoring multiple ways of knowing.

Finally, this book is a milestone for us. The project began long before we ever considered editing a book on the topic. Chapter 20, written by Ayele and colleagues, gives an account of the central axis of this journey: the art and health promotion sessions held at international conferences on health promotion organized by the International Union for Health Promotion and Education (IUHPE). These sessions saw their beginnings when we turned a perceived obstacle into an opportunity and asked ourselves, "How could we talk about health without using words?" It was in these sessions that we began to glimpse the metaphor of "tools and bridges" to explain how the arts might provide unique opportunities for health promotion. Tools enable and support action, they make tasks easier, they smooth challenges, and they file rough edges. Bridges allow us to access hard-to-reach places, cross rough terrain, and reduce distance. Through our own diverse collaboration in planning and facilitating these sessions, we saw the potential for arts to act as precise tools to address complex health promotion issues, and to act as bridges—across language and connecting people to one another in their humanity—to promote health and to fight inequity and health disparities. We hope this book reflects this journey while inspiring critical, creative, and transformative practices.

References

Bauer, G. R. (2014). Incorporating intersectionality theory into population health research methodology: Challenges and the potential to advance health equity. *Social Science & Medicine, 110*,
10–17. https://doi.org/10.1016/j.socscimed.2014.03.022.
Bell, L. A., & Desai, D. (2011). Imagining otherwise: Connecting the arts and social justice to
envision and act for change: Special issue introduction. *Equity and Excellence in Education,
44*(3), 287–295. https://doi.org/10.1080/10665684.2011.591672.
Boal, A. (1995). *The rainbow of desire: The Boal method of theatre and therapy.* London:
Psychology Press.
Cameron, M., Crane, N., Ings, R., & Taylor, K. (2013). Promoting well-being through creativity:
How arts and public health can learn from each other. *Perspectives in Public Health.* https://
doi.org/10.1177/1757913912466951.
Carson, A. J., Chappell, N. L., & Knight, C. J. (2007). Promoting health and innovative health promotion practice through a community arts centre. *Health Promotion Practice, 8*(4), 366–374.
https://doi.org/10.1177/1524839906289342.
Chandanabhumma, P. P., & Narasimhan, S. (2019). Towards health equity and social justice: An
applied framework of decolonization in health promotion. *Health Promotion International,*
daz053. Advance online publication. https://doi.org/10.1093/heapro/daz053.
Chatterjee, H. J., Camic, P. M., Lockyer, B., & Thomson, L. J. M. (2018). Non-clinical community interventions: A systematized review of social prescribing schemes. *Arts & Health, 10*(2),
97–123. https://doi.org/10.1080/17533015.2017.1334002.
Chilcote, R. L. (2007). Art therapy with child tsunami survivors in Sri Lanka. *Art Therapy, 24*(4),
156–162. https://doi.org/10.1080/07421656.2007.10129475.
Clift, S., & Camic, P. M. (2016). *Oxford textbook of creative arts, health, and wellbeing:
International perspectives on practice, policy and research.* Oxford: Oxford University Press.
Clift, S., & Hancox, G. (2010). The significance of choral singing for sustaining psychological
wellbeing: findings from a survey of choristers in England, Australia and Germany. *Music
Performance Research, 3*, 76–96.
Cohen, G., Perlstein, S., Chapline, J., Kelly, J., Firth, K. M., & Simmens, S. (2007). The impact of
professionally conducted cultural programs on the physical health, mental health, and social
functioning of older adults—2-year results. *Journal of Aging, Humanities, and the Arts, 1*(1–2),
5–22. https://doi.org/10.1080/19325610701410791.
Corbin, J., & Bonde, L. T. (2012). Intersections of context and HIV/AIDS in sub-Saharan Africa:
What can we learn from feminist theory? *Perspectives in Public Health, 132*(1), 8–9. https://
doi.org/10.1177/1757913911430909.
Corbin, J. H., Jones, J., & Barry, M. M. (2016). What makes intersectoral partnerships for health
promotion work? A review of the international literature. *Health Promotion International,*
daw061. https://doi.org/10.1093/heapro/daw061.
Craemer, R. (2009). The arts and health: From economic theory to cost-effectiveness. *UNESCO
Observatory, Faculty of Architecture, Building and Planning. The University of Melbourne
Refereed E-Journal, 1*, 4.
Crenshaw, K. (1990). Mapping the margins: Intersectionality, identity politics, and violence
against women of color. *Stanford Law Review, 43*(6), 1241–1300. https://heinonline.org/HOL/
P?h=hein.journals/stflr43&i=1257. Accessed 21 February 2020.
CSDH (Ed.). (2008). *Closing the gap in a generation: Health equity through action on the social
determinants of health: Commission on Social Determinants of Health final report.* Geneva:
World Health Organization, Commission on Social Determinants of Health.
Czyzewski, K. (2011). Colonialism as a broader social determinant of health. *International
Indigenous Policy Journal; London, 2*(1). https://doi.org/10.18584/iipj.2011.2.1.5.
Davies, C., Knuiman, M., & Rosenberg, M. (2015). The art of being mentally healthy: A study to
quantify the relationship between recreational arts engagement and mental well-being in the
general population. *BMC Public Health, 16*(1), 15. https://doi.org/10.1186/s12889-015-2672-7.

Daykin, N., Orme, J., Evans, D., Salmon, D., McEachran, M., & Brain, S. (2008). The impact of participation in performing arts on adolescent health and behaviour: A systematic review of the literature. *Journal of Health Psychology, 13*(2), 251–264. https://doi.org/10.1177/1359105307086699.

DeGruy, J. (2005). *Post traumatic slave syndrome: America's legacy of enduring injury and healing.* Milwaukie: Uptone Press.

Djurichkovic, A. (2011). *Art in prisons: A literature review of the philosophies and impacts of visual art programs for correctional populations (No. 3).* Broadway NSW: UTS ePRESS.

Fancourt, D., & Finn, S. (2019). *What is the evidence on the role of the arts in improving health and well-being? A scoping review (2019).* Copenhagen: WHO Regional Office for Europe (Health Evidence Network (HEN) synthesis report 67).

Fraser, A., Bungay, H., & Munn-Giddings, C. (2014). The value of the use of participatory arts activities in residential care settings to enhance the well-being and quality of life of older people: A rapid review of the literature. *Arts & Health, 6*(3), 266–278. https://doi.org/10.1080/17533015.2014.923008.

Freire, P. (1970). *Pedagogy of the oppressed.* New York: Herder and Herder.

Frishkopf, M., Hamze, H., Alhassan, M., Zukpeni, I. A., Abu, S., & Zakus, D. (2016). Performing arts as a social technology for community health promotion in northern Ghana. *Family Medicine and Community Health, 4*(1), 22–36. https://doi.org/10.15212/FMCH.2016.0105.

Gussak, D. (2007). The effectiveness of art therapy in reducing depression in prison populations. *International Journal of Offender Therapy and Comparative Criminology, 51*(4), 444–460. https://doi.org/10.1177/0306624X06294137.

Hallam, S., Creech, A., Gaunt, H., Pincas, A., Varvarigou, M., & McQueen, H. (2011). *Music for Life project: The role of participation in community music activities in promoting social engagement and well-being in older people.* Sheffield: University of Sheffield.

Huss, E., Kaufman, R., Avgar, A., & Shuker, E. (2016). Arts as a vehicle for community building and post-disaster development. *Disasters, 40*(2), 284–303. https://doi.org/10.1111/disa.12143.

Jackson, C. J., Mullis, R., & Hughes, M. (2010). Development of a theater-based nutrition and physical activity intervention for low-income, urban, African American adolescents. *Progress in Community Health Partnerships: Research, Education, and Action, 4*(2), 89–98. https://doi.org/10.1353/cpr.0.0115.

Jensen, A., & Bonde, L. (2018). The use of arts interventions for mental health and well-being in health settings. *Perspectives in Public Health, 138*(4), 209–214. https://doi.org/10.1177/1757913918772602.

Kilroy, A., Garner, C., Parkinson, C., Kagan, C., & Senior, P. (2007). *Towards transformation: exploring the impact of culture, creativity and the arts of health and wellbeing.* Manchester: Arts for Health, Manchester Metropolitan University. http://e-space.mmu.ac.uk/24673/. Accessed 15 January 2020.

McDonald, M., Antunez, G., & Gottemoeller, M. (2007). Using the arts and literature in health education. *International Quarterly of Community Health Education, 27*(3), 265–278. https://doi.org/10.2190/IQ.27.3.f.

McKay, F. H., & McKenzie, H. (2018). Using art for health promotion: Evaluating an in-school program through student perspectives. *Health Promotion Practice, 19*(4), 522–530. https://doi.org/10.1177/1524839917735076.

McPhail-Bell, K., Fredericks, B., & Brough, M. (2013). Beyond the accolades: A postcolonial critique of the foundations of the Ottawa Charter. *Global Health Promotion, 20*(2), 22–29. https://doi.org/10.1177/1757975913490427.

Menzies, P. (2008). Developing an Aboriginal healing model for intergenerational trauma. *International Journal of Health Promotion and Education, 46*(2), 41–48. https://doi.org/10.1080/14635240.2008.10708128.

Österlind, E. (2008). Acting out of habits—Can theatre of the oppressed promote change? Boal's theatre methods in relation to Bourdieu's concept of habitus. *Research in Drama Education: The Journal of Applied Theatre and Performance, 13*(1), 71–82. https://doi.org/10.1080/13569780701825328.

PAHO. (2009). *Declaración de Lima sobre arte, salud y desarrollo*. PAHO.

Preti, C., & Welch, G. F. (2011). Music in a hospital: The impact of a live music program on pediatric patients and their caregivers. *Music and Medicine, 3*(4), 213–223. https://doi. org/10.1177/1943862111399449.

Raw, A., Lewis, S., Russell, A., & Macnaughton, J. (2012). A hole in the heart: Confronting the drive for evidence-based impact research in arts and health. *Arts & Health, 4*(2), 97–108. https://doi.org/10.1080/17533015.2011.619991.

Salazar, X., & Olivos, F. (2014). *Artivismo. Cambio Social y Activismo Cultural. Seminario de Debate*. Lima: IESSDEH; UPCH. https://es.scribd.com/doc/282435382/Artivismo-pdf. Accessed 19 February 2020.

Sanmartino, M. (coordination). (2015). Hablamos de Chagas. Aportes para (re)pensar la problemática con una mirada integral. Contenidos: Amieva, C., Balsalobre, A., Carrillo, C., Marti, G., Medone, P., Mordeglia, C., et al. Buenos Aires: CONICET

Shand, M. (2014). *Understanding and building resilience with art: A socio-ecological approach.* Joondalup: Edith Cowan University. Retrieved from https://ro.ecu.edu.au/theses/1402/.

Spencer, G., Corbin, J. H., & Miedema, E. (2019). Sustainable development goals for health promotion: A critical frame analysis. *Health Promotion International, 34*(4), 847–858. https://doi. org/10.1093/heapro/day036.

Stuckey, H. L., & Nobel, J. (2010). The connection between art, healing, and public health: A review of current literature. *American Journal of Public Health, 100*(2), 254–263. https://doi. org/10.2105/AJPH.2008.156497.

Thebault, Reis, Andrew Ba Tran, and Vanessa Williams. (2020). The Coronavirus Is Infecting and Killing Black Americans at an Alarmingly High Rate. *Washington Post*, April 7, 2020, sec. National. https://www.washingtonpost.com/nation/2020/04/07/coronavirus-is-infecting-killing-black-americans-an-alarmingly-high-rate-post-analysis-shows/. Accessed 20 April 2020.

van der Kolk, B. (2015). *The body keeps the score: Brain, mind, and body in the healing of trauma (reprint edition)*. New York: Penguin Books.

Ward, A. (2013). Understanding postcolonial traumas. *Journal of Theoretical and Philosophical Psychology, 33*(3), 170–184. https://doi.org/10.1037/a0033576.

White, M. (2006). Establishing common ground in community-based arts in health. *Journal of the Royal Society for the Promotion of Health, 126*(3), 128–133. https://doi. org/10.1177/1466424006064302.

World Health Organization. (1948). Constitution of the World Health Organization. http://apps. who.int/gb/bd/PDF/bd47/EN/constitution-en.pdf?ua=1. Accessed 20 February 2020.

World Health Organization. (1986). The Ottawa Charter for Health Promotion. https://www.who. int/healthpromotion/conferences/previous/ottawa/en/. Accessed 20 February 2020.

World Health Organization. (2018). Disability and health. https://www.who.int/news-room/factsheets/detail/disability-and-health. Accessed 18 February 2020.

Part II
Arts and Health Promotion: Tools and Bridges for Practice

Chapter 2
Drawing as a Salutogenic Therapy Aid for Grieving Adolescents

Masego Katisi, Philip Jefferies, and Mpho Sebako

2.1 Introduction

Drawing can improve sensory motor skills, encourage the use of imagination, help to develop creativity, and above all presents a fun and enjoyable pastime (Vendeville et al. 2018). However, beyond play and skill development, it is an important method of communication and a tool for exploring complex and difficult issues, which may be more challenging with younger individuals (Pifalo 2007; Ugurlu et al. 2016). Drawing can also assist as a therapeutic aid in the identification of pathways to good health and well-being, such as enabling young people to map and reflect on their local supportive resources, in turn enabling a more positive reappraisal of their situation (Campbell et al. 2010; Campbell et al. 2015). The first chapter of this volume (see Chap. 1), describes the potential for the Arts and health promotion in a broad treatment, this chapter focuses specifically on the salutogenic qualities of drawing.

M. Katisi (✉)
Western Norway University of Applied Sciences, Faculty of Health and Social Sciences, Bergen, Norway
e-mail: Masego.Katisi@hvl.no

P. Jefferies
Resilience Research Centre, Faculty of Health, Dalhousie University, Halifax, NS, Canada
e-mail: philip.jefferies@dal.ca

M. Sebako
Ark and Mark Trust, Gaborone, Botswana
e-mail: msebako@arkandmark.org

© The Author(s) 2021
J. H. Corbin et al. (eds.), *Arts and Health Promotion*,
https://doi.org/10.1007/978-3-030-56417-9_2

19

2.2   The Context

In sub-Saharan Africa, the scourge of HIV/AIDS causes over 380,000 deaths per year. The infection rate in the region continues to increase, and UNAIDS records that 18.7 million (half of the HIV/AIDS infected population) live in East and Southern Africa (UNAIDS 2019). Many children have watched their parents suffer through this debilitating illness, and many have also witnessed their final moments. In addition to the trauma caused by the death of a parent, many of these children also experience subsequent challenges like stigma, poverty, abuse (sexual, emotional, and/or physical), and relational and educational issues (Meissner et al. 2017; Thamuku and Daniel 2013; Wakhweya et al. 2008; Xiaoming et al. 2015).

In a review of studies exploring the mental health of children affected by HIV/AIDS in sub-Saharan Africa, Skovdal (2012) determined that the majority focused on distress and reports of stress and depression, which were related to the burden of caring for ailing parents and the need to look after younger siblings (Cluver et al. 2007; Toska et al. 2016). However, clinicians who focus on distress risk pathologizing children's social experiences, and others have established that activities such as caring for others and performing home chores are seen by affected children as good training and competence building (Daniel et al. 2007; Skovdal and Daniel 2012). Thus, an alternative perspective that focuses on the strengths and positive supports despite adversity can elucidate social and psychological pathways to resilience.

Furthermore, while many interventions have been established to support orphaned children in Africa (Deininger et al. 2003; Heath et al. 2014; Schenk 2009; Strebel 2004), there is a lack of knowledge exploring how drawing could be used in these settings as an additional tool to help children process their grief and other challenges they have experienced and continue to experience (Thamuku and Daniel 2013), and also how drawing may be used to identify the support and resources children can draw on to build and maintain their resilience.

2.3   Theoretical Framework

This study uses the Sense of Coherence (SOC) from the salutogenic framework of health promotion to explore the use of drawings by grieving adolescents in Botswana. Antonovsky (1996) describes SOC as a global orientation that derives from one's confidence that both internal and external environments are predictable, resources are available, and problems are simply challenges worthy of investment and engagement. An individual's SOC is divided into three parts, each on a continuum (Fig. 2.1). The first is *comprehensibility*, meaning that one comprehends or evaluates their life situation as understandable and resolvable. The second component is *manageability*, which is the extent to which one believes that the resources around them can help address their life stressors. The third component is *meaningfulness*, which is a motivational component describing one's positive emotional

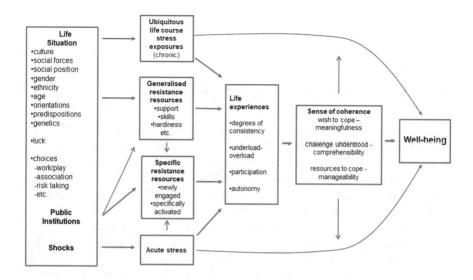

Mittelmark MB (2013). Resources for Health in the Salutogenic Model: Specific Resistance Resources contra Generalised Resistance Resources in the Context of Health Promotion Practice and Research. *Netherlands Congres Volksgezondheid 2013*, 3 April, 2013.

Fig. 2.1 The salutogenic model of health and sense of coherence. (Adapted from Mittelmark 2013, with permission from Antonovsky)

tendencies toward their life situation. It means believing that things make sense and that one's actions in relation to their situation can make things better.

As is shown in Fig. 2.1, SOC links with the availability of resources (termed *Generalized Resistance Resources*, or GRR) (Mittelmark and Bull 2013). GRRs strengthen one's SOC, and a strong SOC influences the ability to manage one's life situation and move toward health (Antonovsky 1996). Reciprocally, a stronger SOC helps individuals to navigate and negotiate for these GRRs (Mittelmark 2017) and to address their challenges and move toward health. When one has a strong SOC, that individual is likely to be able to confront and manage challenges more effectively (Mittelmark 2017; Mittelmark and Bull 2013).

The role of SOC in supporting people's movement toward health has been investigated by researchers across many life settings (Darkwah et al. 2017; Jellesma et al. 2006; Løndal 2010; Mayer and Krause 2011; Nammontri et al. 2013; Ray et al. 2009). For instance, Elfassi et al. (2016) found that adolescents' coping capacities shift from mainly depending on primary external-behavior-oriented sources of support to their internal capacities. However, they acknowledged that regardless of adolescents' growing cognitive strength, the availability of resources in and around the home environments still remain key in helping them see life challenges as more comprehensible, manageable, and meaningful. Similarly, Braun-Lewensohn et al. (2017) reviewed studies of SOC in childhood and families, finding that predictors of children's psychosomatic complaints were mostly related to resources in their environment, including ill health of mothers, weak social relations with peers, and unsupportive school environments. Both internal and external resources are therefore key in enhancing children's SOC.

2.4 The Intervention: Balekane EARTH

This study is part of a larger project exploring the effectiveness of the Balekane EARTH program in Botswana. "Balekane" is a Botswanan/Setswana word for the participants of the program, meaning "age-mates," and EARTH is an acronym for Empathy-based, Action-orientated, Relationship-building, Transformative, Healing therapy. The program is designed to offer psychosocial treatment and support for adolescents aged 12–15 who have experienced significant trauma (most often the loss of parent(s) due to HIV/AIDS). The program initially runs for 14 days at wilderness camps where young people engage in individual and group therapy. The camps are organized in such a way that therapy is complemented by team building activities through the use of high and low ropes challenge courses; enactment of rites of affirmation to mark group and individual progress; and safari drives to learn about animal behavior and apply reflectively to own behaviors. The program then continues for 3 years with services provided to the participants back in their home communities. Further information about the program can be found in Katisi et al. (2019).

During the camps, at about halfway through the therapy sessions, drawings are introduced together with written and verbal narration to help the young people process their grief. Individual-focused narrative therapy about the drawings and the experience of the drawing process then follows. The sessions conclude with group narrative therapy in the final days of the camp. The therapies involving the drawings focus on both what the child has drawn and constructive resolutions about challenges that the drawings and the drawing process indicate.

2.4.1 Method

The art therapy workbook used for eliciting drawings was an adapted version of Margie Heegaard's *When Someone Very Special Dies: Children Can Learn to Cope with Grief* (Heegaard 1996). This locally adapted workbook was given the title *Grieving Someone Special* and consists of 25 pages of prompts for content, including sketching, coloring, and sometimes writing. For instance, one page reads: "Life is full of changes: There have been a lot of changes where I live. Draw or write to show a change that concerns you the most." Another reads: "People in the community participate in funerals. This is what they do." Another prompts: "Different feelings are allowed. Sometimes I feel..."

When engaging with the workbook, participants sit alone under a tree of their choice and draw in peace under non-intrusive supervision. After completion, they discuss their drawings and drawing experience privately with their social workers. When they are ready, they share some of their experiences and discuss strategies to resolve difficulties as a group.

The drawings in this chapter come from 15 adolescents aged 12–15 years who selected pictures they were happy for us to share. We analyzed these drawings as well as others in their workbook along with their written and verbal narrations. Their data was complemented by two young adults, aged 22 and 25, who completed the program when they were 18 and were willing to share their stories. The participants also took part in focus group discussions at the end of the camps, and we include some content from these discussions in our analysis of the drawings. Further insight comes from interviews with, and observations from, four social workers who undertook the therapy with the participants.

2.4.2 Data Analysis

To analyze the data (including drawings, captions, narrations, and other sources of information), we used thematic content analysis (Attride-Stirling 2001). We utilized a hybrid approach by first deductively drawing codes from the data that linked to qualities associated with an SOC, and then inductively abstracting basic themes, organizing themes, and global themes. The first author (MK) performed the analysis, which then involved the social workers affirming that the themes were appropriate representations (i.e., member checking).

Our analysis is structured around the concepts of *comprehensibility, manageability*, and *meaningfulness* from the salutogenic model. These three concepts are interlinked and not easily separable as stand-alone themes. However, in the salutogenic framework above, the "life course stress exposures" and "generalized resistance resources" are more concrete and distinguishable when describing participants' situations. We therefore categorized these descriptions using three global themes: (1) *stressors*, (2) *resources*, and (3) *strategies*. It is also important to note that the participants conveyed painful experiences, resources, resolutions, and hope in mixed and overlapping ways. Lastly, we identified global themes as a whole using the SOC concepts of *comprehensibility, manageability*, and *meaningfulness*.

Ethical approval for this research was granted by Botswana's Ministry of Local Government. We acquired written consent from participants, social workers, and caregivers, which was provided in the weeks prior to the wilderness camps and included permission to publish drawings. Pseudonyms were used to maintain confidentiality, and identifying details (like names) were removed from the drawings. As the participants were recounting painful memories, we ensured these discussions took place in a therapeutic environment where they had access to qualified professional support.

2.5 Findings

2.5.1 Stressors

The drawings that the participants shared indicated different challenging issues that seemed to be ongoing stressors in their lives. These stressors included witchcraft, sudden death, death due to illness, suicide, and poverty.

2.5.1.1 Witchcraft

Several of the participants reported that witches tormented them, both in dreams and in waking life. Some described their belief that the reason their parents got sick and died was because they (parents) were bewitched. For example, the drawing below (Fig. 2.2) was created by Leila, a 15-year-old girl, under the prompt asking, "What happens during funerals?" The witches, drawn wearing black church clothes, were neighbors who were also members of the church and involved in conducting the funeral. Leila expressed that these three neighbors were too controlling during the funeral, instructing the family on how and where the burial should be and being involved in family rituals. During individual and group therapy, Leila explained that

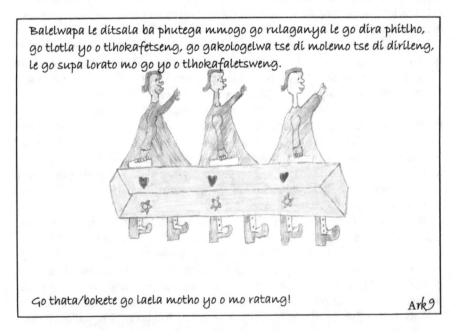

Fig. 2.2 Leila's depiction of witchcraft (the caption reads: "During the funeral, relatives and friends gather together to arrange for burial."). (Reproduced with permission from Ark and Mark Trust, Botswana. Copyright © 2021 Ark and Mark Trust. All rights reserved)

her family told her that the witches later dug up and took away the casket from the graveyard and that no one could return it. This was something that caused her great distress, as she felt that she could not visit her mother's "empty" grave. She felt like she lost her mother twice.

During the focus groups, Leila explained that the three hearts and flowers on the casket were her own expressions of love toward her mother. She used these symbols to depict her feelings but also to explain that her love moved together with her mother's body, wherever the witches took it. She remained concerned and upset about not knowing where her mother had been taken. Leila also struggled to complete the picture, skipping to different pages before returning to the picture to continue. At one point she abandoned the workbook, appearing tense, and requested a break. She later shared her feelings about drawing during focus group discussions: *"I felt scared again by the witches. I don't know them exactly, but I guess they are...some of our neighbors. ...It was hard. I was able to talk about it [the picture] during group discussions after talking for a long time with my social worker. It was...not easy before..."*

2.5.1.2 Sudden Death

The participants used drawings to express love, a sense of oneness with their late parents, and expressions of shock. The latter was related to unexpected death, even in cases where the adolescents were aware that their parents were sick. In some drawings, color and the positioning of figures indicated experiences of trauma that still lingered. Several participants drew themselves as comparably small figures and at a distance away from the body of the parent when expressing sudden deaths.

Tracy, a 14-year-old girl who lost her mother unexpectedly, explained that her picture reflected her shock and helplessness, which she continued to feel. Her drawing portrays herself viewing her mother's corpse (Fig. 2.3). When asked why she drew herself with no hands, she said, *"In this picture, I am holding my hands behind. You cannot see them. I hold my hands back when I do not know what to do. I am shocked here, you see...my mother died...suddenly."* Like Leila, Tracy decorated the blanket covering her late mother with flowers. She explained that the flowers demonstrated her love for her mother. In another drawing, she drew and described taking flowers to her mother's grave, particularly on occasions when she was mistreated at home. She colored herself and her mother with similar colors because it showed they are one and they need each other. She also explained that the line in between them is a curtain that was in the house when she viewed her corpse, a symbol of separation.

Like Leila and others, Joseph (age 17) drew himself and his late mother quite small on the page (Fig. 2.4). When asked about this, he explained that smallness was an expression of confusion, shock, and immense helplessness. *"I felt like nobody,"* he said. It is important to note that not every detail or characteristic is symbolic or representative of something. For example, when asked about his use of colors, Joseph said that there was no particular reason for this choice.

Mo go botlhe ba losika ba ba suleng, yo o neng a le botlhokwa thata mo go nna ke _____.

Setshwantsho se, se supa ka fa a tlhokafetseng ka teng, ka fa go nkamileng ka teng.

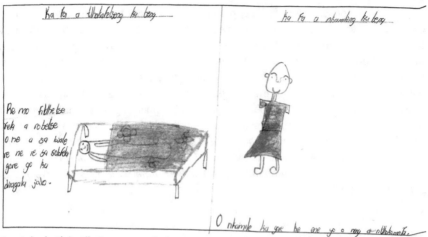

Ka fa a tlhokafetseng ka teng

Ka fa a nkamileng ka teng

Re mo fitlhetse feela a robetse o ne a se bwale re ne re sa bolela gore go ka diragala jalo.

O nkamile ka gore ke ene yo o neng a ntlhokomela.

Go ntsha kutlobotlhoko ya gago ke nngwe ya ditsela tsa go e fokotsa.

Fig. 2.3 Tracy's depiction of the sudden death of her mother (the caption reads: "Among all that have died, the most important person was…my mother. She just died in sleep. She was not ill… This hurt me the most…she was the only one taking care of us."). (Reproduced with permission from Ark and Mark Trust, Botswana. Copyright © 2021 Ark and Mark Trust. All rights reserved)

The social workers reported that many participants who lost their parents saw them deteriorate daily. Several of them expressed that it was painful to watch their parents—some of whom experienced excruciating pain—struggling with their sickness. One participant explained that they used to sneak out from school to check on their ailing mother at home. The children felt fear and helplessness, and this lingered with them long after the passing of their parents.

Peter (Fig. 2.5) was a 15-year-old participant who appeared particularly traumatized by the sudden death of his mother. He said, *"I cry. I cry always. They say a boy is not supposed to cry but I cry a lot. It scares me to have these thoughts. It is because I want to see my mother. I want her to help me. I cry when I think like this. See, my tears are like rain…"* Peter cried a lot during the early sessions, but the social workers suggested that he seemed happier afterwards. During focus group discussions, Peter said, *"I do not cry a lot now. I talked a lot. Maybe I need to talk a lot so that I don't cry a lot. I need help from someone else. I realize my late mother cannot help."*

Crying seemed to trigger crying. One social worker shared that others in the group cried when they saw others cry. *"During this session, one child started crying when sharing her story. One more followed and suddenly almost all were crying except for a few boys. We had to end the session after everyone felt relieved… They*

Mo go botlhe ba losika ba ba suleng, yo o neng a le botlhokwa thata mo go nna ke _____ .

Setshwantsho se, se supa ka fa a tlhokafetseng ka teng, ka fa go nkamileng ka teng.

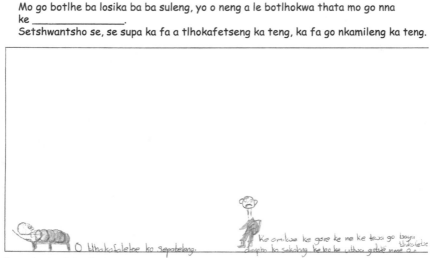

Go ntsha kutlobotlhoko ya gago ke nngwe ya ditsela tsa go e fokotsa.

Fig. 2.4 Joseph's depiction of his mother's death (the caption reads: "She died at the hospital. What hurts me the most is that I was told of her death the same day I got presents for doing well at school."). (Reproduced with permission from Ark and Mark Trust, Botswana. Copyright © 2021 Ark and Mark Trust. All rights reserved)

preferred not to share any more of their stories until the following day. Crying gave them a relief, then they were ready to share more experiences the following day."

2.5.1.3 Ghosts and the Dead

One 13-year-old boy, Thomas, simply wrote, *"You cannot help me…"* He did not draw any pictures in his workbook and instead wrote long narrations about a "thokolosi" (ghost) that visited him all night and tormented him. He explained how this caused him difficulties in school. He described the thokolosi as hairy and animalistic in figure and movement. In his dreams, it always opened its mouth wide to scare him. He believed the thokolosi was a figure representing an angry dead relative. When asked why he did not draw the thokolosi, he exclaimed, *"No, I can't draw it. It would come to life…. No, I can't. It will scare me."* Other participants also feared drawing figures related to trauma, believing that doing so could make them real— like bringing relatives back from the dead, which would not be a positive experience. In these instances, although drawing may not be possible, the lack of drawing itself prompts discussion of challenging issues which would not otherwise come up.

During one-on-one sessions, it emerged that Thomas's main concern was not the thokolosi or how it looked, but rather how he was treated at school by his classmates due to his lack of sleep. He wrote, *"…they call me 'setotwane,' the one who does not sleep at night, because I sleep in class. Please auntie (name of social worker), help*

Bangwe ba ikutlwa ba le nosi ebile ba na le bodutu mo ba feletsang ba eletsa go swa. Tshwantsha o supe gore o ikutlwa jang.

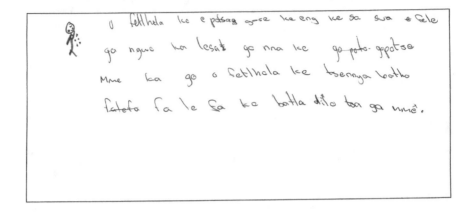

Loso ga le itlhophelwe. Ikgethele go tshela botshelo jo bo siameng.

Fig. 2.5 Peter's self-portrayal of him crying (the caption reads: "I always wonder why I cannot just die so that I stop continuously thinking about my mother."). (Reproduced with permission from Ark and Mark Trust, Botswana. Copyright © 2021 Ark and Mark Trust. All rights reserved)

me, I do not want to be called 'setotwane.'" When the social worker tried to address the thokolosi, Thomas pleaded with her just to help him sleep, believing that only his pastor could help him deal with the thokolosi.

Some participants were able to draw figures of the dead that they dreamt or thought about. In Fig. 2.6, Tracy (who also drew Fig. 2.3) drew her mother and herself again, seemingly without hands. Tracy explained that the absence of hands symbolizes helplessness because they miss each other but cannot meet and hug each other again. She also explained that they are both wearing red because they are both experiencing pain in the world of the dead and the living.

2.5.1.4   Caregiver Suicide

A number of participants drew pictures depicting the suicide of a parent or caregiver. Some had committed suicide to end the pain they were experiencing. Other times, caregivers took their own lives because they felt unable to care for family members.

Some participants described being tormented by the suicide of their parents and caregivers. For instance, 15-year-old Raymond focused his attention on the body of his uncle (Fig. 2.7). He colored the body and rope with close attention to detail, shading and giving relief to different parts. In contrast, little attention was given to the tree, which he did not give color to at all. The social worker later recounted what

Ditshwantsho tse di tshosang di tla mo dikakanyong le mo ditorong tsame dinako di ngwe. Tshwantsha/kwala o supa toro kgotsa dikakanyo tse di tshosang tse o kileng wa nna le tsone.

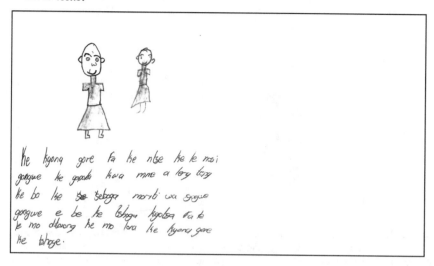

Go a thusa go dira ditshwantsho tseo mo pampiring o bo o buisanya le mongwe ka tsone.

Fig. 2.6 Tracy's depiction of seeing the dead (the caption reads: "I often see a figure of my mother when I am alone and thinking about her. Sometimes I see her in my dreams. I get scared when this happens."). (Reproduced with permission from Ark and Mark Trust, Botswana. Copyright © 2021 Ark and Mark Trust. All rights reserved)

Raymond had told her—that his uncle was the center of his life and that he cared deeply about him. Raymond expressed that his uncle's clothes were very vivid in his memory, and that the imagery sometimes disturbed his thinking and his concentration at school.

According to his social worker, Raymond described all the good things his uncle used to do to support him after his mother's death. He explained that after his uncle committed suicide, he had no support. He said he felt helpless and at one time attempted suicide on the same tree. He showed the social worker the scars on his neck from the failed attempt.

One participant, Thabo (age 13), drew his late mother who committed suicide (Fig. 2.8). He used the same colors in another picture of his family home burning down (Fig. 2.9). When asked to talk about the colors, such as why he drew his mother in red, he said, "...*death is just like fire. It takes away life. Blood and fire are red.*" He also said that blue marked significant things that were problems in his life. The blue tree and the blue on the house (reminding him of the damage) were things that continued to disturb him.

Mongwe yo ke neng ke mo rata o tlhokafetse. Setshwantsho sa
motho yo ke se:

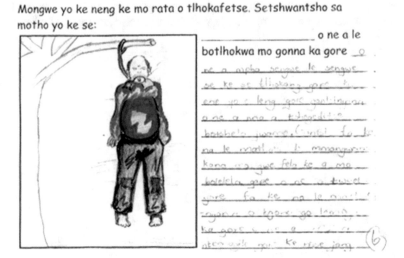

_____ o ne a le
botlhokwa mo gonna ka gore _o .

Fig. 2.7 Raymond's depiction of the suicide of his uncle (the caption reads: "My uncle had my life in his hands. He provided everything for me, I used to tell him when [my] aunt troubled me…but now he is gone."). (Reproduced with permission from Ark and Mark Trust, Botswana. Copyright © 2021 Ark and Mark Trust. All rights reserved)

2.5.1.5 Poverty

Many of the young people revealed their economic status through drawings, and several conveyed changes in this status after the loss of their parents. Some became poor as a result of losing a breadwinner, while others' property and inheritance were seized by older relatives, knowing that the children would be powerless to stop them. Their sudden absence of financial support led to a shortage of food, health care, clothing, and other basic needs.

The change to poorer conditions constantly reminded 13-year-old Tracy of her late mother (Fig. 2.10). She explained that the big house her mother built still exists and is used by other extended members of the family, despite cracks in the walls. She was moved to sleep in a smaller (mud) house, where she felt unsafe because the door could not be locked. According to the social worker, Tracy cried a lot when talking about this, saying, *"It exposes us to risks. I want to live in my late mum's big house."*

Throughout her narrations, Tracy mentioned God as her source of strength but explained that her grandmother and aunt tried to stop her from attending church, saying she would bring bad spirits into the family. This caused her some distress, as she would frequently attend church with her late mother and felt blocked from continuing this ritual and engaging with this source of support.

Mo go botlhe ba losika ba ba suleng, yo o neng a le botlhokwa thata mo go nna ke_____

Setshwantsho se se supa fa a tlhokafetseng ka teng, ka fa go nkamileng ka teng.

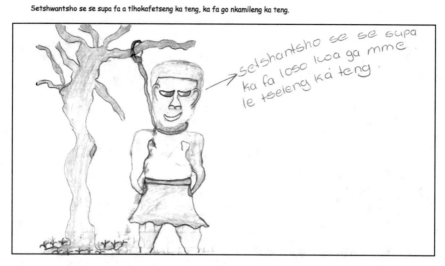

Go ntsha kutlobotlhoko ya gago ke nngwe ya ditsela tsa go e fokotsa.

Fig. 2.8 Thabo's depiction of his mother's suicide (the caption reads: "This picture shows how my mother died."). (Reproduced with permission from Ark and Mark Trust, Botswana. Copyright © 2021 Ark and Mark Trust. All rights reserved)

2.5.2 Resources and Strategies

Through the process of drawing and reflecting on their drawings, the participants identified several external resources that could help them manage challenges in their lives. Of these resources, relationships were cited as critical. They referred to peers at the camp, relatives, social workers, other staff at the camp, community chiefs, teachers, friends, and neighbors. Those most commonly discussed are explored below.

2.5.2.1 Peers

Peers were described as a strong source of support at the camp. The group sessions encouraged sympathy and empathy among the participants when they listened to each other talking about their drawings: *"I listened to others talk about their problems. I am not the only one... We all need help."* Not only did this process facilitate a greater sense of kinship, it was also described as cathartic. Leila said, *"...I mean, when others shared stories about witchcraft then I felt free but not totally free. I shared some bits...and we cried together...then I was a little relieved... After listening to other children, I felt better..."* Many of the participants also mentioned that

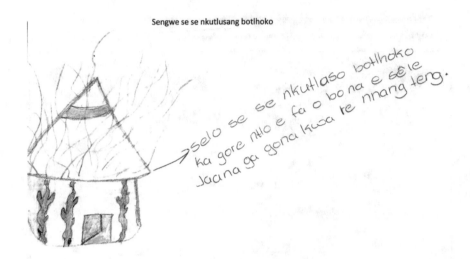

Sengwe se se nkutlusang botlhoko

Go tshwantsha kutlobotlhoko go fokotsa botlhoko

Fig. 2.9 Thabo's depiction of his house burning down (the caption reads: "What hurts me the most is that we have no place to live. As you can see, our house is burnt down by fire."). (Reproduced with permission from Ark and Mark Trust, Botswana. Copyright © 2021 Ark and Mark Trust. All rights reserved)

they would continue talking to others from the camp after the end of the camp if they felt sad.

2.5.2.2 Relatives

Relatives were seen as a source of stress and a source of strength at the same time. Many of the young participants were abused by relatives yet still looked to them for support, suggesting these perceptions could come at different times: *"They are not always bad"*; *"I can talk to them when they are happy"*; *"It seems I am bothering my relatives…I will not give up, sometimes they listen."*

Following drawing and discussions, some suggested that a change in a relationship with caregivers could be possible: *"I live with my aunt. I will tell her that I told the social worker (about the witches). She may not be happy with me. But she loves me a lot. Maybe we can talk together more about this."*

2.5.2.3 Social Workers

Many of the participants described a closer connection to their social worker following the camp. Peter, who had previously expressed wishing to die, wrote, *"I now have a plan. When I am in pain and need help, I would like to talk to my social*

Go nnile le diphetogo tse dintsi kwa ke nnang teng. Tshwantsha kana o kwale o supa phetogo e e go tshwentseng thata.

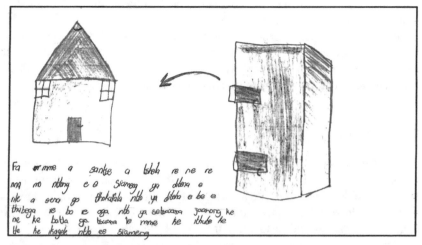

Batho ba le bantsi ba tlhaloganya ka mathata a gago, gape ba leka go go thusa.

Fig. 2.10 Tracy's depiction of the change in her housing (the caption reads: "When my mother was still alive, we had a decent home. She had built us a nice house. After her death, the house cracked and fell apart. We then built a traditional round mud house. I want to be like my mother, to get educated and build a good house for myself."). (Reproduced with permission from Ark and Mark Trust, Botswana. Copyright © 2021 Ark and Mark Trust. All rights reserved)

worker. She is a nice person." A greater connection with the social worker appeared to be established through the process of drawing and discussion, leading to this new source of support for the individual: "*I have been very angry with uncle. I felt better after discussing this picture with the social worker. I have to do something to get more help so that the lost house is replaced…I have hope…*"

2.5.2.4 Community Leaders

Traditional leaders (chiefs) were described as being helpful in resolving issues of abuse, mitigating property grabbing by relatives, and tracing absent fathers (a common issue in the region): "*The chief of my village supports children… Last year he came here, with my sister's group. I think I can talk to him when I have problems. [Like] if they [caregivers] beat me again.*" Through drawing, the adolescents described knowing more about what they could talk to their community leaders about in order to try to receive assistance or resolve conflicts.

2.5.2.5 Community Members

Participants also considered the community as helpful in stressful times. Some referred to neighbors who were also their relatives and expressed that they could be good sources of support. Raymond, who had attempted suicide on the same tree his uncle used, was rescued from the tree by community members. Reflecting on this incident gave him hope that there were others out there who cared about him. He said that this led him to seek help from teachers at school.

2.5.2.6 Spirituality

After drawing their experiences and describing past and ongoing challenges, some of the children described how God and going to church could help them manage these difficulties. Thomas, the one tormented by a thokolosi, believed his pastor's prayers would keep the monster at bay, while others suggested that God and being a good Christian would keep them insulated from the dangers of witches and witchcraft.

2.6 Discussion

Drawing, as employed in this context, appears to work well when used in conjunction with written and verbal narratives. It appears to achieve what other types of approaches could miss (Vendeville et al. 2018), such as when the participants felt unable or unwilling to bring up issues in group or individual sessions but were able to draw them. Through drawing, the participants disclosed suppressed traumatic experiences: suicide attempts, wishes to die, hallucinations, experiences at graveyards, scary dreams, beliefs and trauma connected to witches and ghosts, visits by the dead, and ongoing abuse. If used with care and skill, drawing can be a safe way of delving deeper into one's inner experience. (Rubin 2011). Not only does drawing serve as a powerful communication tool for challenging incidents, it also helps convey and release suppressed emotions (Bonoti and Misalidi 2015).

Lev-Wiesel and Liraz (2007) argue that when drawing is used before verbal narrations, it encourages children's communication of traumatic experiences. In their study, children who lived with drug-addicted fathers drew scary eyes, undernourished skeletal fathers, and instruments connected to drug use. After drawing, these children were able to describe their drawings verbally, indirectly conveying their traumatic experiences, while the control group who did not draw had difficulty expressing similar emotionally provoking experiences. However, some have argued that drawing becomes easier for individuals to engage in if they follow narrative approaches first (Farokhi and Hashemi 2011; Malindi and Theron 2011). For instance, when other therapeutic approaches like group discussions, drama, or individual therapy are used before drawings, they prepare children to freely use drawings to express hidden emotions that they may struggle to convey (Dalley and Case 2014). Indeed, when first devising the Balekane EARTH program, Thamuku and Daniel (2013) explored different therapeutic approaches and noted that in the initial group work, the participants tended to prefer to discuss their general social challenges, and that this gentle introduction helps to softens their "hard shell" of grief. Once this shell was opened, it permitted access to more challenging issues, which can be reached through the use of drawings (Thamuku and Daniel 2013). This reflects the findings of others who have emphasized that effective therapy is cumulative, starting with the less sensitive issues before progressing to those that are more sensitive; the foundational steps help participants to open up slowly (Bonoti and Misalidi 2015; Farokhi and Hashemi 2011; Thamuku and Daniel 2013).

In the present study, we established that drawing was introduced on the seventh day of therapy, after several narrative sessions. But narratives were also used after the drawing experience to discuss what was in the drawings. Therefore, the EARTH program seems flexible in the sequence of verbal narratives and drawing. Most of the participants were able to draw, narrate, and explain painful emotions connected to traumatic experiences, but the order and unlocking mechanism behind these steps varied among the participants; some drew in the beginning in order to be able to talk about an issue, while others struggled to draw if issues were not broached and worked through verbally first. It is possible that those who only wrote narratives in their workbooks could have been asked to go back and draw after verbal therapy sessions with their social workers. This underscores the importance of using drawing as an additional and complementary tool in therapeutic programs and encourages using it flexibly with discussion.

The theory of salutogenesis provides a framework to systematically and critically examine the health-promoting benefits of drawing. In this discussion, we reflect on the key findings from the drawings and the experiences of the drawing process using the concepts of *comprehensibility*, *manageability*, and *meaningfulness*.

2.6.1 Comprehensibility

During group narratives about their drawings, hearing the stories of the other adolescents helped participants understand their own experiences. For example, Leila helped others feel able to express their experiences with witchcraft. One of the social workers described how, in one group session, the crying of one participant gave permission for others to cry and release suppressed pain. These examples show that adolescents were able to connect and deal with past terrors. Narratives on drawings enabled them to comprehend that their own feelings are "normal" and okay to express—that others have similar pain (Anolak et al. 2018). Given the widespread beliefs about witchcraft that persist in sub-Saharan Africa, Leila's story is, unfortunately, not uncommon (Mills 2018).

Our analysis of the participants' drawings and their accompanying narratives indicates that the the comprehension of their problems was influenced by how they experienced loss, grief, and trauma; by the availability of resources around them; and by their opportunities to navigate to access those resources. In their narratives, some expressed that they had already accessed help—for example, seeing social workers. Others started taking action by talking to friends and other adults at the camp.

Regardless of their extreme emotional challenges, the participants seemed to have an understanding that their situations were resolvable. Initially, some appeared more helpless and others were more optimistic, while many moved back and forth between pain and progress to health through the 14 days of the camp. In the case of the latter, the SOC was not experienced as a continuum, as reflected in Fig. 2.1, but rather as a dynamic movement between comprehension, stress, and well-being. Most young people seemed to go back and forth between their challenges and strategies to get back home and use resources. Their hope was linked both to resources they had previously known were available and to ones they had newly learned about. Some had attempted to use resources such as family, friends, and professional services like social workers before the camp; although these young people were still experiencing the same challenges, they would not give up. Their drawings showed that the camp experience strengthened them to persist or to try again in other ways. Many believed they could solve the intangible with the abstract—for example, addressing witchcraft experiences with their belief in God.

2.6.2   Manageability

When people show hope, and when their perceptions of stressors are tied with the availability of resources, it indicates the manageability of situations, hence movement toward health (Darkwah et al. 2017). In this study, drawing helped to activate positive internal resources, with the participants often saying that the drawing process itself gave them a sense of relief and release. Some mentioned that while drawing their traumatic experiences, they felt pain, missed their late parents, cried, and felt fear, but at the end of the process they felt a relief from their hearts. This fits with an understanding of the cathartic properties of drawing (Bonoti and Misalidi 2015).

Art and writing has empowering effects (Garista et al. 2019; Thamuku and Daniel 2013), and this was reflected in our findings, where participants consistently reflected on sources of support. They noted a network of resources: peers at the camps, relatives, camp and local social workers, teachers, traditional leaders, neighbors, and the broader community. Writing and talking about such strategies appeared to support them as they drew hurtful experiences. In particular, peer and group work helped them realize that they shared experiences of loss, fear, abuse, and pain with others. A sense of support and greater manageability materialized when others were seen to cope with their difficulties.

Some participants were already aware of resources and had used them before the camp, but through drawing they became aware of additional resources available to them. They also gained knowledge about different ways to use the resources they had tried before, such as getting support from caregivers when relationships were strained.

2.6.3 Meaningfulness

Drawing helped the young people to make sense of the distressing experiences related to the loss of parents and caregivers, and, once clarified, they became active participants in the process to discover solutions to their challenges. Their motivation to participate in sessions and take action was linked to the existing resources that the program seemed to make possible for them to access. The social workers reported a positive change in those who were withdrawn—even in those who were initially wishing to die. Many participants became optimistic about their futures by the end of the camp and described positive next steps and longer-term plans. The young adults who participated were examples of this positive change, having become successful and active members of their communities. These ideas are further explored in the final chapter of this volume (*see* Chap. 21), which suggests a theoretical framework for conceptualizing some of these meaning-making dynamics.

2.7 Conclusion

For adolescents in stressful situations, drawing is a tool that can help them move toward greater health and well-being. Using a salutogenic lens, our findings reveal that drawing can be beneficial in helping young people communicate complex emotional stressors and map different resources that they have around them. Drawing has empowering effects, promotes creativity, and can help young people visualize strategies to manage their traumatic experiences.

However, we found that when young people experience trauma, they do make efforts to access existing resources, even before therapy, indicating that they should not be pathologized as only weak, stressed, or depressed. Therapeutic programs should embrace and build on these existing resources and identify those that may be present but troubled or unused. Drawing presents an important tool for such discovery and communication, both for the individual and the practitioner.

References

Anolak, H., Watt, B., & Thornton, C. (2018). Guided imagery and music (GIM) combined with music, drawing and narrative (MDN) as an intervention for reducing perinatal anxiety. *Women and Birth, 31*, S30–S31. https://doi.org/10.1016/j.wombi.2018.08.095.

Antonovsky, A. (1996). The salutogenic model as a theory to guide health promotion. *Health Promotion International, 11*(1), 11–18. https://doi.org/10.1093/heapro/11.1.11.

Attride-Stirling, J. (2001). Thematic networks: An analytic tool for qualitative research. *Qualitative Research, 1*(3), 385–405. https://doi.org/10.1177/146879410100100307.

Bonoti, F., & Misalidi, P. (2015). Social emotions in children's human figure drawings: Drawing shame, pride and jealousy. *Infant and Child Development, 24*(6), 661–672.

Braun-Lewensohn, O., Idan, O., Lindström, B., & Margalit, M. (2017). Salutogenesis: Sense of coherence in adolescence. In B. M. Maurice, S. Shifra, M. E. F. Georg, J. M. Bauer, M. P. Jürgen, et al. (Eds.), *The handbook of salutogenesis* (pp. 123–136). New York: Springer.

Campbell, C., Skovdal, M., Mupambireyi, Z., & Gregson, S. (2010). Exploring children's stigmatisation of AIDS-affected children in Zimbabwe through drawings and stories. *Social Science & Medicine, 71*(5), 975–985. https://doi.org/10.1016/j.socscimed.2010.05.028.

Campbell, C., Andersen, L., Mutsikiwa, A., Madanhire, C., Skovdal, M., Nyamukapa, C., et al. (2015). Re-thinking children's agency in extreme hardship: Zimbabwean children's draw-and-write about their HIV-affected peers. *Health & Place, 31*, 54–64. https://doi.org/10.1016/j.healthplace.2014.09.008.

Cluver, L., Gardner, F., & Operario, O. (2007). Psychological distress amongst AIDS-orphaned children in urban South Africa. *Journal of Child Psychology and Psychiatry, 48*(8), 755–763. http://onlinelibrary.wiley.com/store/10.1111/j.1469-7610.2007.01757.x/asset/j.1469-7610.2007.01757.x.pdf?v=1&t=jb6gxz29&s=502102d3302afc31e8af9b99cdffbd48e93105ef.

Dalley, T., & Case, C. (2014). *The handbook of art therapy*. East Sussex: Routledge.

Daniel, M., Apila, H. M., Bjorgo, R., & Lie, G. T. (2007). Breaching cultural silence: Enhancing resilience among Ugandan orphans. *Ajar-African Journal of Aids Research, 6*(2), 109–120. https://doi.org/10.2989/16085900709490405.

Darkwah, E., Asumeng, M., & Daniel, M. (2017). Caring for "parentless" children: An exploration of work stressors and resources as experienced by caregivers in children's homes in Ghana. *International Journal of Child, Youth and Family Studies, 8*(2), 59–89. https://doi.org/10.18357/ijcyfs82201717850.

Deininger, K., Garcia, M., & Subbarao, K. (2003). AIDS-induced orphanhood as a systemic shock: Magnitude, impact, and program interventions in Africa. *World Development, 31*(7), 1201–1220.

Elfassi, Y., Braun-Lewensohn, O., Krumer-Nevo, M., & Sagy, S. (2016). Community sense of coherence among adolescents as related to their involvement in risk behaviors. *Journal of Community Psychology, 44*(1), 22–37. https://doi.org/10.1002/jcop.21739.

Farokhi, M., & Hashemi, M. (2011). The analysis of children's drawings: Social, emotional, physical, and psychological aspects. *Procedia-Social and Behavioral Sciences, 30*, 2219–2224.

Garista, P., Pocetta, G., & Lindström, B. (2019). Picturing academic learning: Salutogenic and health promoting perspectives on drawings. *Health Promotion International, 34*(4), 859–868.

Heath, M. A., Donald, D. R., Theron, L. C., & Lyon, R. C. (2014). AIDS in South Africa: Therapeutic interventions to strengthen resilience among orphans and vulnerable children. *School Psychology International, 35*(3), 309–337. https://doi.org/10.1177/0143034314529912.

Heegaard, M. E. (1996). *When someone very special dies: Children can learn to cope with grief*. Minneapolis, MN: Woodland Press.

Jellesma, F. C., Rieffe, C., Terwogt, M. M., & Kneepkens, C. M. F. (2006). Somatic complaints and health care use in children: Mood, emotion awareness and sense of coherence. *Social Science & Medicine, 63*, 2640–2648. https://doi.org/10.1016/j.socscimed.2006.07.004.

Katisi, M., Jefferies, P., Dikolobe, O., Moeti, O., Brisson, J., & Ungar, M. (2019). Fostering resilience in children who have been orphaned: Preliminary results from the Botswana Balekane EARTH program. *Child & Youth Care Forum, 48*, 585–601.

Lev-Wiesel, R., & Liraz, R. (2007). Drawings vs. narratives: Drawing as a tool to encourage verbalization in children whose fathers are drug abusers. *Clinical Child Psychology and Psychiatry, 12*(1), 65–75. https://doi.org/10.1177/1359104507071056.

Løndal, K. (2010). Children's lived experience and their sense of coherence: Bodily play in a Norwegian after-school programme. *Child Care in Practice, 16*(4), 391–407. https://doi.org/1 0.1080/13575279.2010.498414.

Malindi, M., & Theron, L. (2011). Drawing on strengths: Images of ecological contributions to street child resilience. In L. C. Theron, C. Mitchell, J. Stuart, & A. Smith (Eds.), *Picturing research drawings as visual methodology* (pp. 105–118). Rotterdam: Sense Publishers.

Mayer, C. H., & Krause, C. (2011). Promoting mental health and salutogenesis in transcultural organizational and work contexts. Taylor & Francis Online. https://doi.org/10.3109/0954026 1.2011.636549.

Meissner, R. J., Ferguson, J., Otto, C., Gretschel, P., & Ramugondo, E. (2017). A play-informed, caregiver-implemented, home-based intervention for HIV-positive children and their families living in low-income conditions in South Africa. *World Federation of Occupational Therapists Bulletin, 73*(2), 83–87. https://doi.org/10.1080/14473828.2017.1375068.

Mills, J. (2018). Witchcraft, witches, and violence in Ghana. Taylor & Francis Online. https://doi. org/10.1080/00083968.2018.1439280.

Mittelmark, M. B. (2017). *Introduction to the handbook of salutogenesis. The Handbook of Salutogenesis* (pp. 3–5). New York: Springer.

Mittelmark, M. B., & Bull, T. (2013). The salutogenic model of health in health promotion research. *Global Health Promotion, 20*(2), 30–38. https://doi.org/10.1177/1757975913486684.

Nammontri, O., Robinson, P. G., & Baker, S. R. (2013). Enhancing oral health via sense of coherence: A cluster-randomized trial. *Journal of Dental Research, 92*(1), 26–31. https://doi. org/10.1177/0022034512459757.

Pifalo, T. (2007). Jogging the cogs: Trauma-focused art therapy and cognitive behavioral therapy with sexually abused children. *Art Therapy, 24*(4), 170–175. https://doi.org/10.1080/0742165 6.2007.10129471.

Ray, C., Suominen, S., & Roos, E. (2009). The role of parent's sense of coherence in irregular meal pattern and food intake pattern of children aged 10–11 in Finland. *Journal of Epidemiology & Community Health, 63*(12). https://doi.org/10.1136/jech.2008.085100.

Rubin, J. A. (2011). *The art of art therapy: What every art therapist needs to know*. London: Routledge.

Schenk, K. D. (2009). Community interventions providing care and support to orphans and vulnerable children: A review of evaluation evidence. *AIDS Care, 21*(7), 918–942. http://www. tandfonline.com/doi/pdf/10.1080/09540120802537831?needAccess=true.

Skovdal, M. (2012). Pathologising healthy children? A review of the literature exploring the mental health of HIV-affected children in sub-Saharan Africa. *Transcultural Psychiatry, 49*(3–4), 461–491. https://doi.org/10.1177/1363461512448325.

Skovdal, M., & Daniel, M. (2012). Resilience through participation and coping-enabling social environments: The case of HIV-affected children in sub-Saharan Africa. *African Journal of AIDS Research, 11*(3), 153–164. https://doi.org/10.2989/16085906.2012.734975.

Strebel, A. (2004). *The development, implementation and evaluation of interventions for the care of orphans and vulnerable children in Botswana, South Africa and Zimbabwe: A literature review of evidence-based interventions for home-based child-centred development*. Cape Town: HSRC Publishers.

Thamuku, M., & Daniel, M. (2013). Exploring responses to transformative group therapy for orphaned children in the context of mass orphaning in Botswana. *Death Studies, 37*(5), 413–447. https://doi.org/10.1080/07481187.2012.654594.

Toska, E., Gittings, L., Hodes, R., Cluver, L. D., Govender, K., Chademana, K. E., et al. (2016). Resourcing resilience: Social protection for HIV prevention amongst children and adolescents in Eastern and Southern Africa. *African Journal of AIDS Research, 15*(2), 123–140. https://doi.org/10.2989/16085906.2016.1194299.

Ugurlu, N., Akca, L., & Acarturk, C. (2016). An art therapy intervention for symptoms of post-traumatic stress, depression and anxiety among Syrian refugee children. *Vulnerable Children and Youth Studies, 11*(2), 89–102. https://doi.org/10.1080/17450128.2016.1181288.

UNAIDS. (2019). Global HIV & AIDS statistics—2019 fact sheet. Available at https://www.unaids.org/en/resources/fact-sheet.

Vendeville, N., Blanc, N., & Brechet, C. (2018). Tears for girls and teeth for boys: The influence of gender on children's depiction of sadness and anger in their drawings. *Educational Psychology*, 1–18. https://doi.org/10.1080/01443410.2018.1461810.

Wakhweya, A., Dirks, R., & Yeboah, K. (2008). Children thrive in families: Family-centred models of care and support for orphans and other vulnerable children affected by HIV and AIDS. *AIDS JLICA.*

Xiaoming, L., Peilian, C., Lorraine, S., Lucie, C., & Bonita, S. (2015). Psychological resilience among children affected by parental HIV/AIDS: A conceptual framework. *Health Psychology and Behavioral Medicine, 3*(1), 217–235. https://doi.org/10.1080/21642850.2015.1068698.

Chapter 3
Promoting Spiritual Health: Using Poetry as a Coping Strategy for Iranian Women Post-divorce

Fatemeh Zarei

3.1 Divorce as a Complex Life Event

Divorce has many facets. In the legal sense, divorce is defined as the end of the formal contract of a marriage (Putnam 2011). Scholars use the term to refer to a couple's separation and as a socially constructed experience that affects the whole family (Harold and Leve 2018; Leturcq and Panico 2019; Xerxa et al. 2019). Depending on the social and cultural context, the divorce process can be more or less complicated and stressful. In Iran, the process is extremely complex for women. First, a submission of a divorce registration request might not be accepted if submitted by a woman; the experience of filing is determined by the petitioner's gender role (Habibi et al. 2015). Ending a marriage might be simple and quick, or it might be time-consuming, overwhelming, and tedious. Although divorce laws continue to favor men, women are increasingly initiating divorces (Moghadam 2004). While inequity exists in the structures determining legal divorce proceedings, this increase serves as a sign that traditional marriage is changing as women gain equality. According to a study that explored the perspectives of women who experienced Iran's judiciary in divorce proceedings, custody and dowry concerns, and family court alimony, Iranian women identified low levels of legal awareness, the experience of post-divorce poverty, and low self-esteem because of the patriarchal hegemonic structure as the major barriers in their access to family justice (Bahar et al. 2018).

F. Zarei (✉)
Department of Health Education and Health Promotion, Faculty of Medical Sciences, Tarbiat Modares University, Tehran, Iran
e-mail: f.zarei@modares.ac.ir

© The Author(s) 2021
J. H. Corbin et al. (eds.), *Arts and Health Promotion*,
https://doi.org/10.1007/978-3-030-56417-9_3

41

3.1.1 Divorce in Iran

Over the last two decades, divorce rates in Iran have been rising (Bolhari et al. 2012). In 2009, the divorce rate was 17%, rising to 29% 8 years later in 2017 (Jafarian Dehkordi and Amiri 2018). During the years 2004–2010, most of the women in Iran experiencing divorce were aged 20–24 years, while the average age for men was 25–29 years (Jafarian Dehkordi and Amiri 2018). These figures reflect that Iranian women get married younger and also experience divorce earlier than men.

3.1.2 Factors Contributing to Divorce

Research has identified numerous factors contributing to divorce, including economic, psychosocial, and social issues (Ardi and Maizura 2018; Pirak et al. 2019; Raley and Sweeney 2020). Financial difficulties such as rising costs of housing, high unemployment rates, and inflation can contribute to divorce. Economic hardship adds stress and increases the risk of marital conflict and the likelihood of marriage dissolution (Sadeghi and Agadjanian 2019). Other risk factors are psychosocial and social, including a lack of compatibility and understanding, not meeting partners' psychological needs, domestic violence, personality conflict, gender inequality, problems with children, lack of responsibility, family interference, cultural differences, education level differences, drugs and alcohol use, infidelity, and sexual dissatisfaction (Jafarian Dehkordi and Amiri 2018).

3.2 Post-divorce Life Among Iranian Women

In Iran, as in several other contexts, divorce represents a family and social crisis. Divorce causes family imbalances and a loss of family stability, and often damages family members' health and psychological well-being (Robinson 2018). The impacts of divorce are not necessarily felt equitably by all family members. Indeed, Iranian studies have shown that divorced women may face far more challenges and obstacles than divorced men (Bahar et al. 2018; Nikparvar et al. 2017; Pirak et al. 2019; Zagami et al. 2019) and experience more problems such as depression, social isolation, and poverty that threaten their well-being (Zare et al. 2017). Context also plays a role in the socially constructed meaning of divorce. For instance, in Iran, research has found that the stigma assigned to a divorced woman can impact her social dignity and can lead to her exclusion from society (Zare et al. 2017; Zarei et al. 2017). Iranian women often experience divorce as a socially excluding process. They may experience post-divorce discrimination when seeking occupational opportunities, weakened social ties, lack of family and social support, social and family ostracism, and health issues (Merghati-Khoei et al. 2014).

On a personal level, divorce also affects Iranian women's sexual well-being. Findings from a study in Iran by Zarei et al. (2013) revealed how societal discrimination, women's perceptions, and post-divorce life experiences combine to informally regulate women's sexual lives and silence the expression of their sexuality. The study found that women's sexuality is highly influenced by societal scripts and by the expectation for women that post-divorce life should proceed without expression of their sexuality. The authors argued that the root of the regulatory and ideological ambivalence toward divorced women's sexuality lies in the male-dominant structure of Iranian society. In a culture where silence, sexual purity, chastity, and women's sexual repression are highly valued, few women will risk their social reputation. Instead, they conform their sexual lives to fit the dominant framework of society, and their sexual health and well-being is ignored. The lived experiences of Iranian women reveal that divorce is a much more complicated issue than the simple separation of two people, and goes beyond individualistic and psychological outcomes (Pirak et al. 2019). Therefore, identifying, understanding, and planning for divorce and its resulting consequences require a deeper and more deliberate view that is informed by these lived perceptions and experiences.

3.2.1 Post-divorce Life Adjustment: Developing Personal Skills

Developing personal skills is one of the five key action areas for health promotion identified in the Ottawa Charter to empower individuals to give them more control over their health (World Health Organization 1986). Developing personal skills includes the development of health literacy, basic motor skills, and an awareness of the connections between risk behaviors and disease. It encourages protective behaviors and builds knowledge to better navigate the health system and to analyze health information critically. However, developing personal skills is not just about physical health, specific skills, and knowledge. It also aims to promote lifelong learning that enables individuals to harness health as a resource for their lives. This implies that knowledge and skills relevant to social settings, family contexts, spiritual issues, life purpose, and mental and emotional stability are all components of personal skill development (World Health Organization 1986)

As the number of marriages ending in divorce in Iran has increased, post-divorce life adjustment has become a major concern for a larger number of impacted women. Any support for this transition requires attention to socio-cultural and psychological perspectives to ensure culturally appropriate coping strategies. Commonly prescribed strategies such as stress management, relaxation methods, yoga, and meditation (Rosario and Leite 2019) may support psychological well-being; however, these strategies offer little support for coping with the complex cultural concerns divorced women might face in Iran. In other words, a new perspective about post-divorce life difficulties may be needed to provide a more holistic and effective personal coping strategy.

3.3   Meaning-Making and Spiritual Health: An Under-examined Concept in Health Promotion

A spiritual engagement with the world can be important for human health (Kristeller 2010). Life satisfaction is one aspect of spiritual health, and finding meaning in life events can be a pathway toward life satisfaction (Linley and Joseph 2011; Steger and Frazier 2005). In general, spiritual engagement includes a sense of connection to something greater than oneself, and it typically involves a search for meaning in life (Mueller et al. 2001).

The *existential paradigm* and *Logotherapy approach* as a treatment in psychiatry suggest that the primary motivational force of an individual is to find meaning in life. The prominent leaders of existentialism—such as Viktor E. Frankl in 1946, Erich Seligmann Fromm in 1953, and Irvin Yalom in 1980—argued that existentialism is a philosophy that emphasizes the individual's existence, freedom, and choice. *Existentialism* is the view that human beings define their own meanings in life, and try to make rational decisions despite living in an irrational universe. According to the *Logotherapy approach* introduced in 1946 by Frankl, meaning in life can be discovered in three different ways: (1) by creating a work or doing a deed; (2) by experiencing something or encountering someone; and (3) by the attitude we take toward unavoidable suffering, asserting that "everything can be taken from a man but one thing: the last of the human freedoms—to choose one's attitude in any given set of circumstances" (Frankl 1967, p. 138–142)

Given the social context, stigma, and suffering many Iranian women endure after divorce, a strategy for promoting meaning-making and spiritual health, rather than stress reduction activities done in isolation, might better equip them to transition to their new lives.

3.3.1   Art as an Effective Personal Development Strategy

Art is the expression or application of human creative skill and imagination. Art produces ideas and artifacts to be appreciated primarily for their beauty or emotional power (Davies et al. 2015; see also Chap. 1, in this volume). Poetry is one of the literary art forms. Marjorie Perloff, the American poetry scholar and critic, said "poetry compares present to past, divulges some hidden emotion, or comes to a new understanding of the situation" (Perloff 2002, p.7–43). This means that poetry conjures images in the mind and creates new ways to experience the world and express thoughts. One can convert these mental images into meaningful and understandable concepts.

Given these attributes, poetry is an art form particularly suited to affect awareness, attitude, and beliefs at both individual and societal levels. Kazemek et al. (2004) explored an ongoing project where, through poetry, oral history, and storytelling, children and young adults with particular emotional and learning needs were connected to older mentors. The research highlights the literary and personal benefits for all the participants in intergenerational exchanges facilitated through engagement with the arts. Art has been significant in human societies throughout history. It is rooted in culture and reflects the values and beliefs of the culture that produced it. Known as the birthplace of poetry (Roohollah 2018; Rypka 2013), poetry has been a significant outlet for emotional and thought expression in Iran since ancient times. Iranian poets, such as Hafez, Saadi, Ferdowsi, and Rumi, are known globally for writing poetry that conveys love and resentment, anger and frustration, as well as other feelings linked to private or national interests (Sen Nag 2019).

Rumi, in particular, has remained relevant over time. The French Iranologist Henri Massé (1886–1969), in comparing the four Iranian poets mentioned above to other well-known poets, concluded that Rumi cannot be compared to anyone in this world (Ghahremani 2016; ParsToday 2017; Rozina 2017). Yosefi, an Iranian literary critic, in the book *Cheshmeh Roshan [Bright Fountain]*, points out that "Rumi is unique and will remain unique. He is not only a poet but rather a sociologist and especially a psychologist who exactly knows human nature..." (Yosefi 2018, p. 207).

3.3.1.1 The Work of Rumi

Jalāl ad-Dīn Muhammad Rūmī, also known popularly as Rumi (1207–1273), was a thirteenth-century Persian poet, jurist, Islamic scholar, theologian, and Sufi mystic. Rumi's works are written mainly in Persian, but occasionally he also used Turkish, Arabic, and Greek in his poems.

During the last 25 years of his life, Rumi composed over 70,000 verses of poetry collected in six distinct volumes. His poetry illuminates a diversity of topics, covering deep philosophical and mystical issues; fiery expressions of passionate love filled with yearning and desire; and more didactically framed verses filled with anecdotes, lessons for living, moral stories, stories from all three Abrahamic religions, popular topics of the day, and even satirical tales.

Rumi proposes that the difficulties humans encounter and overcome can lead to growth while encouraging a letting go of dependency. In other words, breaking from the shackles of our ego [egoistic attachments] may promote growth. While promoting spiritual reflection, Rumi's poems transcend religion and ethnicity. Lastly, Rumi's poems are mystical[1] (De Bruijn 2014; Lewis 2014)—that is, his poems embrace spiritual concepts that involve the contemplation of an individual's understanding of and connection to meaning beyond themselves (Yosefi 2018).

---

[1] One of the most helpful expressions of the internal experiences of a mystic is mystical poetry. By nature, a mystic can access a state of consciousness beyond humanity's usual consciousness.

3.4 Describing the Initiative

The present chapter describes a creative initiative that involved using the poetry of Rumi to promote health and well-being through meaning-making for Iranian women during their transition to post-divorce life. The general goal of the project was to promote and develop personal skills among divorced women through poetry reading sessions, which focused on the works of Rumi. The philosophy behind the initiative was to introduce Rumi's poetry to divorced women to encourage broadening their perspectives about the problems presented in post-divorce life and to help them explore the meaning of their life events and their futures.

In 2016, a group of 25 divorced women aged 25–55 were recruited to participate in the project through a safe-community center, established in 2010, in the west part of Tehran. The eligibility requirements for participation were being legally divorced, literate, and living in Tehran. Participants in the study had at least a high school education. Most were living in rental houses alone, and a few of were living with their relatives at the time of conducting the current project. The women mainly resided in district 21 of Tehran[2] and were referred to "The Office of Vice President for Women and Family Affairs" to be provided with ongoing financial support. Those eligible for this social program were facing unemployment, poverty, being a single parent, and being divorced or widowed. In addition to providing financial support, this safe-community center gives workshops for developing life skills, as well as psychological counseling.

The intervention included 15 one-hour sessions held weekly and conducted in Persian. The participants were encouraged to speak freely and share their perceptions of Rumi verses. The meetings were led by two health promotion experts and a Persian literature specialist with expertise on interpretation of Rumi's poems. Each session consisted of reading Rumi's poetry and then engaging in a dialogue on relevant concepts such as meaning of life, contentment, and acceptance and how those concepts were connected with post-divorce life. The Persian literature specialist read the poems and highlighted some of the relevant concepts contained in the verses for 15 minutes. Each participant was provided with a copy of *Masnavi,* a poetry book by Rumi, to follow along with the literature instructor. Then, in collaboration with the health promotion specialists, the participants extracted the underlying meanings from the poems and interpreted them for 30 minutes. The last 15 minutes of each session were allotted to the sharing of participants' own experiences. In this last part, as participants described their stories, other participants often took part in this emotional storytelling by showing feelings such as excitement and empathy, and sometimes even crying. At the end of each meeting, the literature specialist would often introduce a relevant book or novel to improve the participants' understanding of the concepts discussed. A novel[3] by the Turkish author Elif Shafak, which discusses a compelling, dramatic, and exuberant account of how love works in the world, was also read by the participants.

---

[2] Tehran is divided into 22 districts.

[3] *The Forty Rules of Love,* a novel about Rumi's life.

3.5   Iranian Women Post-divorce: Lived Experience

The following results describe the lived experiences of women who shared their stories of post-divorce life in our meeting sessions.

One prominent theme in the early discussions centered on the women's feelings of unfairness toward their situation. These participants lamented their experiences of separation, divorce, and its consequences. They described feeling that divorce was a disaster that had ruined their lives and that no reconstruction was ever possible. Consequently, these women felt hopelessness toward the future and resisted the idea of reconstructing their attitudes about their post-divorce life.

> Divorce is like a robber that destroys life and cannot make this life again (35-year-old divorced woman).

Moreover, they revealed that one of the more frequent feelings they experienced was hopelessness.

> When I got divorced, I had no hope to continue life. My daughter, my friends, all abandoned me. You know why, because I was not credible anymore (40-year-old divorced woman).

Shock, fear, anxiety, depression, anger, frustration, and bitterness are difficult and common feelings in post-divorce life (Ardi and Maizura 2018). When it comes to divorce and hopelessness, participants expressed a feeling of being powerless, unable to change the way things were.

The fear of living alone after divorce was one of the most common psychological concerns expressed by the participants. They believed it would be very difficult to afford daily expenses and to perform their daily activities.

> After divorce I began living with my old mother. My only wish is to die before her. If she dies before me, I will have no one to talk with, as my family died in Bam earthquake (39-year-old divorced woman).

Negative thoughts are a normal part of divorce (Ardi and Maizura 2018). Even in the best of times, all people have negative thoughts. However, in the case of getting divorced, negative thoughts and rumination can take over. These people become trapped in a world of fears.

> What if this happens or that happens? Of course, this [divorce] is something really, really unfortunate (34-year-old divorced woman).

Participants believed that divorce would stigmatize them socially. Feelings of fear of social labels originating from the cultural concept of divorce was another obstacle they described.

> I think divorce is a type of disease, like cancer. So, merely being a divorcee is not a sufficient justification for labeling. I will be stigmatized for divorce as well (35-year-old divorced woman).

It seems that some psycho-socio-cultural predisposing factors affect post-divorce life. In other words, the participants believed that their life after divorce had been influenced by their lived experiences, including feelings of frustration, hopelessness, stigmatization, and isolation. Thus, familiarizing them with post-divorce coping strategies incorporating a spiritual perspective would be helpful.

3.5.1 Meaning-Making: Engaging with Rumi

One theme explored in many ways in Rumi's poetry is that finding meaning in life provides satisfaction. In other words, a divorced woman who can find meaning in her unavoidable suffering can begin to move on and see purpose for her life in the future. Satisfaction with herself and her life can then emerge and lead to a sense of peace and well-being.

3.6 Participants' Experiences in the Program

We asked participants at the end of each session to provide feedback on their feelings and perceptions. Two primary questions were asked. We categorized participant's perceptions in three ways according to logotherapy approach (see Sect. 3.3) which focused on developing participant's personal skills in health promotion area.

The Attitude Toward Divorce
The first related to their feelings and perceptions of the significance derived from Rumi's poetry: Is divorce still a misfortune?

> …Rumi's poetry has [an] effect on me. I found that every event on Earth is purposefully designed. Separation and divorce are no exception to this rule for me (37-year-old divorced woman).

Other women responded:

> Honestly, I was never sure I could stand on my feet again after I got divorced. I had a lot of problems (after the divorce). Now I found that divorce has taught me a lesson. So I would rather accept all outcomes from divorce—loneliness, stigma, and even rejection—because in Rumi's poems I realized that even a misery is the basis for self-development and growth (41-year-old divorced woman).

> …recently I found that's why nothing ever made me contented. I carried prejudice about the meaning of divorce. I had perceived divorce from my family's perspective. They still find divorce taboo. Now I feel free and think of the divorce as a magic box that should be explored (40-year-old divorce woman).

Experiencing Divorce
We also asked them to describe their experiences related to divorce and explain their reflections after considering and discussing Rumi's poetry.

> …Looking deeper into this experience, I find that before the divorce, my relationship with my daughter had faded because my mind was so busy and focused on my relationship with my ex-husband. But the divorce made me pay more attention to my daughter and listen to

her more. I have to appreciate this experience [Divorce] because it highlighted the role of motherhood in me. (39-year-old divorce woman)

Well, I believe there were a lot of possibilities for my personal development after my divorce. I continued my education and attended university. Actually, 'divorce' was meaningful for my life (44-year-old divorced woman).

Goal Setting

Actually, I don't have a particular job right now and I live with my old mother. I always wanted to be a hairdresser, but my ex-husband objected. I'm going to learn a hairdressing course so I can make money. (43-year –old divorce woman)

I am a young woman and I am capable of childbearing. I can help an infertile couple have children by donating my eggs [ovules]. I couldn't have children because my husband was infertile. We tried several treatments, but they were fruitless. Lastly, we decided to get divorce. Now I think I can be mother of several children if I stop being selfish. (34-year –old divorce woman)

3.7 Conclusion

Health has cultural dimensions, and addressing an individual's health challenges through means of empowerment and behavior change without acknowledging cultural components is unproductive (Norbeck and Lock 2019). Undoubtedly, the process of empowering individuals through culturally sensitive health education in creative and indirect ways can be effective. As theorized in Chap. 21 of this volume, art that is rooted in history and culture can provide a pathway to wellbeing by supporting understanding of oneself in relation to one's context and to a sense of broader meaning. Poetry and literature are powerful tools in teaching health concepts due to their cultural and metaphorical nature. In fact, developing personal skills is assumed to improve health directly by facilitating an informed use of health care and indirectly by encouraging healthy habits and behaviors (Mirowsky 2017).

Returning to the concept of existentialism, this program supported participants as they discovered their own meanings in post-divorce life in three ways: by motivating them to create or act; by helping them accept or cope with difficulties and stressors; and by modifying their attitudes and perceptions of their experience of suffering after divorce. The incorporation of art in this program supported participants in developing a belief that life satisfaction is one aspect of spiritual health, and finding meaning in life events such as divorce can be a pathway toward life satisfaction. The women identified and accepted the difficulties they experienced while finding meaning from post-divorce suffering. Participants reported experiencing a greater sense of peace, tranquility, and well-being, and an openness to envisioning a purpose for the future. This program stimulated dialogue about coping strategies for life post-divorce through the explanation and interpretation of concepts explored in the verses. This project revealed that the use of art, and poetry specifically, can be a viable approach to promoting health among Iranian women who have experienced divorce.

References

Ardi, Z., & Maizura, N. (2018). The psychological analysis of divorce at early marriage. *International Journal of Research in Counseling and Education, 2*(2), 77–82. https://doi.org/10.24036/0026za0002.

Bahar, M., Hamedanian, F., Farajiha, M., & Golpaygani, T. S. (2018). Women's access to family justice in Iran: Exploring the main barriers. *Pertanika Journal of Social Sciences & Humanities, 26*(T), 147–164. http://psasir.upm.edu.my/id/eprint/66251/1/JSSH%20Vol.%20 26%20%28T%29%20Feb.%202018%20%28View%20Full%20Journal%29.pdf#page=161.

Bolhari, J., Ramezan Zadeh, F., Abedininia, N., Naghizadeh, M. M., Pahlavani, H., & Saberi, M. (2012). The survey of divorce incidence in divorce applicants in Tehran [Persian]. *Journal of Family and Reproductive Health, 6*(3), 129–137. http://jfrh.tums.ac.ir/index.php/jfrh/article/view/156.

Davies, C., Knuiman, M., & Rosenberg, M. (2015). The art of being mentally healthy: A study to quantify the relationship between recreational arts engagement and mental well-being in the general population. *BMC Public Health, 16*(1), 15. https://doi.org/10.1186/s12889-015-2672-7.

De Bruijn, J. T. P. (2014). *Persian Sufi poetry: An introduction to the mystical use of classical Persian poems*. UK: Routledge.

Frankl, V. E. (1967). Logotherapy and existentialism. *Psychotherapy: Theory, Research & Practice, 4*(3), 138–142. https://doi.org/10.1037/h0087982.

Ghahremani, Z. (2016). RUMI. Web log post. https://zoeghahremani.com/2016/01/15/rumi/.

Habibi, M., Hajiheydari, Z., & Darharaj, M. (2015). Causes of divorce in the marriage phase from the viewpoint of couples referred to Iran's family courts. *Journal of Divorce & Remarriage, 56*(1), 43–56.

Harold, G. T., & Leve, L. D. (2018). Parents as partners: How the parental relationship affects children's psychological development. In A. Balfour, M. Morgan, & C. Vincent (Eds.), *How couple relationships shape our world: Clinical practice, research, and policy perspectives* (pp. 25–56). New York: Routledge.

Jafarian Dehkordi, S., & Amiri, M. (2018). Divorce: An international multi-dimensional challenge [Persian]. *International Journal of Epidemiologic Research, 5*(2), 64–66. https://doi.org/10.15171/ijer.2018.14.

Kazemek, F., Wellik, J., & Zimmerman, P. (2004). Poetry, storytelling, and star-making: An intergenerational model for special education. *Journal of Poetry Therapy, 17*(1), 1–8. https://doi.org/10.1080/08893670410001698523.

Kristeller, J. L. (2010). Spiritual engagement as a mechanism of change in mindfulness-and acceptance-based therapies. In R. A. Baer (Ed.), *Assessing mindfulness and acceptance processes in clients: Illuminating the theory and practice of change* (pp. 155–184). Oakland: New Harbinger Publications.

Leturcq, M., & Panico, L. (2019). The long-term effects of parental separation on childhood multi-dimensional deprivation: A lifecourse approach. *Social Indicators Research, 144*(2), 921–954. https://doi.org/10.1007/s11205-018-02060-1.

Lewis, F. D. (2014). *Rumi—Past and present, east and west: The life, teachings, and poetry of Jalâl al-Din Rumi*. Oxford: Oneworld Publications.

Linley, P. A., & Joseph, S. (2011). Meaning in life and posttraumatic growth. *Journal of Loss and Trauma, 16*(2), 150–159. https://doi.org/10.1080/15325024.2010.519287.

Merghati-Khoei, E., Solhi, M., Nedjat, S., Taghdisi, M. H., Zadeh, D. S., Taket, A. R., et al. (2014). How a divorcee's sexual life is socially constructed and understood in the Iranian culture.

Journal of Divorce & Remarriage, 55(5), 335–347. https://doi.org/10.1080/10502556.2014.
921968.

Mirowsky, J. (2017). *Education, social status, and health.* London: Routledge.

Moghadam, V. M. (2004). Women in the Islamic Republic of Iran: Legal status, social positions, and collective action. Paper presented at the "Iran After" conference for the Woodrow Wilson International Center for Scholars.

Mueller, P. S., Plevak, D. J., & Rummans, T. A. (2001). Religious involvement, spirituality, and medicine: implications for clinical practice. Paper presented at the Mayo Clinic proceedings.

Nikparvar, F., Stith, S., Myers-Bowman, K., Akbarzadeh, M., & Daneshpour, M. (2017, December 1). Theorizing the process of leaving a violent marriage and getting a divorce in Tehran. *Journal of Interpersonal Violence.* https://doi.org/10.1177/0886260517746184.

Norbeck, E., & Lock, M. (2019). *Health, illness, and medical care in Japan: Cultural and social dimensions.* Honolulu: University of Hawaii Press.

ParsToday.(2017).WorldliteratureindebtedtoFarsilanguageandliterature.Retrievedfromhttps://parstoday.com/en/radio/iran-i63133-world_literature_indebted_to_farsi_language_and_literature

Perloff, M. (2002). 21st-century modernism: The new. *Poetics,* 7–43.

Pirak, A., Negarandeh, R., & Khakbazan, Z. (2019). Post-divorce regret among Iranian women: A qualitative study. *International Journal of Community Based Nursing and Midwifery, 7*(1), 75. https://doi.org/10.30476/IJCBNM.2019.40848. https://www.ncbi.nlm.nih.gov/pubmed/30643835.

Putnam, R. R. (2011). First comes marriage, then comes divorce: A perspective on the process. *Journal of Divorce & Remarriage, 52*(7), 557–564. https://doi.org/10.1080/10502556.2011.6 15661.

Raley, R. K., & Sweeney, M. M. (2020). Divorce, repartnering, and stepfamilies: A decade in review. *Journal of Marriage and Family, 82*(1), 81–99. https://doi.org/10.1111/jomf.12651.

Robinson, M. (2018). *Divorce as family transition: When private sorrow becomes a public matter.* New York: Routledge.

Roohollah, R. (2018). Ralph Waldo Emerson's immersion in Saadi's poetry. *World Scientific News, 92*(2), 283–293.

Rosario, J., & Leite, J. (2019). Standardization method for teaching yoga meditation and asanas: A case study. *MOJ Clinical & Medical Case Reports, 9*(1), 9–12. https://pdfs.semanticscholar.org/8896/16e45181bc4f0434d0b311f025250d940af8.pdf.

Rozina, A. (2017, January 5). The erasure of Islam from the poetry of Rumi. *The New Yorker.* Retrieved from https://www.newyorker.com/books/page-turner/the-erasure-of-islam-from-the-poetry-of-rumi.

Rypka, J. (2013). *History of Iranian literature.* New York: Springer Science & Business Media.

Sadeghi, R., & Agadjanian, V. (2019). Attitude and propensity to divorce in Iran: Structural and ideational determinants. *Journal of Divorce & Remarriage, 60*(6), 479–500. https://doi.org/10.1080/10502556.2019.1586228.

Sen Nag, O. (2019). The culture of Iran. Retrieved from worldatlas.com/articles/the-culture-of-iran.htm

Steger, M. F., & Frazier, P. (2005). Meaning in life: One link in the chain from religiousness to well-being. *Journal of Counseling Psychology, 52*(4), 574–582. https://psycnet.apa.org/doi/10.1037/0022-0167.52.4.574.

World Health Organization. (1986, November 21). The Ottawa charter for health promotion: First international conference on health promotion. Geneva: WHO.

Xerxa, Y., Rescorla, L. A., Serdarevic, F., Van IJzendorn, M. H., Jaddoe, V. W., Verhulst, F. C., et al. (2019). The complex role of parental separation in the association between family conflict and child problem behavior. *Journal of Clinical Child & Adolescent Psychology, 49*(1), 79–93. https://doi.org/10.1080/15374416.2018.1520118.

Yosefi, G. H. (2018). *Cheshme-Roshan* [Persian]. Tehran: Elmi.

Zagami, S. E., Roudsari, R. L., Janghorban, R., Mojtaba, S., Bazaz, M., Amirian, M., et al. (2019). A qualitative study of the challenges experienced by Iranian infertile couples after unsuccessful assisted reproductive technologies. *International Journal of Womens Health and Reproduction Sciences, 7*(3), 331–338. https://doi.org/10.15296/ijwhr.2019.55.

Zare, S., Aguilar-Vafaie, M. E., & Ahmadi, F. (2017). Perception of identity threat as the main disturbance of Iranian divorced women: A qualitative study. *Journal of Divorce & Remarriage, 58*(1), 1–15. https://doi.org/10.1080/10502556.2016.1257902.

Zarei, F., Merghati Khoei, E., Taket, A. R., Rahmani, A., & Smith, T. G. (2013). How does divorce affect Iranian women's sexual well-being? *Journal of Divorce & Remarriage, 54*(5), 381–392.

Zarei, F., Solhi, M., Merghati-Khoei, E., Taghdisi, M. H., Shojaeizadeh, D., Taket, A. R., et al. (2017). Development and psychometric properties of social exclusion questionnaire for Iranian divorced women. *Iranian Journal of Public Health, 46*(5), 640–649. https://www.ncbi.nlm.nih.gov/pmc/articles/PMC5442277/.

Chapter 4
Student Creativity and Professional Artwork in a School Food Intervention in Denmark

Dorte Ruge

4.1 Introduction

Schools are important health settings for children (Jensen and Simovska 2005; SHE Network 2018; Simovska 2012). Impacted by national, regional, and school policies, the experience of health—and particularly nutrition—in schools is entirely subject to the strength of those policies. In Denmark, as in many other countries such as Norway, New Zealand, and Australia, there is no national school food program to ensure proper nutrition during the school day for all students. Parents and caregivers in Denmark are required to prepare and pack lunch and an afternoon snack for students on a daily basis (Sabinsky 2013).

Given the diverse circumstances in which children live, the effect of this policy impacts health and learning inequitably. Students from vulnerable families are more likely to bring insufficient meals from home to school, if they bring any meals at all (Rasmussen et al. 2019). The general legislation for Danish schools, in Danish: Folkeskolen (Retsinformation 2018), prescribes that food and meal systems in schools "can" be supported by municipal systems (Stovgaard et al. 2017). However, the reliance on caregivers to provide food results in a food environment based on "free-choice" (Stovgaard and Wistoft 2018). This can be characterized as a result of a market-driven neoliberal approach, in which families are encouraged to buy all of their food in the supermarket. This situation leads to a certain "supermarketization" of the way that food is organized and talked about in schools. The packed lunch is "from supermarket" and reflects the social status of the family. The quality of the packed lunch varies a lot, and sometimes it is not even brought to school, not eaten in school, or not stored at the right temperature. Furthermore, the packed lunch is often not adequate to cover the nutritional needs for students (Sabinsky 2013; Stovgaard and Wistoft 2018).

D. Ruge (✉)
University College Lillebelt, Odense, Denmark
e-mail: doru@ucl.dk

© The Author(s) 2021
J. H. Corbin et al. (eds.), *Arts and Health Promotion*,
https://doi.org/10.1007/978-3-030-56417-9_4

This system in Danish schools is especially unfortunate for students from disadvantaged and immigrant families (Brembeck 2009; Rasmussen et al. 2019). In 2014, Denmark engaged in national school reform to improve learning and well-being for all students (Danish Ministry of Education 2019; Simovska et al. 2015). Consequently, school days became longer, and teaching became more goal-oriented. However, research documents report that students are hungry during the school day, as the packed lunch is insufficient to cover their needs (Ruge 2015; Ruge et al. 2017; Stovgaard and Wistoft 2018). The national Health Institute of Public Health, that monitor the Danish HB report on child health in schools, documented that socioeconomic factors greatly determine inequality in health among children and youth in Denmark (Rasmussen et al. 2019).

This situation gives rise to various "local level solutions" that aim to reduce inequity through health promotion initiatives around nutrition practices and food environments in schools. In the absence of appropriate national policy and public school food initiatives, local initiatives have sought to fill the nutritional gap experienced by students in Danish schools. The project "LOMA-lokal mad" (in English: LOMA-local food) represents a municipal- and school-driven example that included an art-based approach. The overall aim of the project was to reduce inequity in health and learning via student development of food- and health-related action competence through participatory food- and creative arts activities (Jensen and Simovska 2005; Ruge 2015; see also Chap.1, in this volume). Its main activities encompassed student participation in planning, cooking, and serving food for peers. The approach integrated cross-curricular and project-oriented activities, including students interacting with food within an art-based, creative universe. From 2015 to 2017, 2754 students in primary and secondary levels from five schools in four municipalities participated in the project.

The aim of this chapter is to present findings from a single case study (Yin 2006) of the LOMA-local food (LOMA) project from 2015 to 2017. The chapter focuses on the integration of student creativity and professional artwork as an element in the LOMA project. The research question was formulated as follows: "How did the combination of teachers' didactic work, student creativity, and professional artwork support motivation, improve relations, and nurture the development of shared ownership among students in the LOMA project?"

4.2   Background

The first LOMA school in Denmark—Nymarkskolen in Svendborg—initiated the process of combining student creativity and artwork with school food activities back in 2012.[1] During this year, a group of secondary students (aged 13–14) in the art class "Art and Graphic Design" collaborated in groups and developed an

---

[1] Nymarkskolen in the Municipality of Svendborg from 2011 to 2013.

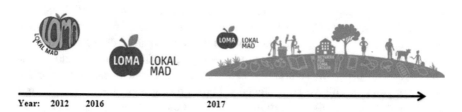

Year: 2012   2016   2017

Fig. 4.1 Timeline for the development process from the initial LOMA logo made by students at secondary level to the LOMA universe

appropriate LOMA logo. The art teacher supervised the process and applied a democratic approach that encouraged student creativity. By the end of the course, student groups compared their suggestions and collectively decided on one logo that encompassed both a positive health message and a learning message (Ruge 2015; Ruge et al. 2016). The LOMA project received additional funding in 2014 because of positive results from this first LOMA school (Ruge 2015). The objective was a scaling-up of the LOMA approach to five more schools.[2] Originally, the pencil-drawn illustration developed by the students at Nymarkskolen was intended to be the logo to be used across all of the six schools in the project. However, it turned out to be too difficult to reproduce the hand-drawn analog logo for letterhead, digital homepage, print, social media, online educational materials, certificates, and other shared items. Consequently, the project management team and the steering group (consisting of headmasters from all schools) contacted a professional artist[3] to develop a graphic design for a logo, based on the original. It was the intention to use it in the "LOMA universe" to inspire students' creative imaginations and involvement in the activities. (See the logo development process in Fig. 4.1.)

The LOMA universe was a visual environment for the school setting that supported and communicated the LOMA school "ethos" and invited students to engage in educational activities, not only in a physical way (e.g., cooking) but also in a creative and imaginative way with ideas and visions. During 2015–2016, the artist developed the LOMA universe in collaboration with the project management team, the steering group, and teachers.

In the first stage, the new logo was created and modified for multiple format use. The "looking glass" and other smaller details from the initial hand-drawn logo were difficult to transfer to the new logo, and it was with regret that the steering group decided to eliminate them. While disappointed, they acknowledged that the colors in the new logo were brighter, the writing of the name was more distinct, and the new logo was more versatile for sharing across media platforms. In the second stage, the initial vision from the participants was to form a tree with multiple LOMA apples, one for each school. However, this endeavor suffered similar problems with the reproduction of smaller details in the different formats and required creative

---

[2] Supported by Nordea-fonden. See more at www.lomaskole.dk
[3] The name of the Danish professional artist is M. Madsen.

modification. Through an interactive process between the artist and participants, the idea of depicting the LOMA universe as a curved surface of the Earth with one-dimensional figures was put forward. Through a participatory dialogue, the result was a simplistic depiction of an integrated ecosystem with inhabitants and natural and cultural artifacts. The central elements were the Earth, the tree, the sun, the sky, the school, and the collaborating students. In the green ground, there were multiple analog and digital "tools for learning," such as a book, bread, an apple, a fish, a plate, a fork and knife, an iPad, and a looking glass. Later, the artist added other human elements (e.g., a teacher and a farmer) and some animals with supportive functions in the universe. In the third stage, the focus was on not "overloading" the universe and instead leaving open space for student interpretation, imagination, and creativity. In the beginning of 2016, LOMA teacher-training courses introduced teachers to the graphic design of the LOMA universe. Teachers were trained in pedagogical and didactical methods to support student creativity and to encourage students to use their imagination to invent "food stories" inspired by the LOMA universe illustration. Responding positively to these ideas, teachers requested larger posters depicting the LOMA universe to use as a shared frame for class activities in school.

4.3 Conceptual Framework

The conceptual framework for the health promotion efforts of the program was based on the Ottawa Charter and its description of the fundamental resources for health: "*peace, shelter, education, food, income, a stable ecosystem, sustainable resources, social justice and equity. Improvement in health requires a secure foundation in these basic prerequisites*" (WHO 1986, p. 1). Since 1986, this statement has been widely accepted and integrated in global public health definitions and strategies (White et al. 2013). The Ottawa Charter also forms the foundation for various health promotion settings, including promoting healthy food consumption in early-life settings such as schools and kindergartens, since eating patterns formed in childhood tend to track into adulthood (Langford et al. 2014; SHE Network 2018; WHO 2018). Furthermore, the WHO suggests the application of an educational approach to health promotion. This case applies social constructivist theory to the relationship between health promotion, art-based student creativity, food, and learning as social practice in schools (Jensen and Simovska 2005; Ruge 2015; Vygotsky 2004; WHO 1986). Following this, cultural norms structure social practices such as food growing, food preparation, food procurement, and food consumption. Furthermore, cultural norms at home, in school, and in social media shape the way students in school relate to food. As a social practice, food in schools can be integrated with other social practices and guided by teachers' didactic work in curriculum activities such as cooking, health education, and science.

In this study, there was a special focus on how artwork in curriculum and food activities was integrated into the LOMA project. By including art, teachers' didactic work encouraged student creativity. This approach is supported by the theory of Vygotsky that emphasizes the importance of nurturing creativity in children. (Vygotsky 2004). According to Vygotsky (2004), not only art teachers but also professional artists can contribute to the cultivation of student creativity in schools. In support of including professional artists in educational activities, Dewey (2005) has stated that the experience of art will accentuate the quality of belonging to a large whole: the universe in which we live (Dewey p. 214).

For comparison, the Nottingham Apprenticeship Model is an example of how a systematic and structured partnership on "learning for the arts" between professional artists and schools can contribute to student creativity and "revitalize education in the arts" and other creative activities as well (Griffiths and Woolf 2009, p. 17–18). In the Nottingham project, artists led the activities, whereas teachers led the activities in the LOMA project. The advantage of teacher-led activities is that the teacher is not a "passive spectator," but rather is embedded in the school so the activities can continue after the artist has left the school. This difference is fundamental for the distribution of roles and responsibilities between teachers and artists—and for student outcomes. If teachers select a didactical model that encourages creative imagination in artwork, teacher-led activities will support the development of student creativity, critical thinking, and positive relations between students and teachers.

This approach is also supported by the works of Freire (2018), who emphasized how a dialogical approach to education encourages people to use their creative power as they develop the ability to critically reflect on challenges in life (Freire 2018). For schools, Freire described the importance of dialogical, problem-posing, and collaborative pedagogical methods as opposed to mainstream 'banking' educational methods with the aim of promoting critical awareness among students.

In a twenty-first century educational context, the work of Fullan and Langworthy on new pedagogies also emphasizes the importance of dialogical, visionary, and collaborative approaches in school:

> We need our learning systems to encourage youth to develop their own visions about what it means to connect and flourish in their constantly emerging world and equip them with the skills to pursue those visions. This expansive notion, encompassing the broader idea of human flourishing, is what we mean by "deep learning." (Fullan and Langworthy 2013)

In conclusion, creative collaboration between teachers and students is linked to critical thinking about the possibility of change. In the case of LOMA-project the creative collaboration is linked to the request for more sustainable and climate-friendly food systems via local food sourcing and cooking. Based on this understanding, this chapter will describe and analyze a specific case from the LOMA project. The categories for analysis are divided in the physical, organizational, didactical, and socio-cultural dimensions, to analyze school foodscapes (Dolphijn 2004; Ruge 2015).[4]

---

[4]For clarification: In the following analysis, the term "LOMA universe" represents the graphic design (cf. Fig. 4.1). The term "LOMA foodscape" represents the total educational setting at the school as a whole.

4.4   Planning and Conducting LOMA Teaching

The LOMA approach seeks to integrate food activities into the general curriculum and into educational activities. Importantly, this approach centers LOMA teaching as important for all activities in the LOMA project. Often primary- and secondary-level schools planned a number of 'LOMA weeks' for the whole school year. In a LOMA week, schools applied a project-oriented approach in which teachers could collaborate on LOMA themes across subjects throughout all five school days. The LOMA project consultants initiated planning of the LOMA weeks during school-based training for teachers. In addition to teachers, teacher assistants and kitchen managers also participated as "educators" in the training activities. The teacher-training course encompassed theory and methods in LOMA pedagogy and didactics (see Table 4.1). The training included an action-learning element, in which

Table 4.1 The modules in the "LOMA education model" for teachers

Module 1. Introduction to theory and methods
Duration: 1 day at the school
Theory about school foodscapes: How to reflect on and change a foodscape at school?
The local perspective on cooking, learning, and sharing meals and local sourcing of food for school meals
Transformative learning—basic elements
Involvement of students and encouraging student creativity and collaboration
Introduction to the graphic design of the "LOMA universe"
How to include the ideas and the graphics made by professional artists in LOMA activities?
Children's own foodscapes
Didactics and learning goals in cross-curricular and problem-based activities
How to collaborate with a farm? Farm excursion for staff with educational focus
Module 2. Teacher-teams plan their own LOMA week
Duration: 1 day at the school
Teacher teams, select subjects and learning goals and integrate student creativity in educational activities. Decisions made on art forms and student outputs
Meeting with students to invite them to participate in planning of LOMA week
Contact collaborators and organize logistics and plans for teamwork (online)
Establish heterogeneous groups across classes (teacher task)
Plan workshops, farm visits, and menus. Send information to parents 2 weeks in advance
Module 3. Teacher-teams conduct a LOMA week with students
Duration: 5 days at the school for teachers and students
Excursion for students to a local farm. Reflections before, during, and after in relation to learning goals for 'LOMA-week'
Conduct workshops with students. Rotations during the week: all groups work 1 day in each of the workshops from 8 AM to 2 PM
Each day, the student groups and their teachers share a joint meal at lunch prepared by students, teachers, and the kitchen manager: todays cooking-team
Dissemination of student artwork and other creative products from student groups; sharing artwork among student groups. Often using ICT or exhibitions in the hall
Inviting "friendship classes," school management staff, or parents for a meal. Visit from LOMA project management team, evaluations, team reflections, and "lessons learned"
Evaluation with students, colleagues, and consultants. Sharing knowledge with the following teacher-team for the next 'LOMA-week' at the school

teachers were encouraged to work dialogically? as a social learning group, or a "community of practice" (Fullan and Langworthy 2013; Ruge et al. 2016; Wenger et al. 2002). The implication of this was that all participants were "learners" and all contributions were welcomed without regard to professional status. Teacher-teams often used a five-day workshop model for a LOMA week. All teachers were able to attend during their regular teaching schedule, and this facilitated a thematic, project-oriented, didactical model for students' work. Over 5 days, all students worked in shifts in all five workshops. The workshop on "cooking a joint meal for peers" was compulsory for teachers to include in the plan.

4.5   Case Study of a LOMA Week in a Primary School

The categories for analysis of this case focus on the organizational, didactical, socio-cultural, and physical dimensions, drawing on the conceptual framework previously described for analyzing "LOMA school foodscapes" (Dolphijn 2004; Ruge 2015). The objects, events, and activities in these different dimensions comprised the following:

(a) **Organizational dimension:** During teacher training modules, eight teachers, one kitchen manager, and one teacher assistant planned their LOMA week. They divided six classes of first-graders (aged 6–7 years) into four working groups across classes (110 students total) in order to improve interaction, collaboration and positive relations among students. All working groups spent 1 day in each workshop during the week.

(b) **Didactic and socio-cultural dimensions:** Teachers represented in total more than 20 different school subjects, because each teacher could teach three different subjects. The team had to decide on a joint cross-curricular theme for the project before they chose the subjects and learning goals. In this case, they agreed on "Apple" as a theme that functioned as an overall frame that was open for student creativity and suggestions from teachers and the kitchen staff. Five workshops were established, with each workshop covering two subjects. In the "Language & Media" workshop (see Figs. 4.2 and 4.3, teachers encouraged students to use "child spelling," where the students imagined the best way to spell the word. Students seemed confident with this and were not embarrassed about eventual errors. As a way of supporting student recognition and ownership, teachers used the LOMA logo on the board and on student materials. All students and all teachers shared and enjoyed the food that students cooked each day during the LOMA week. The kitchen manager adjusted the food production to primary level of competences.

(c) **Physical dimension:** In the "Art & Science" workshop, students learned about the LOMA universe and the importance of trees, especially apple trees. Pupils followed the botanical development from seed to tree. They cut apples, picked the seeds, and learned how to plant them. They imagined how trees would grow on Earth and made drawings of this. Students worked in smaller groups to produce food-art pictures from fresh carrots, apples, and other vegetables. They took digital photos of their food-art and presented them to peers by the end of the workshop and on posters in the hall (see Figs. 4.2 and 4.3). Students archived photos on iPads to share with parents. In the "Language & Media" workshop, students created books with narratives based on their own experiences and learning. They used their photos from other workshops or they visited the other groups and took photos of peers "in action" (see Fig. 4.4).

Based on data from each dimension, there are indications of how the combination of teachers' didactic work with professional artwork (the logo and framing of the "LOMA universe") and student creativity (students' own artwork) supported recognition and motivation among students, such as when they created their "vegetable-art" pictures. Furthermore, students developed knowledge (e.g., about trees) and skills (e.g., cutting apples). Students also seemed to develop self-esteem and an ownership in the form of being proud to show their joint artwork to other peers and to the whole school. The following transcript of data is based on a semi-structured focus group interview (Kvale 2008) with students, who had engaged in digital creative learning activities by using their Ipad (cf. Fig. 4.4).

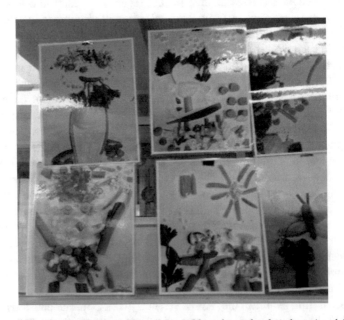

Figs. 4.2 and 4.3 Pictures of "vegetable-art" created by primary level students (aged 6–7 years) and shared on posters in the hall and online via iPads and smartboards

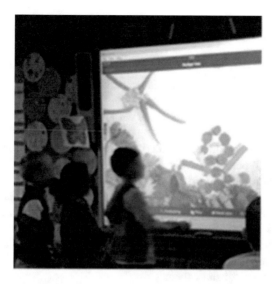

Figs. 4.2 and 4.3 (continued)

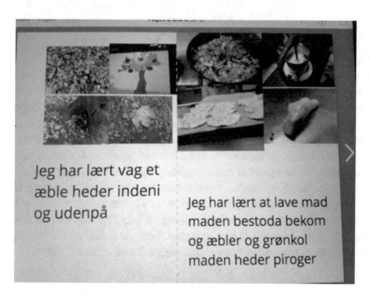

Fig. 4.4 Student creativity via digital "journal books" made on iPads with students' own photos from the LOMA project. Translation of text in 'child-spelling': *"I have learned wat an apple is caled inside and outside. I have learned to cook… the food was made of apples and green-cabage and was caled piroger"* (in child-spelling)

I = interviewer;
R3, R4, R5 = student respondents (aged 6 years)

I: What did you do today?
R4:   Hmm…It's a "book creator," it's called…
I: What is it all about, can you tell me?
R4:   Yes, you can make a lot of books with it.
I: How is that?
R4:   You can take pictures and video, and then you can insert it, because there is lots of pages and such. We have made our journal book /*on it*/.
I: What is it used for, that journal book?
R3:   I think you can make as many pages as you like. You can also make recordings of sounds and much more [*doing gestures with hands to illustrate*].
I: What should it be used for?
R5:   It will be used to show all the other primary classes and the pre-primary classes, and I believe the other classes, too.
I: What are you going to show them?
R5:   Show them the book.
I: What is it about?
R5:   It's about what we have made. We have made food in "Nature and Technology" and in "Danish" and "Mathematics."
I: So these are the subjects that have been involved this week?
R4:   - yes, and "Food."

The voices of these three respondents represent the larger group of students as "one student voice." Considering this, there are indications that students did improve their relations with one another during participation in the variated "LOMA foodscape"—both in the smaller group ("what *we* have made") and also by a shared ownership with the larger group ("show *all the other* primary classes"). Students seemed conscious about their own creative contribution and how this was a connection to the "larger whole"—to the school community. They also seem to have gained self-esteem and pride in showing their creative work to other students. Finally, students seemed to have developed basic knowledge about food, as well as insight into how food was integrated with other subjects in school. Based on data from the various dimensions, there are indications of students feeling a shared responsibility and ownership toward the whole "LOMA school foodscape" that seems to make sense to them.

4.6   Evaluation of Case Study

The research question for this study focused on how the combination of teachers' didactic work, student creativity, and professional artwork supported motivation, improved relationships, and nurtured the development of a shared ownership among participants in the LOMA project.

Based on results from analysis of the representative single-case at the primary level in one of the LOMA schools, there are indications that the combination of teachers' didactic work with professional art and student creativity, supported improved relations, well-being and the development of a shared ownership among students. It seems as if creativity had been cultivated with good results during the project. Additionally, students seemed to have developed components of action competence with regard to food and health in the form of new knowledge and skills, self-esteem, experience with real-life challenges, and experience with collaboration (Jensen and Simovska 2005; Ruge 2015).

The program theory of the LOMA project was evaluated by The Danish Evaluation Institute from 2015 to 2017. They concluded that student and teacher participation led to improved relations, and development of shared ownership in the health-promoting "learning environment" and to an experience of "enthusiasm" (Danish Evaluation Institute 2017). The overall framing of the project by the shared logo and the visual "LOMA universe" seems to have supported these findings. In Denmark, the notion of "enthusiasm" among all students is not often connected to school activities. Children in primary school often report feel "bored" in traditional Danish and Math classroom lessons, and so the cultivating of enthusiasm and creativity through shared ownership in a collaborative, varied learning environment is meaningful (Nielsen et al. 2017, p. 16).

Based on the findings in this case study, there are indications that teachers are adept at including student creativity in their didactic work on health promotion. However, they may need support and inspiration from professional artists to achieve learning goals and to improve well-being. There are also indications from this study that when teacher-teams collaborate in stronger professional learning groups, they can design and create learning environments that encourage student creativity and forms of "deep learning" (Fullan and Langworthy 2013). These results are supported by the general evaluation by the Danish Evaluation Institute. In addition to the recognition of improved relations among students, the Danish Evaluation Institute emphasized that the collaborative and creative approach in the LOMA-project also seemed to have improved relations among staff as well.

4.6.1   Limitations and Implications

There are limitations to this study that could have benefitted from analysis of multiple cases. Certainly, there was a variety of results from the participating schools, and some schools responded to the idea of the "LOMA universe" in a more positive way than others. Art teachers especially showed positive agency and interest, which could have been further examined. Sometimes the informal hierarchies among teachers had a strong influence on the planning of workshops, which meant that ideas to enhance student creativity did not gain support from colleagues. This is an argument for initially establishing a special "bond" between the external artists and the art teachers during teacher-training modules.

Implications for future research suggest that action-research approaches are needed to develop research designs based on social constructivist theory and critical social theory. Holistic, action-learning designs that can capture development and changes both in the "whole school system" and for the "whole human being," among students and teachers alike. Unfortunately, the current challenges to planetary health and sustainable development are closely linked to human health. Therefore, creative imagination and critical thinking are in demand for the future worldwide. A holistic and integrated approach to food in schools might be a good way to promote health, well-being, and sustainable development in practice.

4.7   Conclusion

Healthy food in schools should not only be about food, nutrition, taste, programs and systems. Food in schools should include teachers' planning of dialogical learning processes from a problem-based and project-oriented didactic approach, that provide space for creative imagination and critical thinking. Currently, the notions of "healthy eating", "food literacy" and "food technology" tend to have a reductionist and hegemonic influence on school food discourse (Traverso-Yepez and Hunter 2016). As in other settings and in related general understandings of health (see Chap. 21, in this volume), these notions and approaches to school food provision seem to be predominantly based on individualized, market-oriented, and "Western" conceptions. The findings support the notion that it is important to scaffold teachers in how to didactically include student creativity in health promotion activities and other similar initiatives. Doing so is a way to support and stimulate participation not only of "the student as taster," "the student as eater," and/or "the student as consumer or producer," but especially of the "whole creative and learning human being." There are indications that the 'whole school' and 'whole system approach' might benefit from applying a "fully human" Freirean perspective in an updated version, aimed at "deep learning." This could be advantageous not in order to individualize the challenges in health, but rather to give teachers the opportunity to invite children and adolescents into dialogical learning processes as "whole" human beings with creativity, multiple competences, emotions, bodily and emotional needs, skills, backgrounds, and identities.

Acknowledgments I would like to thank the students, teachers, kitchen managers, and headmasters who made this study meaningful and possible. I am also grateful to artist Marie Madsen for her collaboration and creative contribution to the LOMA-local food project.

References

Brembeck, H. (2009). Childrens' becoming in frontiering foodscapes. In A. James, A. Kjørholt, & V. Tingstad (Eds.), *Children, food and identity in everyday life*. New York: Springer.
Danish Evaluation Institute. (2017). Evaluation of the LOMA project. Evaluation report. https://www.eva.dk/grundskole/evaluering-projektet-loma. Accessed Nov 2018.

Danish Ministry of Education. (2019). Agreement on school reform 2013. Available online. https://eng.uvm.dk/primary-and-lower-secondary-education/the-folkeskole/about-the-folkeskole. Accessed Nov 2019.

Dewey, J. (2005). Art as experience. In S. D. Ross (Ed.), *Art and its significance: An anthology of aesthetic theory*. Albany: State University of New York Press.

Dolphijn, R. (2004). *Foodscapes: Towards a Deleuzian ethics of consumption*. The Netherlands: Eburon Publishers.

Freire, P. (2018). *Pedagogy of the oppressed*. USA: Bloomsbury Publishing.

Fullan, M., & Langworthy, M. (2013). *Towards a new end: New pedagogies for deep learning*. Seattle: Collaborative Impact.

Griffiths, M., & Woolf, F. (2009). The Nottingham apprenticeship model: Schools in partnership with artists and creative practitioners. *British Educational Research Journal, 35*(4), 557–574.

Jensen, B. B., & Simovska, V. (2005). Involving students in learning and health promotion processes—clarifying why? what? and how? *Health Promotion & Education, 12*(3–4), 150–156.

Kvale, S. (2008). *Doing interviews*. Thousand Oaks: Sage.

Langford, R., Bonell, C. P., Jones, H. E., Pouliou, T., Murphy, S. M., Waters, E., et al. (2014). The WHO Health Promoting School framework for improving the health and well-being of students and their academic achievement. *Cochrane Database of Systematic Reviews*, (4), CD008958.

Nielsen, C. P., Keilow, M., & Westergaard, C. L. (2017). Elevernes oplevelser af skolen i folkeskolereformens tredje år. VIVE Report (in English: Student experience of school in the third year of 2014 reform). Available online. https://www.vive.dk/da/udgivelser/elevernes-oplevelser-af-skolen-i-folkeskolereformens-tredje-aar-en-kortlaegning-6832/. Accessed Nov 2018.

Rasmussen, M., Kierkegaard, L., Rosenwein, S. V., Holstein, B. E., Damsgaard, M. T., & Due, P. (2019). Skolebørnsundersøgelsen 2018: Helbred, trivsel og sundhedsadfærd blandt 11-, 13-og 15-årige skoleelever i Danmark (in English: Health behaviour in school-aged children: students aged 11, 13 and 15 years in Denmark). http://www.hbsc.org/

Retsinformation. (2018). Legislation of public schools. Folkeskoleloven. https://www.retsinformation.dk/Forms/r0710.aspx?id=196651. Accessed Nov 2018.

Ruge, D. (2015). *Integrating health promotion, learning and sustainable development* (Dissertation). University College Lillebelt and Aalborg University.

Ruge, D., Nielsen, M. K., Mikkelsen, B. E., & Bruun-Jensen, B. (2016). Examining participation in relation to students' development of health-related action competence in a school food setting: LOMA case study. *Health Education, 116*(1), 69–85.

Ruge, D., Puck, M., & Hansen, T. I. (2017). Report 1. Foreløbige resultater fra analyse af LOMA intervention (in English: Preliminary results from analysis of LOMA intervention). Quantitative methods. University College Lillebelt, Department of Pedagogy and Society, Odense.

Sabinsky, M. S. (2013). Healthy eating at schools. How does a school food program affect the quality of dietary intake at lunch among children aged 7–13 years? DTU, Denmark.

SHE Network. (2018). Schools for health in Europe. http://www.schools-for-health.eu/she-network. Accessed May 2019.

Simovska, V. (2012). What do health-promoting schools promote? Processes and outcomes in school health promotion. *Health Education, 112*(2), 84–88.

Simovska, V., Nordin, L. L., & Madsen, K. D. (2015). Health promotion in Danish schools: Local priorities, policies and practices. *Health Promotion International, 31*(2), 480–489.

Stovgaard, M., & Wistoft, K. (2018). Rammer for mad og måltider i skolen—en forskningsrapport (in English: Framing food and meals in school—report from intervention study). Aarhus University-DCA-Nationalt Center for Fødevarer og Jordbrug.

Stovgaard, M., Thorborg, M. M., Bjerge, H. H., Andersen, B. V., & Wistoft, K. (2017). Rammer for mad og måltider i skolen: en systematisk forskningskortlægning (in English: Framing food and meals in school: a systematic review). Aarhus University-DCA-Nationalt Center for Fødevarer og Jordbrug.

Traverso-Yepez, M., & Hunter, K. (2016). From "healthy eating" to a holistic approach to current food environments. *SAGE Open, 6*(3), 2158244016665891.

Vygotsky, L. S. (2004). Imagination and creativity in childhood. *Journal of Russian & East European Psychology, 42*(1), 7–9.

Wenger, E., McDermott, R. A., & Snyder, W. (2002). *Cultivating communities of practice: A guide to managing knowledge.* Boston: Harvard Business Press.

White, F., Stallones, L., & Last, J. M. (2013). *Global public health: Ecological foundations.* New York/Oxford: Oxford University Press.

World Health Organization. (1986). The Ottawa charter for health promotion. http://www.who.int/healthpromotion/conferences/previous/ottawa/en/. Accessed May 2019.

World Health Organization. (2018). Global school health initiative (Health Promoting Schools partnership). http://www.who.int/school_youth_health/gshi/en/. Accessed May 2019.

Yin, R. (2006). *Case study research: Design and methods. Applied social research methods series* (Vol. 5, pp. 25). London: Sage Publications.

Chapter 5
Creatively Healthy: Art in a Care Home Setting in Scotland

Gillian C. Barton

5.1 Introduction

In 2017, the UK All-Party Parliamentary Group (APPG) on Arts, Health, and Wellbeing published *"Creative Health: The Arts for Health and Wellbeing,"* providing compelling evidence on how the arts and culture can make a positive impact in tackling health inequalities and improving health, well-being, and quality of life for people of all ages. Within this report, Sir Michael Marmot, director of the Institute of Health Equity, University College London, acknowledges this by stating: "The mind is the gateway through which the social determinants impact upon health and this report is about the life of the mind. It provides a substantial body of evidence showing how the arts, enriching the mind through creative and cultural activity, can mitigate the negative effects of social disadvantage (p. 2)." The growing awareness of the powerful contribution that the arts can make to support health and well-being across age groups is leading health and social care professionals to seek practical guidance and support in developing appropriate evidence-based programs.

This chapter describes an arts-based initiative in a care home setting in Scotland that was designed to promote health and well-being through creative expression, social inclusion, and the aesthetic beautification of space for residents ranging in age from 48 to 100, 50% of whom have been diagnosed with dementia. The project was designed to involve residents, their families, and staff to promote inclusion, create a piece of public art, and provide lasting memories.

G. C. Barton (✉)
Healthy Workstyles Consultancy, Aberdeen, UK
e-mail: hello@healthyworkstyles.com

© The Author(s) 2021
J. H. Corbin et al. (eds.), *Arts and Health Promotion*,
https://doi.org/10.1007/978-3-030-56417-9_5

5.2 Art, Health, and Well-being

The term "*the arts*" commonly includes diverse forms of expression such as poetry, storytelling, drama, theater, music, visual arts (such as painting and sculpture), and cultural pursuits including visiting museums and art galleries. The value of the arts in the promotion of health and well-being is increasingly being recognized both within the "medical model" and more recently within non-medical settings (Seligman 2011). "*Art therapy*" over the past decade has been used in health care settings as a therapeutic tool for an array of health conditions including mental illness, cancer, autism, pain management, and dementia, and is only delivered by qualified art therapists (Elkis-Abuhoff and Morgan 2019). Such therapies are described by the British Association of Art Therapists (BAAT 2018) as strategies within the wider field of psychotherapy, which incorporate art and creative expression as the primary tool for communication. Art is not used for diagnosis but as a mechanism for processing emotions and experiences, which may be confusing or distressing to talk about.

Coburn et al. (2017) suggest that health, well-being, and the environment are symbiotic and that by working strategically, sustainable health-promoting environments can influence people's well-being. With the increasing need for prevention of ill health, the value of beautiful spaces on improving health and well-being has the potential to support individuals and society as a whole (Coburn et al. 2017). Good environmental design can enable healthier lifestyles and improved well-being, and there is the potential to achieve substantial long-term savings in health and social care costs as a result (CABE 2009; Coburn et al. 2017; Jones and Yates 2013). The beautification of living and recreational spaces has long been recognized, dating back to the Palaeolithic age with cave drawings. There were also early indications of the benefits of art in relation to health, although these ideas came from philosophers rather than physicians (Fancourt 2017). The benefits of art, creativity, and culture are associated with many factors, including supportive environments both indoors and outdoors, thus offering an innovative approach to public health by providing restorative and regenerative opportunities (Chatterjee et al. 2018; Cutler 2013; see also Chap. 1, this volume). The powerful impact of beautiful spaces on healing and well-being is gaining recognition with the term "*Healing Built Environment*" (HBE), used to describe "...healthcare buildings that (1) reduce the stress levels for all healthcare building users; and (2) promote health benefits for users" (Zhang et al. 2018, p. 747).[1] This is a relatively new area of research, and Zhang and colleagues propose a concept called the "*environment-occupant-health framework*" (E-O-H) that they suggest could be of value to a wide range of profes-

---

sionals, offering the opportunity to "…provide a common language between clinicians, planners, designers and patients when a healthcare building/space is built or refurbished" (Zhang et al. 2018, p. 761).

In 2017, Age UK created an *"Index of Wellbeing in Later Life"* to provide a comprehensive and systematic way to measure well-being for adults over the age of 60, examining five key domains: personal, social, health, resources, and local. The most notable finding was that creative and cultural participation contributed most significantly to well-being out of all 40 factors explored (Green et al. 2017). The Index also clearly demonstrated that "…the importance of maintaining meaningful engagement with the world around you in later life—whether this is through social, creative or physical activity, work, or belonging to some form of community group" is vital to well-being (Green et al. 2017, p. 12).

5.3 Social Isolation and Loneliness

There are many reasons why people become isolated. In addition to those associated with becoming elderly, Wilkinson and Pickett (2018) suggest these reasons include societal changes, family breakdowns, ill health, and financial difficulties. A recent report suggests that socially isolated people are 3.5 times more likely to enter local-authority-funded residential care (No Isolation, 2019).

There is now a growing body of evidence demonstrating the effect that isolation and loneliness have on mortality, indicating comparability with risk factors like smoking and obesity. Loneliness can affect both physical and mental health with an increased risk of coronary heart disease, stroke, cognitive decline, depression, and dementia (Aiden 2016; Holt-Lunstad et al. 2010; Valtorta et al. 2016). In the UK alone, there are over 1.2 million chronically lonely people, and this number is set to rise with the aging population (Age UK 2016). It is evident that being part of a social network and having a sense of belonging and self-worth are crucial for health and well-being regardless of age. Owen (2014, p. 27) suggests that "…the sense of loneliness that manifests itself in care homes often begins when older people are still living in their own homes." A study conducted in England between 2002 and 2015 exploring loneliness in the care home found that by tackling loneliness in the aging population, well-being could be enhanced, thus delaying and potentially reducing the demand for residential care (Hanratty et al. 2018).

5.4 The Aging Population, Dementia, and Alzheimer's Disease

The United Nations (2018) estimated that in 2017, 13% (962 million) of the global population was over the age of 60. The UK Office of National Statistics (ONS) reports that its country's population is growing due, in part, to aging, and that the percentage of people over age 65 is increasing, estimating that it will continue to grow to almost a quarter of the population by 2045. This aging population boom, however, presents new challenges. Dementia is regarded as one of the biggest twenty-first-century health and social care issues (ONS 2017). The World Health Organization defines dementia as "...a syndrome in which there is deterioration in memory, thinking, behavior and the ability to perform everyday activities" (WHO 2017 para. 1–2). The most common type of dementia is found in those diagnosed with Alzheimer's Disease. In the UK, 850,000 people are affected by Alzheimer's Disease including 40,000 people under the age of 65, and the incidence of dementia is predicted to increase to 1.6 million by the year 2040 (The Alzheimer's Society 2018). The impact of the disease on people's lives has been explored through in-depth interviews with carers and dementia sufferers (Carter and Rigby 2017). The research highlights that dementia is still misunderstood and viewed negatively, potentially increasing feelings of low self-worth and isolation for both sufferers and carers. The Alzheimer's Society urges everyone, not only health and social care providers, but society as a whole, to recognize the problem and for substantial funding to be allocated for research and improved social care provision.

5.5   The Arts and the Care of Older Adults

The importance of health promotion and disease prevention in the aging population is fundamental, and the arts can play a significant role by reducing social isolation, increasing confidence, improving mobility, and building community capacity (Age UK 2017). Positive well-being can lead to more fulfilling and flourishing communities that can in turn delay or indeed prevent entry into the care home setting by enabling individuals to remain at home (Windle et al. 2016). Aging can lead to a range of health challenges including dementia, brittle bones, changing gait, diminished eyesight, hearing loss, and reduced self-confidence as a result (Oliver et al. 2014). A report published by Collective Encounters 2013 —"*Arts and Dementia: bringing professional arts practice into care settings*"—highlights the extensive research undertaken in exploring the benefits of engaging with participatory arts in the social context; it demonstrates the benefits of participatory arts in providing creative activities, facilitating social interaction, enabling choice, and supporting personal development within social care settings for dementia sufferers.

The value of art and creativity in the care home setting is recognized as being of importance to residents' physical and mental well-being and their overall quality of life. Taking part in activities, whether familiar or new, provides opportunities to gain knowledge, boost confidence, and connect in different ways (Speer and Delgado 2017). Such activities are not only rewarding but also offer feasible ways of providing excellence in care (Cutler et al. 2011). Creativity has no barriers, is inclusive, is non-judgmental, and offers individuals and communities unique opportunities to participate regardless of age, disability, social challenges, and gender (Potter 2016). The use of arts in health has flourished over recent decades, and its potential is gaining recognition for what was once regarded as a fringe activity (Fancourt 2017). Health promotion enables people to increase control over and improve their health and well-being in a wide variety of ways, and participation in the arts gives individuals the opportunity to socially connect, learn new skills, and most importantly express themselves creatively (APPG 2017; Fancourt 2017; WHO 1986).

5.6 The Project: "Tree of Many Colours"

5.6.1 The Care Home Setting

The village of Aboyne, Aberdeenshire, Scotland was the geographic location for this innovative outdoor art project. Aboyne is situated within the Marr area, which is one of six administrative areas within Aberdeenshire Council, with a population of 2910, of which 16.7% is over the age of 65 (Aberdeenshire Council 2016). Aboyne is one of three villages that encompasses Royal Deeside, and its economy is largely dependent on land-based enterprises, agriculture, and tourism.

The idea for the project evolved after Michelle Riddock, the manager of Allachburn Care Home in Aboyne, and her assistant managers visited a new purpose-built residential care home. To assist with the transition process, the manager of the new care home engaged an artist to help residents express how they felt about leaving their previous residential care home and moving to the new one. The project was titled "*Moving Out, Moving In,*" and a unique canvas was created capturing residents' feelings, interests, memories, and personalities. It was this project that inspired the assistant managers to explore a creative outdoor project for Allachburn.

5.6.2 Project Aim and Objectives

The aim of the project was to offer residents and staff a meaningful, stimulating, and creative experience. The project had three main objectives:

1. To explore whether participation had any impact on the health and well-being of residents and staff
2. To increase staff awareness of the value of arts-based activities in delivering participant-centered care
3. To raise awareness of the project within the wider community through engagement and sponsorship

5.6.3 Project Team

The project took more than six months of planning, involving the leadership and collaboration of the following partners:

- Michelle Riddock, Allachburn Care Home Manager (and other Allachburn staff)
- Gil Barton, Facilitator and Health and Well-being Consultant
- Ian Robertson, Artist
- Margaret O'Connor, Chief Executive at Art in Healthcare (AiH), a charity based in Edinburgh
- Beth Bidwell, Ceramic Technician at Scottish Sculpture Workshop (SSW), Lumsden, Aberdeenshire

Gil Barton had been asked to assist with ideas for a creative outdoor project through her volunteer role as trustee of a local charity (Mid Deeside Community Trust).

5.6.4 Funding

The funding for the project was a combination of sponsorship; fundraising by the Care Home Family (CHF); and the goodwill of staff, family, and friends. The available funding was insufficient to cover the full costs and as a result, the project team agreed to run this as a pilot project, absorbing any outstanding costs.

5.6.5 Project Planning

The manager of Allachburn was open to ideas and innovative in her approach to running the home, which was a key factor in the development stages. One of the critical aspects of a successful arts-in-health project is positive engagement with participants and staff, which can be challenging particularly within a health care setting and/or when working with a vulnerable group of individuals (The Welsh NHS Confederation 2018). The early involvement of the CHF resulted in much interest, and this engagement brought the project to life during the planning phase. The manager consulted with residents, their families, and staff to determine if there was interest; once interest was established, a Residents' Representative Group was formed called "*Allachburn Art Project*". Any health and safety considerations should be addressed at the early outset of the planning stage to ensure adoption of safe practices (Fancourt 2017), and the Representative Group and project team worked together to ensure this.

The facilitator, being locally based, liaised with all partners to ensure the project was on track. Working in Aberdeenshire rather than Edinburgh or Glasgow was new for AiH, and it was important that the facilitator liaised effectively with all partners.

The artist was not locally based, presenting a further logistical challenge. Concise project planning was necessary, and the construction of a logic model framework ensured that the key components were integrated and outcomes were focused (Cohen et al. 2014; Fancourt 2017). To ensure maximum opportunity for participants, a total of eight workshops were planned throughout August on Tuesdays and Wednesdays from 10–12 AM and 2–4 PM each day. In planning the workshops, it was important to take into account the normal routines and regular activities of the care home itself.

5.6.6 Practical and Creative Considerations

The most suitable medium for the project was clay, requiring extensive planning by the artist, and this was where the support of the ceramic technician was crucial. Practically, it was important that the tiles were of a regular thickness for aesthetic reasons and to ensure consistent results in the glazing and firing processes. The outdoor display would be exposed to the elements; therefore, to weatherproof it, the clay needed to be coarse and reinforced with sandy grout. The client group lacked the dexterity required to manipulate large lumps of clay; consequently, the artist prepared over 80 rolled clay slabs. The preparation, glazing, and firing of the clay required round trips of over 140 miles by the artist, which was not only time consuming but costly. The artist was able to stay overnight in Allachburn, which was practically, financially, and logistically advantageous. These "hidden" costs can often be overlooked, and it is important to consider these in the planning stages.

5.6.7 Project Evaluation

Project evaluation was undertaken using a combination of qualitative and video-based observational research (VOR) through questionnaires, semi-structured interviews, and video capture. The purpose of the evaluation was to determine whether the aim and objectives of the project had been met. The use of video recording was primarily aimed at producing an informal short video of the project journey for residents and their families with an iPad used by staff and the facilitator during the workshops. Although this may have provided future promotional, evidential, or educational material, there was no budget for the production of a professional film.

In this instance, there was no formal sampling method utilized due to the nature of the project; it was a convenience sample restricted to the CHF aiming to cover as many participants as possible. The participants were care home residents and their families, staff, and their children. Residents chose independently to attend, and those with dementia were involved along with the support of family members or staff.

The workshops ran during school holiday time, providing opportunities for children to be involved. For those who were unable to give informed consent for participation and the evaluation, family members were involved in any decision making (see Fig. 5.1). A short questionnaire previously developed by AiH for a dementia event in 2017 was utilized, consisting of ten open and closed questions; these questionnaires were completed at the beginning and end of the workshops. Semi-structured interviews were conducted by Gil Barton with the care home manager, the AiH chief executive, and the artist (Fig. 5.2).

5.6.8   Results

A total of ten questionnaires were completed by eight residents and two staff members. Completion of the questionnaire by residents was challenging despite support by the facilitator and staff. Twenty residents participated throughout the workshops, although some only stayed for a short time due to their health conditions. Three residents consistently attended every session, and one of their nieces came to each morning workshop. Twelve staff members completed tiles while assisting residents, and nine children took part.

Thematic analysis of the questionnaires (Ritchie and Lewis 2011) highlighted five main themes as detailed in Fig. 5.3.

Fig. 5.1 Project participants

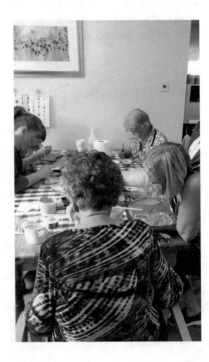

Fig. 5.2 Tree of many colours ceramics

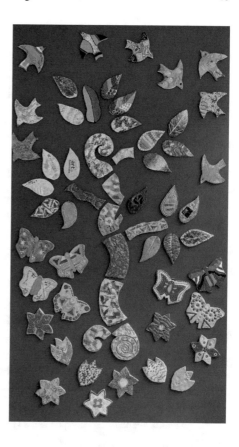

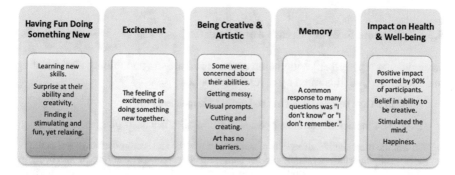

Fig. 5.3 Five main themes identified by participants

5.6.8.1   Theme 1: Having Fun Doing Something New

There was much fun and laughter throughout the project by both residents and staff, evident in the video footage. Some residents, while not actively participating, were content watching the workshops, and running these over two consecutive days each week for a month allowed the team to establish familiarity with residents and staff. The artist commented:

> "The project really came to life with the involvement of youngsters—children of staff members or relatives of the residents—which also seemed to be the catalyst that encouraged more of the staff members to join in. This sparked a busy, positive atmosphere with a range of ages from very young to elderly engaged side by side, slightly curious about the novelty of the situation and seemingly delighted just to be having fun making something together."

A staff participant (Respondent #8) said:

> "It was SO much fun! Chatting with residents and seeing their creativity! Working with the children, at first everyone was unsure what to do but really everyone put so much in."

5.6.8.2   Theme 2: Excitement

Excitement was a consistent theme throughout the responses, and it was evident that participants were interested, stimulated, and excited about undertaking something new. Having new people in the home appeared to create a different energy, which was reflected in the responses, which characterized the experience by describing it as:

> "… an unusual experience" (Respondent #4)

> "…general buzz" (Respondent #5)

5.6.8.3   Theme 3: Being Creative and Artistic

Respondents reported enjoying being creative and artistic and finding it stimulating and interesting, as illustrated by several comments:

> "Belief that I can be creative, art has no barrier." (Respondent #8)

> "I did that. I'm not really an artistic person, but I did enjoy that one!" (Respondent #3)

> "One of the most significant aspects of this project was the real sense of achievement in the participants when they eventually saw the dull, earthy materials they had worked with being transformed into the bright glowing display of the finished work." (Artist)

5.6.8.4 Theme 4: Memory

Unsurprisingly, some of the participants were unable to recall having taken part in the creative activities without prompting. One example of this was a resident (Respondent # 6) who participated in two workshops creating a flower, stating: "I wasn't involved."

5.6.8.5 Theme 5: Impact on Health and Well-being

The responses to the question regarding impact on health and well-being were all positive, which is contrary to the preceding theme with some participants being unable to recall taking part. It could be assumed that, because most of the questionnaires were completed with the support of staff, when residents were prompted and reminded of what they created they recalled different aspects they had enjoyed. One participant (Respondent #7) highlighted this, saying: "Any activity good for your body [sic]."

5.6.9 Other Captured Qualitative Data

AiH believes that a professional artist working in a social rather than a medical environment is an effective approach, fitting well with the prevention agenda of public health. During an interview with the Chief Executive of AiH, she identified that having no fee was difficult however the project provided an opportunity to enable participatory activity through the workshops led by one of their artists that resulted in 'The Tree of Many Colours'. In addition, AiH were drawn to the 'Healthy Working Lives' agenda that was led by Gil Barton. The commitment of all partners was essential to overcoming any difficulties, and it took creative thinking at times to achieve this.

5.7 Observations and Reflections

During the first workshops, the blank clay slabs were utilized; however, the artist observed that for many, the physical effort of drawing around the template and cutting the shapes was difficult. To alleviate this, in week two the artist adjusted his approach by offering participants ready-made shapes. It became apparent that not only did this increase his interaction with participants, it also enhanced the tactile experience of impressing leaves, seeds, tree bark, and other objects into the regular surface or of making patterns with clay tools, thus encouraging experimentation. The workshops, although slow, were demanding, and the artist's reflection captures this:

"Despite the slow pace of the sessions they were deceptively intense and doing two per day was very tiring, for myself and participants. The most effective time to work seemed to be mid-morning to just before midday. Nevertheless, the later sessions were useful for accommodating the youngsters and staff that participated."

Throughout the workshops, social interaction tended to expand into general conversation, resulting in a more relaxed and sociable atmosphere—particularly when staff dropped in to see what was happening, providing support and encouragement. When staff, relatives, and children joined in, the artist could start allocating tasks to more able participants, and the efforts of the youngsters were a source of real interest to the residents. The assembled pieces needed to dry before the application of colored stains, providing a natural break in the process and allowing for sample preparation between sessions. It was difficult for participants to envisage how the clay and colors would change as the process advanced, and this was helped by having finished glazed and fired examples available.

While there was much joy and laughter throughout the project, one resident found that taking part triggered memories that were upsetting. This female resident initially spent a happy, creative two hours during the first workshop; however, when she returned on the second day, she was despondent, lamenting about her lack of inspiration. Despite support and reassurance, she became tearful and distressed and was taken away from the workshop by staff for a cup of tea. When a family member arrived later, she was able to put this reaction into context, explaining that in the past the resident had baked beautiful wedding cakes, and this experience brought back memories as she grieved for her younger self. The resident did, however, return to a later workshop to paint her two tiles—a butterfly for the tree and a bird for her bedroom door. Recalling happy memories can enhance well-being; yet, as with this situation, reminiscing can also lead to feelings of negativity and loss (Hofer et al. 2017; Speer and Delgado 2017).

The inclusion of children brought an intergenerational aspect to the workshops and created a different dimension, and staff appeared more confident when assisting them, leading to their own creativity. Residents visibly enjoyed having the children working alongside them and sparking new conversations, which can have a positive impact on cognitive processes and creativity (Young et al. 2015). Staff reported anecdotally both during and after project completion that there was such a "buzz" about the project, and it appeared to have brought something special to Allachburn.

As described in the concluding chapter of this book, this arts-based initiative demonstrates the deep and complex interactions art stimulates within health promotion practice. Art increases connections with the self, with others and contributes to environmental beautification (see Chap. 21, this volume). Art activities can connect so viscerally with participants, it can promote profound healing, but may also produce some distress on that journey. It may be important to ensure appropriate support is in place.

5.7.1 Challenges and Considerations

As with any project, there were challenges—mainly funding and the logistics of working effectively as a new partnership, which can take time to develop and over-come. Fancourt (2017) identifies four main partnership models, and in this case the appointment of the artist early on was critical to the project's progression aligning with a Collaborative Design. There were logistical challenges due to the geographi-cal distances between the team and Allachburn, with many of these being borne by the artist, and it was his flexibility, knowledge, commitment, and passion that enabled the project to progress.

The cost of materials and the logistics associated with installing and maintaining the ceramics required specialist input that should not be underestimated. Engagement by the artist early on with the ceramic technician at the SSW led to them taking a keen interest in the project, resulting in significant ongoing in-kind support. The mounting of the individual tiles to the external wall was complex, and Allachburn's handyman was invaluable in formulating an affordable, workable solution.

5.7.2 What Could Be Done Differently?

Just like any project, there are things that could have been done differently; thus, learning by the project team may be useful for others considering similar activities. The evaluation, as it stands currently, has met the project's aim and, broadly, its objectives. Completion of the questionnaire by residents was difficult due in part to the client group, as undertaking any research and evaluation when working with dementia sufferers can be difficult (as evidenced by Chatterjee et al. 2018). The duration of the creative process was another challenging factor, with some residents forgetting they had been involved. Evaluation is something that could be done dif-ferently, particularly when considering future funding for other projects. Given the client group, evaluation methods require flexibility as highlighted by Young et al. (2015) and Fancourt (2017). The filming captured qualitative evidence of participa-tion, emotions, and the process, which will be edited to produce a short video for residents and their families. At this stage, it is unclear whether being involved has had any impact on the health and well-being of staff. If time had allowed, a focus group with staff to explore their involvement in relation to their health and well-being would have demonstrated whether the first objective had been met. Anecdotally, the manager reported that as a result of the project, residents appeared to be more open to new ideas, and staff were more confident and eager to explore other creative activities.

5.8   Conclusion

The benefit of participating in the arts in relation to health and well-being across all ages and abilities is apparent, and this project's aim—"to offer residents and staff a meaningful, stimulating and creative experience"—was clearly met. What started as an idea for a small outdoor art project grew with the collaborative approach taken by the partners and their willingness to work flexibly, regarding it as a "pilot." This flexibility allowed the project to evolve into a significant piece of work. The inclusion of the residents' families and staff brought a different dimension to it and engendered wider interest.

The "Tree of Many Colours" was formally opened by the Provost of Aberdeenshire, Bill Howatson, in February 2019, over a year after project discussions began (see Fig. 5.2). In addition to the ceramic "Tree of Many Colours," a large information sign detailing the project story and credits for each tile is mounted on the front external wall of Allachburn (see Fig. 5.4). It was evident that this artistic venture had brought much happiness and joy to participants, and final thoughts from the artist highlight this:

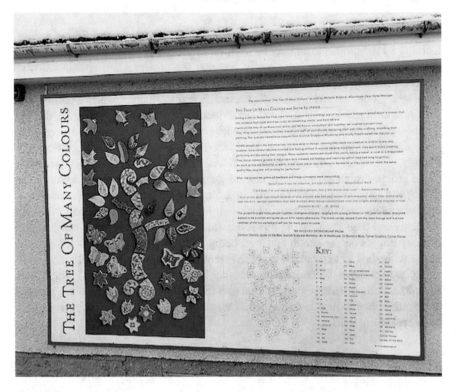

Fig. 5.4 Information sign

"This was probably one of the most rewarding and enjoyable art projects I've been involved with. I'm very pleased that the finished work has been received so positively and my time spent in Allachburn was heart-warming and enlightening."

Acknowledgements I am grateful to everyone who has helped with this project, particularly Michelle Riddock and the staff of Allachburn, Ian Robertson, Margaret O'Connor, AiH, and Beth Bidwell at SSW. Thank you to Karen Hicks, who persuaded me to submit an abstract, and thank you to my reviewers, Val Burnett and Dr. Linda McSwiggan, for their professional peer review. A final thank you goes to my husband, Professor Glenn Iason, for his reviewing, constructive comments, and endless support and encouragement.

References

Aberdeenshire Council. (2016). *Marr area profile*. Inverurie: Aberdeenshire Council. https://www.aberdeenshire.gov.uk/media/18326/marr-profile-2016.pdf. Accessed 25 Oct 2018.

Age UK. (2016). *Dignity in health and social care (England)*. https://www.ageuk.org.uk/globalassets/age-uk/documents/policy-positions/care-and-support/ppp_dignity_in_health_and_social_care_en.pdf. Accessed 28 Nov 2018.

Age UK. (2017). Index of Wellbeing in Later Life. https://www.ageuk.org.uk/our-impact/policy-research/wellbeing-research/index-of-wellbeing/. Accessed 16th September 2020.

Aiden, H. (2016). *Isolation and loneliness: An overview of the literature*. The British Red Cross.

British Association of Art Therapists. (2018). *What is art therapy?* https://www.baat.org/About-Art-Therapy. Accessed 27 Nov 2018.

Carter, D., & Rigby, A. (2017). Turning up the volume: Unheard voices of people with dementia. In *The Alzheimer's Society*. London. https://www.alzheimers.org.uk/about-us/policy-and-influencing/reports/turning-up-volume. Accessed 11 Nov 2018.

Chatterjee, H. J., Camic, P. M., Lockyer, B., & Thomson, L. J. M. (2018). Non-clinical community interventions: A systematised review of social prescribing schemes. *Arts & Health, 10*(2), 97–123. https://doi.org/10.1080/17533015.2017.1334002. Accessed 6 Mar 2019.

Coburn, A., Vartanian, O., & Chatterjee, A. (2017). Buildings, beauty, and the brain: A neuroscience of architectural experience. *Journal of Cognitive Neuroscience*. https://doi.org/10.1162/jocn_a_01146.

Cohen, L., Wimbush, E., Myers, F., Macdonald, W., & Frost, H. (2014). *Optimising older people's quality of life: An outcomes framework. Strategic outcomes model. NHS Health Scotland and Scottish Collaboration for Public Health Research & Policy*. Edinburgh: University of Edinburgh.

Collective Encounters. (2013). *Arts and dementia: Bringing professional arts practice into care settings*. http://collective-encounters.org.uk/. Accessed 27 Nov 2018.

Commission for Architecture and the Built Environment. (2009). *Future health: Sustainable places for health and well-being*. https://www.designcouncil.org.uk/resources/report/sustainable-places-health-and-well-being. Accessed 12 Mar 2019.

Cutler, D. (2013). *Local authorities + older people + arts = a creative combination*. London: The Baring Foundation. Accessed 14 Mar 2019.

Cutler, D., Kelly, D., & Silver, S. (2011). *Creative homes: How the arts can contribute to quality of life in residential care*. London: The Baring Foundation.

Elkis-Abuhoff, D., & Morgan, G. (2019). *Art and expressive therapies within the medical model: Clinical applications*. Abingdon: Routledge.

Fancourt, D. (2017). *Arts in health: Designing and researching intervention*. Oxford: Oxford University Press.

Green, M., Iparraguirre, J., Davidson, S., & Rossall, P. (2017). *A summary of Age UK's index of wellbeing in later life*. London: Age UK. https://www.ageuk.org.uk/our-impact/policy-research/wellbeing-research/. Accessed 13 Mar 2019.

Hanratty, B., Stow, D., Collingridge Moore, D., Valtorta, N. K., & Matthews, F. (2018). Loneliness as a risk factor for care home admission in the English Longitudinal Study of Ageing. *Age and Ageing*. https://doi.org/10.1093/ageing/afy095.

Hofer, J., Busch, H., Poláčková Šolcová, I., & Tavel, P. (2017). When reminiscence is harmful: The relationship between self-negative reminiscence functions, need satisfaction, and depressive symptoms among elderly people from Cameroon, the Czech Republic, and Germany. *Journey of Happiness Studies*. https://doi.org/10.1007/s10902-016-9731-3. Accessed 15 Mar 2019.

Holt-Lunstad, J. H., Smith, T. B., & Bradley Layton, J. (2010). Social relationships and mortality risk: A meta-analytic review. *PLoS Medicine*. https://doi.org/10.1371/journal.pmed.1000316.

Jones, R., & Yates, G. (2013). *The built environment and health: An evidence review*. Glasgow: Glasgow Centre for Population Health. https://www.gcph.co.uk/publications/472_concepts_series_11-the_built_environment_and_health_an_evidence_review. Accessed 12 Mar 2019.

No Isolation. (2019). *The state of social isolation and loneliness in the UK*. https://www.noisolation.com/global/research/the-state-of-social-isolation-and-loneliness-in-the-uk/. Accessed 15 Sept 2019.

Office of National Statistics. (2017, July). *Overview of the UK population*. https://www.ons.gov.uk/peoplepopulationandcommunity/populationandmigration/populationestimates/articles/overviewoftheukpopulation/july2017. Accessed 20 October 2018.

Oliver, D., Foot, C., & Humphries, R. (2014). *Making our health and care systems fit for an ageing population*. London: The Kings Fund. https://www.kingsfund.org.uk/publications/articles/making-care-system-fit-ageing-population. Accessed 3 June 2020.

Owen, T. (2014). Loneliness in care homes. In *Alone in the crowd: Loneliness and diversity*. Campaign to End Loneliness. https://www.campaigntoendloneliness.org/. Accessed 14 Mar 2019.

Potter, S. (2016). *Community programme social impact study evaluation report*. Chichester: Pallant House Gallery.

Ritchie, L., & Lewis, J. (2011). *Qualitative research practice: A guide for social science students and researchers*. London: Sage Publications.

Seligman, M. E. (2011). *Flourish: A visionary new understanding of happiness and well-being*. New York: Simon and Schuster.

Speer, M. E., & Delgado, M. R. (2017). Reminiscing about positive memories buffers acute stress responses. *Nature Human Behaviour*. https://doi.org/10.1038/s41562-017-0093. Accessed 15 Mar 2019.

The Alzheimer's Society. (2018). *Facts for the media: What is dementia?*. https://www.alzheimers.org.uk/about-us/news-and-media/facts-media. Accessed 11 Nov 2018.

The Welsh NHS Confederation. (2018). *Arts, health & well-being*. https://www.nhsconfed.org/-/media/Confederation/Files/Wales-Confed/Literature-review-of-arts-and%2D%2Dhealth-and-wellbeing.pdf. Accessed 14 Sept 2019.

UK All-Party Parliamentary Group on Arts, Health and Wellbeing. (2017). *Creative health: The arts for health and wellbeing*. http://www.artshealthandwellbeing.org.uk/appg-inquiry/. Accessed 9 Nov 2018.

United Nations. (2018). *Ageing*. http://www.un.org/en/sections/issues-depth/ageing/. Accessed 20 Oct 2018.

United Nations Educational, Scientific and Cultural Organization. (2015). *Report of the World Commission on Culture and Development*. https://unesdoc.unesco.org/ark:/48223/pf0000244834. Accessed 28 May 2020.

Valtorta, N. K., Kanaan, M., Gilbody, S., Ronzi, S., & Hanratty, B. (2016). Loneliness and social isolation as risk factors for coronary heart disease and stroke: Systematic review and meta-analysis of longitudinal observational studies. *Heart, 102*, 1009–1016.

Wilkinson, R., & Pickett, K. (2018). *The inner level: How more equal societies reduce stress, restore sanity and improve everyone's wellbeing*. London: Penguin.

Windle, K., George, T., Porter, R., McKay, S., Culliney, M., Walker, J., et al. (2016). *"Staying Well in Calderdale" programme evaluation: Final report*. Lincoln: University of Lincoln.

World Health Organization. (1986). *The Ottawa Charter for health promotion*. https://www.who.int/healthpromotion/conferences/previous/ottawa/en/.

World Health Organization. (2017). *Dementia key facts*. https://www.who.int/news-room/fact-sheets/detail/dementia.

Young, R., Camic, P. M., & Tischler, V. (2015). The impact of community-based arts and health interventions on cognition in people with dementia: A systematic literature review. *Aging & Mental Health*. https://doi.org/10.1080/13607863.2015.1011080.

Zhang, Y., Tzortzopoulos, P., & Kagioglou, M. (2018). Healing built-environment effects on health outcomes: Environment-occupant-health framework. *Journal of Building Research & Information*. https://doi.org/10.1080/09613218.2017.1411130. Accessed 2 March 2019.

Chapter 6
CuidarNos: Art and Social Work to Address Trauma Among Gender-based Violence Advocates After Hurricane María in Puerto Rico

Heriberto Ramírez-Ayala, Elithet Silva-Martínez, and Jenice M. Vázquez-Pagán

6.1 Introduction

On September 20, 2017, one of the most powerful hurricanes in its history impacted Puerto Rico. Close to three million people lost access to basic services such as electricity and clean water. Thousands of families lost their homes, and many communities remained unreachable after a massive collapse in all communications systems throughout the island. Natural disasters result in serious damage to the normal performance of a community, due to the large number of people injured and the considerable loss of human life and property they cause (Park and Duarte 2011). Natural disasters can also affect the health of the people, necessitating not only immediate attention to the victims but also medium- and long-term actions stemming from the absence of basic services, displacement of people or migration, and a lack of food and housing. In the aftermath of María, many faced 12–14-hour lines to access fuel or food. For countless families, the public education system provides access to food for their children, but a great number of schools remained closed due to structural damages or a shortage of staff. This had a negative effect on many children who were unable to access hot meals or drinking water. The combination of these experiences triggered growth in emigration rates to the United States (Delgado 2018), in

H. Ramírez-Ayala (✉)
TIPOS, Toa Alta, Puerto Rico
e-mail: heriberto.educa@gmail.com

E. Silva-Martínez
Beatriz Lassalle Graduate School of Social Work, University of Puerto Rico,
San Juan, Puerto Rico
e-mail: elithet.silva@upr.edu

J. M. Vázquez-Pagán
Department of Social Work, Interamerican University of Puerto Rico, San Juan, Puerto Rico
e-mail: jmvazquez@intermetro.edu

© The Author(s) 2021
J. H. Corbin et al. (eds.), *Arts and Health Promotion*,
https://doi.org/10.1007/978-3-030-56417-9_6

part related to the ongoing economic crisis prior to Hurricane María that intensified in the following several months (Rodríguez-Díaz 2018; Robles et al. 2017).

The United Nations Office for Disaster Risk Reduction (UNISDR 2009) defines "disaster" as follows:

A serious disruption of the functioning of a community or a society at any scale due to hazardous events interacting with conditions of exposure, vulnerability and capacity, leading to one or more of the following: human, material, economic and environmental losses and impacts (pp. 9).

The UNISDR definition recognizes that the impact of a disaster can be localized (e.g., a landslide that blocks access to a rural community) or generalized (e.g., the effects of Hurricane María in Puerto Rico) (Adamson 2018). The magnitude, severity, or sequence of events is what often suggests the most immediate risk of traumatic impact for those caught in the disaster. However, the origin of the disaster, the pre-existing vulnerabilities, and how the disaster develops over time also emerge as determinants of the overall traumatic impact (Adamson 2018).

A study published in 2018 in the New England Journal of Medicine estimated at least 4645 deaths in Puerto Rico were related to the hurricane; yet for many months, the local government assured that the death toll was closer to 64 (Kishore et al. 2018). The authors of the study strongly criticized the methods used to account for these deaths and the lack of transparency by government authorities in Puerto Rico in disclosing information. The people of Puerto Rico experienced great devastation, loss, and trauma after Hurricane María, and this trauma certainly remains present in their daily lives. Almost 2 years after experiencing this socio-natural disaster, many families and communities are still dealing with a lack of access to basic resources such as safe housing and access to health and education, in addition to the repercussions of trauma after such a difficult experience. In 2019, there are many families in urban communities that still live under blue tarps while they wait to save money to

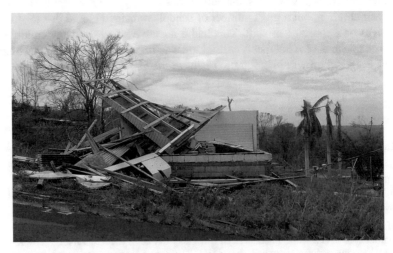

Fig. 6.1 House shattered by the hurricane winds

rebuild their roofs; numerous families in the mountains—especially families headed by women—are still waiting for access to basic services (Fig. 6.1).

A recent study carried out by *Instituto de Estadísticas de Puerto Rico* [Puerto Rico Institute of Statistics] (2016) confirmed that of the 45.1% of the Puerto Rican population living below the poverty line, 46.8% are women. The literature on disasters and violence against women points out that women and girls are more vulnerable to suffering gender-based violence amid disaster, in many cases exacerbated by the lack of access to protection or support at a public level (Cutter 2017; Fisher 2010; True 2016). In addition, there has been limited support for organizations that, with great effort, kept their projects afloat during and after the disaster. Regarding this issue, there is literature on other regions where natural disasters have occurred that show that women live a double disaster and that their losses include intangible dimensions, such as traumatic responses and exacerbation of health conditions including mental health, which could be considered peripheral (Bradshaw and Fordham 2015; Juran and Trivedi 2015). For example, Neumayer and Plümper (2007) highlight that gender differences have an effect in recovery after natural disasters by having a direct link with economic and social inequality as well as with structural violence against women.

Studies have shown the important role of health promotion in recovering a sense of control after a disaster. Jackson et al. (2016) point out that involving disaster victims (including children) in community-based decisions related to health, education, safety, etc. is important and could, in fact, contribute to healing. Collaborating, recognizing strengths and local assets, conducting community-needs assessments, and respecting local knowledge are all part of a continuous system allowing for the promotion of health in disaster situations. In addition, working with pre-existing community centers as trusted places for community services and reconnections can be important after a disaster occurs.

The Ottawa Charter for Health Promotion (WHO 1986) defines "health promotion" as "the process of enabling people to increase control over, and to improve their health." This document is considered important insofar as it recognizes that to achieve a state of complete physical, mental, and social well-being, an individual or group must be able to identify and realize aspirations, satisfy needs, and change or face the environment. It also affirms that health is not only the responsibility of the health sector. It establishes that health promotion policy must combine diverse but complementary approaches that include legislation, fiscal measures, taxes, and organizational changes as part of coordinated action that leads to health, income, and social policies that promote greater equity. As described in Chap. 1 (this volume), arts-based initiatives can be productively used to support and facilitate health promotion by enhancing these intersectoral approaches.

6.2 Seeing a Need

A few days after Hurricane María hit, *Coordinadora Paz para la Mujer (CPM)* [The Puerto Rican Coalition Against Domestic Violence and Sexual Assault] reached out to nearly 40 organizations throughout the island and made the call to support partners who had experienced losses, which included providing shelters for survivors of intimate partner violence and their children. Many of the shelters had already faced major budget cuts. In fact, in 2011, there were close to 15 shelters available, but in September of 2017, only four remained open. Even with several challenges faced by the organizations working with survivors and their children, many returned to rebuild or to provide support with limited resources. Before the hurricane, CPM had been providing support to service providers and community leaders on issues of vicarious trauma, especially due to the alarming number of cases of violence against women. Vicarious trauma involves the indirect trauma that service providers could experience when exposed to the traumatic experiences of their participants. Facing a landscape of devastation from Hurricane María, many advocates and service providers in shelters and other support organizations dealt with the effects of vicarious trauma as well as primary trauma. Following the hurricane, many service providers experienced primary trauma, which consisted of losing their homes, belongings, and even loved ones due to disaster-related factors or being separated due to emigration to the United States. All experienced limited access to basic services such as electricity, running water, and communications, and some even lost their homes and/or family members. At the same time, they were supporting other hurricane survivors who were coping with intimate partner violence, sexual assault, stalking, and sexual harassment in addition to the aftermath of the socio-natural disaster. This scenario led to CPM and the University of Puerto Rico collaborating to develop an art and social work integrated intervention geared toward advocates and service providers to address the combination of primary and vicarious trauma.

In any circumstance related to natural disaster, violence, and/or trauma, service providers experience physical, emotional, and cognitive changes as result of secondary traumatic stress (Naturale 2015; Palm et al. 2004). Violence and trauma can also affect the functioning of their work (Bride 2011). Among the areas affected by stress are the physical, mental, emotional, and behavioral. It has been shown that individual efforts to manage stress are necessary, but probably not enough. In 2011, a study conducted by the American Psychological Association suggested that organizational approaches to stress management are necessary to complement individual approaches; in addition to the efforts made by employees individually, it is important that the organization take comprehensive and structural measures to reduce employee stress and create well-being in the workplace (Cox and Steiner 2013). The results of this study tend to be consistent with the requirements of the Ottawa Charter of Health Promotion (WHO 1986) insofar as they make visible the need for multiple and diverse approaches, at different levels of society, to deal with the stress caused by a traumatic event in life. The *Encuentro CuidarNos,* part of an initiative propelled by CPM after Hurricane María hit Puerto Rico, aimed to support organizational efforts to address and work through primary and secondary traumatic experiences from a diversity of approaches.

Working in the area of gender-based violence requires multidisciplinary approaches to address its complexity and multiple psychological, social, and environmental roots to allow for approaching the problem in a holistic manner. One of the approaches provided by this holistic vision is the "ecological approach" to dealing with violence, instituted by Heise et al. (1994) and based on the work of Bronfenbrenner (1979). This model has been employed by the World Health Organization (WHO) since 2003 and allows violence to be addressed at different levels, namely: the microsocial or individual level; the mesosocial level or the community context; and the macrosocial or institutional level (Olivares and Incháustegui 2011, p. 21–24). Considering these aspects of the ecological model, *CuidarNOS* was designed to meet the personal and professional needs of service providers, as well as those of women survivors of gender violence and their children. Likewise, it sought to meet the organizational needs of the CPM (and the entities that comprise the coalition) to face the changes caused by Hurricane María.

6.3   Encuentro CuidarNOS

The *Encuentro CuidarNOS* is based on an approach consisting of an integrated intervention of art and social work with the goal of meeting the needs of employees as advocates and service providers from different organizations connected to the coalition. As part of its objectives, this initiative sought to address the combination of primary and vicarious trauma and support psychological health and safety in a natural disaster context. *CuidarNOS* was designed to work with the physical, mental, and social aspects of service providers who supported survivors of intimate partner violence as well as with the well-being of the community—particularly women survivors of gender violence, their children, and the work teams within the organizations that provide services to them.

There is a growing body of literature that evidences the benefits of using art as a tool to facilitate reflection as well as to express feelings, promote conversation, and connect with others around us (Karcher 2017; Martinec 2018; Wahl-Alexander 2017). In a project in Sri Lanka related to post-disaster trauma, Huss et al. (2016) highlight how art can be a tool for therapeutic interventions, especially in helping to reconstruct the narrative of the event and in provoking mobilization toward recovery and healing. This element was central to developing the *Encuentro CuidarNOS*. Another important element was acknowledging the neurobiology of trauma and the memory allocated in our bodies. It made us integrate movement as part of the interventions even before repeatedly asking participants to talk about their experiences. In this sense, Wahl-Alexander (2017) touches on how integrative art, physical activity, and somatic healing can be powerful in working in different disaster-related scenarios. As it pertains to other art media such as painting or drawing, we used drawing as a tool for eliciting communication. With his experience of using drawing in a tsunami-related disaster, Alexander (2018) points out that facing disasters and building resiliency requires imagination and refers to multi-dimensional communication through art because it makes it possible to rely exclusively on speech and "objective" understandings of safety. As pointed out by Ahmed and Siddiqi (2006), using art as a tool for therapy "provides a medium for communication and might facilitate the healing of emotional scars" (p. 529).

Before designing the *Encuentro CuidarNOS*, in alliance with CPM and a number of other organizations, the authors had been working directly with communities providing health care and legal aid for families seeking assistance from the U.S. Federal Government and support groups, as well as distributing donations and food. All the towns that we visited had an organization that served survivors of violence at different levels. A month after the hurricane, we started the Purple Caravan, which was composed of volunteers from different disciplines and professions. We also made connections with the organizations that were working directly with the communities dealing with violence against women. In that same week we went back to those communities and had a special gathering with these service providers and/or community leaders through the *Encuentro CuidarNOS*.

The initial purpose of the *Encuentro CuidarNOS* was to provide a safe space for service providers who worked at community-based and non-profit organizations to process their experiences from their own narratives on disaster-related trauma as well as vicarious trauma in working with survivors of intimate partner violence and sexual assault who, simultaneously, experienced disaster-related trauma. We decided to name it an *Encuentro*, or meeting, rather than a workshop or training, given the usual charge given to these terms in the professional arena. The term *Encuentro* laid the ground for an informal setting to share stories that were happening at that moment. Having experienced the hurricane ourselves, we knew that there had not necessarily been an opportunity to process the experience in depth because the island was still in a state of emergency. On the other hand, we were cognizant of the fact that these participants were very clear on their role as service providers, and we were strongly committed to humanizing the *Encuentro* for the participants to allow them to take part as survivors rather than as responders. Between November 2017 and September 2018, we worked with more than 200 advocates and volunteers, with a broad range of professional and personal backgrounds, from more than 15 organizations across Puerto Rico. When analyzing the participants' profiles, we found that there were social workers, psychologists, lawyers, administration officials and staff, legal advocates, child development specialists, educators, interns, volunteers, and community leaders. We visited all the shelters for survivors of intimate partner violence and their children who are part of the coalition of organizations. Also, we visited organizations that provided direct service as well as prevention services and community outreach on topics related to violence against women.

When it came to making the *Encuentro* possible, CPM was instrumental in its implementation. A key factor in gaining access to the groups was that CPM is a very well-respected coalition across the island. Its presence for almost 30 years in addressing intimate partner violence and sexual assault through capacity building, community outreach, and involvement in developing and strengthening social policies based on social justice and human rights has been the foundation of trust for organizations in various communities. In addition, the three of us have been working on the topic of interpersonal violence and violence against women for the past 15 years; therefore, many of the organizations knew us or had previously worked with us.

CPM took on the responsibility of organizing visits to the different organizations and establishing funding for this effort. Staff members established contact with each organization (either by phone or in person, when there was no telephone or digital connection). Given that CPM had also been distributing resources and donations through its Hurricane María Relief Fund, all the organizations were in close communication. In collaboration with CPM and many other allies, the commitment to the recovery of the organizations and the communities where they were situated also motivated us to help organize the Purple Caravan. This initiative gave us first hand access to many of the service providers. We had been working as partners before the *Encuentro*, and this helped in strengthening trust with many of the participants of the program.

6.4 Processing Trauma and Healing Through Art

The American Art Therapy Association (2017) explains that through integrative methods, art therapy engages the mind, body, and spirit in ways that are distinct from verbal articulation alone. Kinesthetic, sensory, perceptual, and symbolic opportunities invite alternative modes of receptive and expressive communication, which can circumvent the limitations of language. Visual and symbolic expression give voice to experience and empower individual, communal, and societal transformation. With this knowledge, we incorporated our expertise in social work and artistic education to face the collective trauma left by Hurricane María. A specialized three-hour *Encuentro* was designed to address the diverse needs, taking into consideration the neurobiology of trauma and its effects.

According to material on the subject, in addition to the effects of trauma on its prefrontal cortex, the brain also undergoes severe structural changes in the hippocampus—the structure that is responsible for the consolidation and organization of memory (Silva-Martinez 2018). Additionally, language is another fundamental area that is affected by trauma. To access memories impacted by trauma and to explore various expressive languages, we created three spaces to address the individual, relational, and collective dimensions. In turn, we selected one or several branches of art that could promote somatic experiences such as body movement, theatrical techniques, drawing, and sound to support healing processes.

The structure of the *Encuentro* combines reflection and play to create a safe space. The authors discussed in advance how to assign which part of the *Encuentro* our partner would be leading. For example, when a creative dynamic was underway, the co-facilitator would be responsible for preparing the materials, participating in the activity, or observing the reactions of the participants. This agreement allowed fluid transitions, kept the space organized, and helped to promote confidence between the facilitator and the group. This body of work involved five phases: harmonization; sensitization; expression; kinesthetic dynamic; and love networks, which consisted of collective exercises that began with the body and transitioned to the spoken word to build hope.

6.4.1 Phases of the Encuentro CuidarNOS

The first part of the *Encuentro* was harmonization, which consisted of two prepara-
tory exercises to foster a climate of trust. After all the participants stated their names
and provided some information about themselves, they were invited to take deep
and conscious breaths, followed by a collective exercise called *el baño* (the bath). In
this theater dynamic, we asked participants to mentally situate themselves in a
waterfall at *El Yunque*, Puerto Rico's beloved national rainforest. The group formed
a circle, and one by one, a person took his or her place at the center of the circle. The
participants who formed the circle would then use their hands to trace the person's
shape, starting with the top of the head and going to the bottom. The movement was
repeated three times and served the purpose of simulating water falling. The participants performed the movement while repeating a slow and calming sound of "shh,"
thus creating the auditory illusion of listening to the sound of a waterfall and being
immersed in water. The intention was to create a state of relaxation, connect with
our roots, and prepare the soul for the next phase of the exercise. Once this phase
was finished, participants expressed feelings of deep relaxation, calmness, and
serenity. After asking participants to become mentally and emotionally present and
inviting them to trust in the process, one of the facilitators provided a brief explanation of the neurobiology of trauma followed by a brief description of the next
exercises.

The second phase—sensitization—aimed to connect participants with their
senses. According to the pioneering work carried out by scientists Linda Buck and
Richard Axel (1991), each olfactory cell has a single receptor, organized by families, which can recognize a specific number of odors. When it perceives one of
them, it sends a signal to different micro-areas of the brain responsible for memory
and interpretation, associating smells with past experiences. In addition to olfactory
stimuli, we also used tactile stimuli. During this phase, the participants remained
seated with their eyes closed and were exposed to various olfactory and tactile stimuli such as containers with soil, stones, cotton, wet towels, air from hand fans, and
water mist with lavender. Because many people drink coffee, and because of its
cultural importance in Puerto Rico, we included coffee in one of the containers.
Many participants commented that they had mental images of their childhood, like
memories of their grandmother preparing coffee. Others mentioned that in the aftermath of the hurricane they drank coffee, while others missed drinking recently
brewed, hot coffee. In addition, as many homes were flooded, participants commented that the tactile stimuli of the wet towels brought back the sensation of
squeezing wet towels during the hurricane.

To retrieve an emotive memory, utilizing a visualization exercise, participants
were invited to breathe deeply and take a journey through their individual memories
of the day Hurricane María hit Puerto Rico. The facilitator guided the experience
with specific questions that emphasized the sense of sight in connection to their
emotions. For example: What clothes were you wearing that day? What were you
doing? Where exactly were you? Did you feel safe? Who accompanied you? Did

you see where the winds or the water came from? At the end of the last question, musical instruments created a symbolic representation of the hurricane. In a subtle way, we used the *kalimba* instrument (*mbira*) to evoke the first drops of water, then wind chimes were introduced, followed by a rain stick to create the atmosphere of rain, the sound of a hand drum, and tree branches. Lastly, we introduced the sound of sheet metal and pieces of wood striking the ground. They represented the materials used to build many of the homes and structures of the island. The drum intensified the beats, raising the rhythm to a climax in unison, the metal sheet and the wood complementing it. Slowly, the intensity of the instruments decreased until culminating with the subtle sound of the *kalimba*, simulating the last drops of rain (Fig. 6.2). The facilitator asked the participants to retrieve a specific memory and emotion that was evoked during the exercise. They were then asked to observe the experience

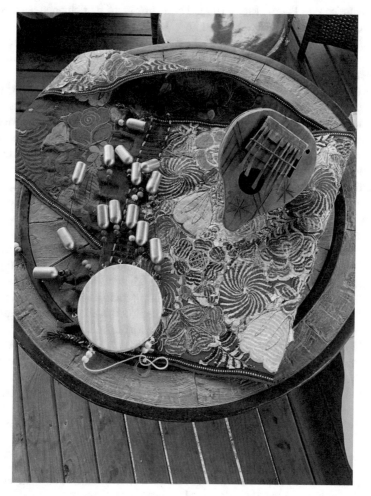

Fig. 6.2 Use of sound to evoke emotive memories

from a distance until they reached the present moment. The facilitator encouraged them to share their experiences in the company of other people and reminded them that they were in a safe place.

The expression phase represents the climactic moment of the *Encuentro*, creating a space for creative expression as a prelude to sharing the experiences. We presented two options. The first was to draw, on paper, the image that most impacted them during the hurricane experience, using two colors that could represent the meaning of this experience. The second option was to choose an object that we had placed on a table related to the experience. On the table we had water bottles, canned food, candles, lanterns, pieces of wood, tree branches, sheet metal, wet towels, a suitcase, and a machete.[1] These objects were commonly used by many when there was no electricity, access to running water, or access to fresh food. The suitcase was placed because of the thousands of people who had emigrated to the United States (Instituto de Estadísticas de Puerto Rico 2017). The majority of participants selected both options, and after they had completed both, we invited them to join a circle so that they could tell their stories. Some of the participants began expressing their emotions, such as desperation, a sense of uncertainty, pain, sadness, and fear, among others.

We observed that during the exercise, empathy was developed and expressed. For example, when participants became overwhelmed with emotion, others offered their support by reaching out their hands or embracing them with a hug. Most participants expressed not knowing how much the hurricane had affected them until the moment they shared their experiences in the circle. Others stated—often in a choked-up voice—that it was in that very moment in the circle that they had heard the stories of their co-workers for the first time, as well as their difficulties, frustrations, and fears that they were still going through. Witnessing and being emotionally present in the story are important to processing the traumatic experience (Silva-Martínez 2018).

The fourth phase—kinesthetic dynamic—proposes returning from emotion to the body through movement. In the exercise titled *Inquilinx* (the tenant), two participants held hands simulating the walls of a home. These two participants represented the right and left walls and in the center, a third participant represented the tenant. One of us facilitated by calling out the right wall, left wall, or tenant. Those who represented the right wall exchanged positions with the others who also represented the right wall in a different home. As they moved through the space, we asked them to use their bodies by moving or even dancing to act out being pushed by the wind. When the facilitator called out the word "hurricane," all participants let go of each other and moved or danced through the space while they created a new formation. The results of the experience were new residences with three walls, single tenants, homes with more than one tenant, or empty houses. In the final part of the exercise,

---

[1] A metal, bladed tool—comparable to a small sword—used by *jíbaros* (Puerto Ricans from the countryside) who work in agriculture. It is quite symbolic of said *jíbaros*, and after the hurricane it was used to cut branches, chop fallen trees, and clear out leftover brush.

we asked participants to remain where they were and look around. We reflected on the new homes and linked them to our experiences after the hurricane. The purpose of the exercise was to understand, from the body, the reconfiguration that we as a country were experiencing: a new landscape, a new social design, a new opportunity to reconfigure our present and future. In all groups, this exercise generated laughter and excitement. Literature related to this topic confirms a positive influence of dance movement therapy (DMT) on the decreasing of trauma-related symptoms (Martinec 2018). These results are explained by the assumption that the use of DMT enhances resilience by including the body in therapeutic process, supports a state of pleasure and satisfaction, mitigates a neurochemical arousal of distress, and finds movement and body-based modalities that are pleasant and acceptable (Martinec 2018).

For the fifth phase, we introduced a discussion on *la brega* (the daily struggle), in which we talked about life after the hurricane and pursued hope as the tenet of the exercises and reflections. First, participants were instructed to use their bodies to give three hugs: a hug to oneself, a hug from heart to heart, and a final hug that involved the whole group in a collective embrace. As we formed a big circle, we told them that in this exercise, everyone would also have an opportunity to fly, which naturally made them doubtful. As we all embraced each other, one of us explained that "flying" consisted of a person holding on to people on each side who would come close enough to have the strength to lift that person up. In this phase of the *Encuentro*, participants being able to suspend themselves in the air one by one while being supported by the shoulders of their co-participants introduced the topic of relying on the power of coming together, despite differences and even tensions among each other.

The purpose of the exercises was to transfer the experience to the body and somatically experience concepts such as affection and support. It encouraged feeling love and provided a concrete experience that participants could remember regarding a support network that sustained them. They were invited to reflect on the feeling of uncertainty after the natural disaster and the need to make a great leap of faith into the new, with the confidence of belonging to a group that supports them. The exercise culminated with giving someone in the group a heart-shaped cushion and sharing words of love and hope with that person (Fig. 6.3). The heart serves as a universal symbol of love and indispensable value to face new realities. This final action helped to exercise gratitude and recognize the importance of humanity in the processes of recovery and resilience. During the exercises, many expressed feeling happy and hopeful in having the emotional tools to build a new destiny.

As we were working with primary and secondary traumatic experiences after the hurricane hit, we emphasized the importance of taking care of the self individually as well as collectively. In order to attend to this, we proposed the game "galactic guardian." This game required each participant to anonymously exchange a piece of paper with the name of a co-worker written on it. Their task was to take care of their co-worker for two weeks. Follow-up was an essential component of this exercise; thus, a month after the workshop, we called participants at the different

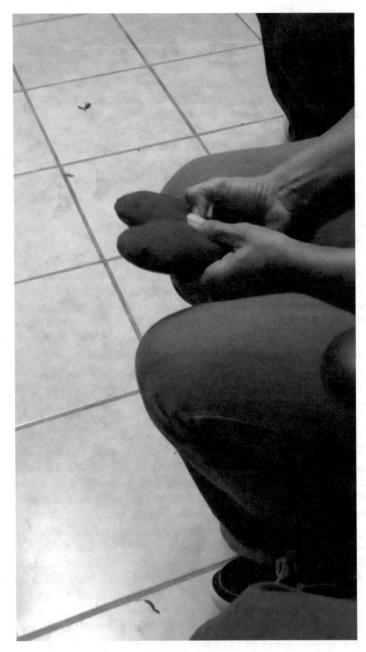

Fig. 6.3 Self-care and collective care through the imagery of love

organizations to share how they took care of each other and what it meant for them to engage in this exercise. Accompaniment throughout the process helped the participants to commit to taking care of each other within the organizational context.

6.5   Encuentro CuidarNOS from the Inside: Experiences of Participants

At every *Encuentro,* we engaged in a debriefing and evaluation at the end of the session. In addition, the participants submitted a written evaluation of their experience. We found that all the participants recognized the importance of setting time aside to process their experiences after the hurricane. In several groups, the participants asked us to return so that other colleagues and partners could be part of the *Encuentro.* The following testimonies illustrate the meaning of the experience for participants:

"Participating in Encuentro CuidarNOS gave a space to breathe and unwind at times when it had been difficult to get it out, and maybe I had not allowed that space. Sometimes, trying to follow the hectic pace of everyday life, it becomes difficult for us to take a space to disconnect, recognize ourselves and allow ourselves to feel and let go. Having this space through CuidarNOS was wonderful with an incredible healing power."

"My experience with CuidarNos was very good, because it was the first time I could open up as I did that day. To be able to have that space and see the perspective from the point of view of my colleagues and how they were impacted my story. After this experience, my colleagues get along very well, we have good chemistry and we can feel confident expressing our feelings… One recommendation is that spaces like these continue to be held. After the hurricane, the statistics of violence and suicide have increased and now any wind that passes by, everyone is waiting. There are still people who have not overcome Hurricane María."

"CuidarNOS was magical, magical in the sense that I could completely transport myself to that day…it has a very substantial part, integrating the arts, sounds, textures. Rather than express it verbally, choosing colors to reflect the feelings and memories of that moment, it was magical. This space was extremely important."

"CuidarNOS was very important and significant, because after Hurricanes Irma and María, it was powerful to take time, a space for us and not devote all our energy, our effort and thought to the community and to other people. It was really the first time we were able to come together for ourselves, between us, embrace each other and listen to our feelings…to listen and to say the things that most impacted us, and those that we would like to see in our work from our perspectives."

"As an artist I like to experiment with the symbol and meaning of things, how objects, sayings or everyday things you can do can transform the meaning of things. When going through the process of CuidarNos, it takes me back to the postulate that I go first, and if I am living and integrating self-care, then I am the living example before other people, as an artist and as an educator community. If you are safe, taken care of and in health, is going to guarantee that this will multiply in the community."

Despite the differences among groups, for many the *Encuentro* meant a valuable opportunity to address the experience of working with others' trauma related to the hurricane as well as to violence, while they dealt with their own experiences of loss. Our analysis of the process leads us to reiterate the need for continued reflection on interventions with service providers, community leaders, and partners using art toward healing and strength.

6.6   Reflections

CuidarNos uses art and movement to enhance services providers' skills in managing the symptoms of trauma and to exercise more control over their own health and environment. The *Encuentro* was a space to connect and collectively process experiences that, as observed in the previous narratives, had not been shared in depth prior to participation. This provided the opportunity to strengthen the relationships at both organizational and personal levels. It also helped to establish grounds for caring at both the individual and collective levels. Self-care was an important element in closing the *Encuentro* experience. Bringing individual self-care to the conversation was as important as discussing collective caring as a tool for humanizing professional interventions, community building, and volunteer work.

At the organizational level, it was important to invite administrators and supervisors to be co-participants with staff. Even though we understood the complexities around bringing them together, especially in cases where they could be facing tensions or conflict, we decided to ask everyone at the organization to attend. The introduction of what the *Encuentro* was about helped in bringing us a bit closer to leveling power imbalances. We were emphatic in the role of the participants, especially in clearly stating the need to trust the process and feel free to engage (or not) in the exercises. At one of the organizations, a staff member preferred not to participate; other than this, we did not encounter opposition or resistance to participate. However, in a couple of cases, it took time for some of the participants to ease into expressing their experiences. At other organizations, staff were unexpectedly upfront regarding tensions with other colleagues.

Each of the organizations that we worked with presented very particular characteristics. The location of the organization and the number of staff and volunteers were one of the major differences in terms of the groups. CPM did its best in making sure that most of its partners had the opportunity to experience the *Encuentro*. A few of the organizations had fewer staff members, so these participants would join others from a sister organization. This changed the dynamic a little, especially in the last part of the *Encuentro*. These cases required a reconfiguration of the exercises, by dividing the group.

The experience of bringing to life the *Encuentro* in partnership with others shows that even with seemingly endless obstacles in recovering, we are reconfiguring the disaster as an opportunity to see ourselves as capable of moving forward collectively. It has allowed us to enable conversations that, although painful, must take place in order to recognize the need for our individual and collective humanity to move toward the development of citizenship and alternative social movements. Today we find fertile ground to join and come closer to healing and transformation.

6.7 Discussion and Conclusion

The experience engaging in a disaster context is multidimensional over time and space. It has been suggested that long-term support is necessary, and that alternative expressions collected over time are useful for disaster awareness and risk reduction education (Alexander 2018). Also, the recovery from trauma may be a shared, community-wide endeavor geared toward individuals, families, and communities receiving services, as well as service providers and supervisors alike (Adamson 2018). In retrospect of the context in which Hurricane María took place—a profound economic crisis, inequality, and violence against women (a serious issue in Puerto Rico)—we needed to address those concerns in the *Encuentro*, as they were pressing issues in the work of the service providers, community leaders, and partners. It is imperative to discuss the social aspect of disasters, and how interventions using art can be very powerful in making such discussions happen. In addressing trauma and healing through a social justice art therapy framework, Karcher (2017) explains the importance of acknowledging that structural, multidimensional factors are interconnected, and that wellness and healing depend on working together to envision transformation and collective healing.

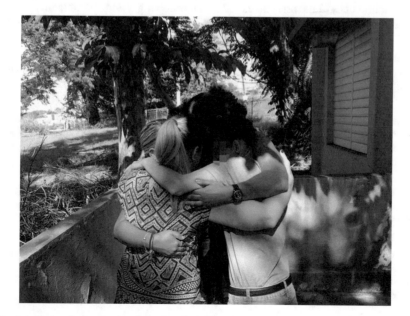

Fig. 6.4 Embracing each other through safe spaces

The *Encuentro CuidarNos* represents an important step in providing a safe space to service providers, partners, and community leaders experiencing physical, emotional, and cognitive changes as a result of primary or secondary traumatic stress in the context of a disaster (Fig. 6.4). This space was built from a feminist perspective and took into consideration the diversity in the narrative and background of each person. Also, the *Encuentro CuidarNos* incorporated intervention to address the combination of primary and vicarious trauma and support psychological health and safety within the context of a natural disaster. As evidenced by Atkins and Burnett (2016) when they examined the relationship between engaging in disaster behavioral health training and interventions in trauma, indeed, individual and collective interventions may help to increase resiliency and reduce burnout among disaster behavioral health providers.

Nevertheless, beyond efforts to develop strategies to manage personal trauma caused by a disaster, organizational initiatives to work with vicarious trauma, and efforts to promote the well-being of communities, permanent organizational efforts are required to address the integral health of the victims. Attention from the state for the development of public and fiscal policies that support the promotion of health from a comprehensive standpoint—including the development of protocols to manage the increase in gender violence after the occurrence of natural phenomena and the granting of adequate funds for organizations that work with this population—is equally necessary.

We discovered that summoning service providers to the *Encuentro* instead of to a traditional training placed the focus of attention on themselves and, as a result, opened a space to become vulnerable, identify emotions, and rely on somatic experiences. This *Encuentro* reaffirmed our belief that processing trauma by integrating different branches of the arts can expedite the following among participants: access to their memories, diverse language to express themselves and identify their emotions, and an overall state of well-being (see also Chap. 21, this volume). Hurricane María awoke our sense of vulnerability. It reminded us that life is ephemeral, that all we truly have is each other, and that we are part of a new social fabric—consolidated into solidarity and both individual and collective well-being.

Acknowledgements This project would not have been possible without the ongoing support of Coordinadora Paz para la Mujer (CPM)—The Puerto Rican Coalition against Domestic Violence and Sexual Assault. To learn more about CPM and their wonderful work, visit www.pazparalamujer.org.

References

Adamson, C. (2018). Trauma-informed supervision in the disaster context. *The Clinical Supervisor, 37*(1), 221–240.

Ahmed, S. H., & Siddiqi, M. N. (2006). Essay: Healing through art therapy in disaster settings. *The Lancet, 368*, S28–S29.

Alexander, R. (2018). Drawing disaster: Reflecting on six years of the Popoki Friendship Story project. *Journal of International Cooperation Studies, 25*(2), 69–96.

American Art Therapy Association. (2017). *About art therapy.* https://arttherapy.org/about-art-therapy/. Accessed 10 Oct 2018.

Atkins, C. D., & Burnett, H. J., Jr. (2016). Specialized disaster behavioral health training: Its connection with response, practice, trauma health, and resilience. *Disaster Health, 3*(2), 57–65.

Bradshaw, S., & Fordham, M. (2015). Double disaster: Disaster through a gender lens. In *Hazards, risks and disasters in society* (pp. 233–251). Oxford: Elsevier.

Bride, B. E. (2011). Collateral damage: The impact of caring for persons who have experienced trauma. (Video). Presentation for the Buffalo Center for Social Research Distinguished Scholar Series, Buffalo, NY. http://www.socialwork.buffalo.edu/resources/product.asp?id=21. Accessed 28 Sept 2018.

Bronfenbrenner, V. (1979). *The ecology of human development: Experiments by nature and design.* Cambridge, MA: Harvard University Press.

Buck, L., & Axel, R. (1991). A novel multigene family may encode odorant receptors: A molecular basis for odor recognition. *Cell, 65*, 175–187.

Cox, K., & Steiner, S. (2013). Workplace wellness. In *Self-care in social work: A guide for practitioners, supervisors and administrators* (pp. 137–158). NASW Press.

Cutter, S. L. (2017). The forgotten casualties redux: Women, children, and disaster risk. *Global Environmental Change, 42*, 117–121.

Delgado, J. A. (2018, September 23). Nearly 200,000 emigrated after María. *El Nuevo Día.* https://www.elnuevodia.com/english/english/nota/nearly200000emigratedaftermaria-2. Accessed 25 Sept 2018.

Fisher, S. (2010). Violence against women and natural disasters: Findings from posttsunami Sri Lanka. *Violence Against Women, 16*(8), 902–918.

Heise L., Pitanguy H., & Germain A. (1994). Violence against women: The hidden health burden. World Bank discussion papers 255.

Huss, E., Kaufman, R., Avgar, A., & Shuker, E. (2016). Arts as a vehicle for community building and post-disaster development. *Disasters, 40*(2), 284–303.

Instituto de Estadísticas de Puerto Rico. (2016). Informe Sobre Desarrollo Humano Puerto Rico. Available at https://www.estadisticas.pr/files/Publicaciones/INFORME_DESARROLLO_HUMANO_PUERTO_RICO_1.pdf. Accessed 8 Oct 2018.

Instituto de Estadísticas de Puerto Rico. (2017). *97 mil personas emigraron a estados unidos en el 2017* [Press release]. https://estadisticas.pr/files/Comunicados/CP_9_13_2018_SDC_1_year_ACS_PRCS_2017.pdf. Accessed 8 Oct 2018.

Jackson, S. F., Fazal, N., Gravel, G., & Papowitz, H. (2016). Evidence for the value of health promotion interventions in natural disaster management. *Health Promotion International, 32*(6), 1057–1066. https://doi.org/10.1093/heapro/daw029.

Juran, L., & Trivedi, J. (2015). Women, gender norms, and natural disasters in Bangladesh. *Geographical Review, 105*(4), 601–611.

Karcher, O. P. (2017). Sociopolitical oppression, trauma, and healing: Moving toward a social justice art therapy framework. *Art Therapy, 34*(3), 123–128.

Kishore, N., Marqués, D., Mahmud, A., Kiang, M. V., Rodriguez, I., Fuller, A., et al. (2018). Mortality in Puerto Rico after Hurricane María. *New England Journal of Medicine, 379*, 162–177.

Martinec, R. (2018). Dance movement therapy in the wider concept of trauma rehabilitation. *Journal of Trauma and Rehabilitation, 1*, 1. Retrieved from https://www.scitechnol.com/peer-review/dance-movement-therapy-in-the-wider-concept-of-trauma-rehabilitation-gmCh.php?article_id=7765.

Naturale, A. (2015). How do we understand disaster-related vicarious trauma, secondary traumatic stress, and compassion fatigue? In G. Quitangon & M. Evces (Eds.), *Vicarious trauma and disaster mental health: Understanding risks and promoting resilience* (pp. 93–110). New York: Routledge.

Neumayer, E., & Plümper, T. (2007). The gendered nature of natural disasters: The impact of catastrophic events on the gender gap in life expectancy, 1981–2002. *Annals of the Association of American Geographers, 97*(3), 551–566.

Olivares, E. y Incháustegui, T. (2011). Modelo ecológico para una vida libre de violencia de género. Comisión Nacional para Prevenir y Erradicar la Violencia contra las Mujeres: México D.F., pp. 21–24. Accessed: http://www.conavim.gob.mx/work/models/CONAVIM/Resource/309/1/images/MoDecoFinalPDF.pdf.

Palm, K. M., Polusny, M. A., & Follette, V. M. (2004). Vicarious traumatization: Potential hazards and interventions for disaster and trauma workers. *Prehospital and Disaster Medicine, 19*(1), 73–78.

Park, E.-K., & Duarte, H. (2011). Epidemiología de desastres naturales. *Revista Tempus Actas de Saúde Coletiva*, 11–18.

Robles, F., Ferré-Sadurní, L., Fausset, R., & Rivera, I. (2017, December 31). Enduring a day of misery in Puerto Rico's ruins. *The New York Times*, p. 16 (originally published October 1, 2017).

Rodríguez-Díaz, C. E. (2018). María in Puerto Rico: Natural disaster in a colonial archipelago. *American Journal of Public Health, 108*(1), 30–32.

Silva-Martínez, E. (2018). *Violencia de género desde un enfoque centrado en trauma* (pp. 7–13). Material educativo elaborado para Coordinadora Paz para la Mujer.

True, J. (2016). Gendered violence in natural disasters: Learning from New Orleans, Haiti and Christchurch. *Aotearoa New Zealand Social Work, 25*(2), 78–89.

United Nations Office for Disaster Risk Reduction (UNISDR). (2009). Terminology. https://www.unisdr.org/we/inform/terminology. Accessed 12 Oct 2018.

Wahl-Alexander, Z. (2017). Promoting emotional recovery following natural disasters through integrative art and physical activity programs. Online Harvard Health Policy Review. Available at http://www.hhpronline.org/articles/2017/10/8/promoting-emotional-recovery-following-natural-disasters-through-integrative-art-and-physical-activity-programs. Accessed 15 Oct 2018.

World Health Organization. (1986). *The Ottawa Charter for Health Promotion*. http://www.euro.who.int/__data/assets/pdf_file/0004/129532/Ottawa_Charter.pdf. Accessed 12 Oct 2018.

Chapter 7
Community Theater for Health Promotion in Japan

Hikari Sandhu, Naoki Hirose, Kazuya Yui, and Masamine Jimba

7.1 Introduction

Health is a resource for everyday life and not the objective of living, states the Ottawa Charter (WHO 1986). Health is a precious resource, and it can advance our well-being. We all have a right to look after our health and well-being, and one potential way to attain that well-being is through art. We are aware of the positive impact of the arts on our being since ancient times and have been using art to support our everyday life (Stuckey and Nobel 2010). Every art medium functions to help us grow, heal, think, and self-actualize (Michalos 2005). This quality of art links to the ultimate goal of health promotion: well-being.

The implementation of arts interventions in the field of health varies from country to country. In the United States, the National Organization of Arts in Health (NOAH) white paper (2017) describes a variety of arts interventions in the health sector, providing examples in five fields: health care facilities, clinical services, caring for caregivers, health science education, and community health and well-being. The various interventions include utilizing arts as therapy, implementing arts for medical education, and promoting arts for health education within community settings (see also Chap. 1). According to White (2009a), policy in the United Kingdom

H. Sandhu (✉) · M. Jimba
Department of Community and Global Health, Graduate School of Medicine,
The University of Tokyo, Tokyo, Japan
e-mail: sandhu@iis.u-tokyo.ac.jp; mjimba@m.u-tokyo.ac.jp

N. Hirose
Global Health Nursing, Graduate School of Biomedical and Health Sciences,
Hiroshima University, Hiroshima, Japan
e-mail: naoki-hirose@hiroshima-u.ac.jp

K. Yui
Department of Community Medicine, Saku Central Hospital, Saku, Nagano, Japan
e-mail: yui@koumi-hp.jp

© The Author(s) 2021
J. H. Corbin et al. (eds.), *Arts and Health Promotion*,
https://doi.org/10.1007/978-3-030-56417-9_7

integrates arts activities with community health to encourage people in the community to engage with health issues. White also introduces the cases of Australia and South Africa in his book, where he describes several examples of how arts-based interventions are used to address community challenges (White 2009b).

As for the impact of arts interventions on our health, one example is the use of art as a tool to promote healthy behavior and lifestyles. For instance, Frishkopf et al. (2016) implemented dancing to promote the importance of sanitization for preventing infectious diseases such as malaria and cholera in Ghana. Another example is where art is used not as a tool but as therapeutic media. Davies et al. (2016) shows the effect of recreational arts interventions on mental well-being in the general population in Australia. These examples show the breadth of art forms and the health fields in which they have been used, encompassing the arts as tools for health promotion, media for therapeutic intervention, and activities for social inclusion (Hamilton et al. 2003).

Arts-based interventions are practiced in settings from a range of different cultural backgrounds. As an example from Asia, Nomura Research Institute& Agency for Cultural Affairs (2015) published a report highlighting the current application of the arts in community settings. The report introduces 63 arts-related programs that aim to tackle social issues in the fields of economics, community environments, education, human rights, and health care. While arts-related programs are being increasingly implemented in community environments to boost economies in low-income communities, eight of the 63 arts-based interventions are being implemented in health care-related fields. These programs were organized to support child victims of natural disasters and pre-dementia members in communities. Not all reports are scientifically evaluated; yet this report does show a level of awareness of the benefit of arts-based intervention in Japan. Other examples exist of how theater has been popular in efforts toward stroke prevention and health education for diabetes patients in hospital settings (Suzuki et al. 2010). Theater workshops have proved effective for medical communication education in general (Ren 2015).

These recent developments build on a long history of such approaches in Japan, although no research reports are available on the earliest arts-based interventions. One grassroots movement that merits attention involved the implementation of arts-based interventions at Saku General Hospital in Nagano prefecture after World War II. Since 1945, the importance of health has been promoted within this farming community by means of live drama performances (Wakatsuki 1971). In 1945, economic events had undermined the importance of health care in the eyes of members of the local farming community. However, participating in health promotion drama events led the farmers to recognize that good health was a vital resource for their well-being and for the activities of their community. Theater-based health promotion provides an opportunity to build empathy and equalize social relations. Because it is audience-centered and engages audiences within the theater work, it also changes people's behavior (Massar et al. 2018). This impact leads to social inclusion in the community (Woodson et al. 2017). Notably, the community learned that the goal was not only to be healthy, but to use that state of health and well-being to live fulfilling lives (Nishirai 1983).

This chapter aims to highlight how theater-based health promotion encouraged medical and health practitioners in resource-limited, rural Japan after World War II, and how works of theater positively transformed community members' mindsets for health promotion.

7.2 The History of Japanese Society and Community Arts

7.2.1 Japanese Community Theater Stages: Eighteenth Century–1920s

In the eighteenth century, before capitalism became mainstream in Japanese society, arts and cultural activities were integrated into daily living and labor within communities. Art was a central aspect of human life. Kabuki (traditional Japanese drama) and Ningyou-jyoruri (puppet plays) developed in the communities around temples or shrines. In the 1800s toward the end of the Edo era, the role of theaters was not only to stage Kabuki or puppet dramas, but also to create a community platform for farmers' businesses. Therefore, the location and function as a community gathering space were important attributes of the stages. Nagano prefecture was particularly attractive, as it is conveniently located in the central part of Japan where many community actors visited and stayed. As a result of these factors, Nagano prefecture had one of the highest numbers of community theater stages in Japan. In the late 1800s, community theater stages in Nagano prefecture changed their role from generating social capital within the community to serving as a stage for dramas. Yet, the dramatic arts remained a community resource and was important into the 1920s to mitigate against the influence of capitalism and provide a voice to farmers.

7.2.2 Taisho Democracy

> Without happiness in society, happiness cannot be ours.
> (Miyazawa 1957, p. 10, translated by the author)

In the 1920s—the Taisho era in Japan— Japanese society was trying to promote democratic rights among its citizens. This movement was triggered by historical events that led to countries using colonialism as a way of showing strength on the international stage. In the West, the United Kingdom had been colonizing and making alliances across the world, and the Ottoman Empire controlled the Middle East; Japan had a chance to join this powerful group of countries by winning the Russo-Japanese War (1904–1905). The victory enabled Japan to stand shoulder to shoulder with the West and led to the formation of alliances with the United Kingdom, the Ottoman Empire, France, and other Western countries (Funabashi 1992).

However, after World War I, many countries, including Japan, experienced hardship due to inflation. The resulting poverty led to the formation of labor unions to protest against political injustice and high unemployment and to stand up for the human rights of citizens. The United Kingdom and other Western countries saw the number of labor strikes increase day by day. In reaction to the carnage of World War I, internationally renowned philosophers and scholars, such as Henri Barubusse and Leo Tolstoy, led the spread of peace movements all over the world. During this period, "proletarianism" became a powerful social movement that encouraged farmers and laborers to unite to change society (Konishi 2015). Within this historical context, in 1920, Japan saw the birth of a major democratic movement, which historians refer to as "Taisho democracy." As part of this movement, Japanese scholars wrote and proliferated philosophy that pitted a cultural movement against the modern civilization that Western counterparts supported (Ito 2003).

The world of the arts followed the same trend during this period. Many scholars considered the arts to be monopolized by the elite classes in society during the rise of capitalism in the early 1900s, and this bred antipathy among proletarian scholars. To counter capitalism, proletarian scholars initiated movements through works of literature to bring the arts back to farmers and laborers. In Japan, scholars followed the book by Romain Rolland, *"Le théâtre du peuple"*, where he focuses on "farmer's arts" to restore the arts (Moriyama 1963). The book was translated into Japanese and had a huge influence on Japanese writers, including Kenji Miyazawa.

7.2.3   Kenji Miyazawa and Farmer's Arts

Kenji Miyazawa (Fig. 7.1) is one of the most famous writers in Japan. Although he only published two books in his lifetime and died when he was 37 years old, he has a legacy of literary work, most of which was edited posthumously. Representative works include *"Gauche de Cellist"* (Miyazawa 1994) and *"Night of the Milky Way Railway"* (Miyazawa 1991).

Miyazawa was born in 1869 in Hananomaki, Iwate prefecture in Japan. He was raised by a pawnbroker father and a Buddhist mother, and although agriculture was the main occupation in his community and most of the community's farmers were impoverished, Miyazawa lived affluently. As he grew up, he struggled with the gap between his living standards and those of the other members of his community. In 1921, at the age of 25, Miyazawa was assigned as a teacher to a farmer's school in Hananomaki. He taught not only agriculture but also literature, philosophy, science, and the arts. In 1922, amidst an agricultural recession as the Taisho democracy was just gaining momentum, farmers in his community raised their voices against sharecropping. Miyazawa was influenced by this proletarian movement and by the agricultural recession.

Miyazawa empowered community farmers to liberate themselves from capitalism. In his work *"Nougyou-geijyutsu"* supposedly written in 1929, he argued that the arts were an integral part of all community activities related to religion, science,

Fig. 7.1 Kenji Miyazawa
(Rinpoo Inc. n.d.)

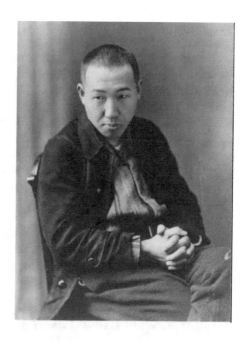

and agriculture, and he emphasized art as the one and only medium that can express a farmer's life ("Farmer's Arts", Miyazawa 1957). This was Miyazawa's approach to community building. Accordingly, when teaching one of his pupils, Jinjiro Matsuda, how to build a truthful farmer's community, he told him: "I have these words for you, be a peasant, do farmer's drama" (Matsuda, as cited by Aikawa 2003, p. 3–5, translated by the author).

Miyazawa foresaw the consequence of the proletarian movement, envisaging the spread of better education, entertainment for farmers, and women's liberation. With this vision in mind, he encouraged Matsuda to build farmer-centered community theater in line with his philosophy of "Farmer's Arts." Matsuda pursued Miyazawa's concept by forming youth circles to improve farmers' lifestyles in Yamagata prefecture, Japan.

7.3 Health Care in Japanese Farming Communities and Saku General Hospital

7.3.1 Health in Japan 1910–1940

In the early 1900s, the health of Japanese farmers depended on their financial status. This was caused by the adverse effects of the worldwide depression, from which the agricultural sector suffered the most. Consequently, the livelihoods of most farmers were damaged or destroyed. Financial stability was a priority over the farmer's health.

The resulting neglect of personal health led to a wide range of issues among Japanese farming communities, including an overall high mortality rate, a high infant mortality rate, and a high rate of tuberculosis (Aoki 2008; Ministry of Health, Labor and Welfare 2014). Despite the farming communities' desperate health care needs, it was difficult for farmers to seek medical care because universal health coverage was not fully operational in those days. The Japanese government had already introduced the idea of universal health coverage, but its coverage did not depend on household income but rather on an individual's occupation. Those who were in charge of managing peasants had to pay 14% of their health care costs from their own pockets; in comparison, the peasants themselves had to pay 22% of their health care costs. Therefore, universal health coverage was financially out of reach for the majority of farmers, who rarely visited medical facilities as a result. Ironically, only when a member of a farming family had died did relatives go to doctors to ask for a death certificate (Fujii 1999a, Fujii1999b).

7.3.2 Health in Usuda Village

In Nagano prefecture, the resources available to agricultural communities were better than those in urban areas, yet the number of health care facilities was still limited. Farmers did not take an interest in their health, a situation that was caused not only by the financial burden of their medical treatment, but was also exacerbated by the history of farmers neglecting their own health since World War I (Fujii 1999a, Fujii1999b). To improve the health of the farming community, farmers needed to improve their health literacy as well as have the opportunity to seek medical attention without incurring overwhelming financial burdens.

Take Usuda village, for example, which was located in South-Saku county, east-central Nagano prefecture. Agriculture was the largest industry—the community consisted mostly of farmers. According to the national survey published in 1940, South-Saku county had 23 physicians and 15 dentists out of 781,111 people (Fujii 1999a). In the case of Usuda village, there were very few general practitioners, and no surgeons were available at any of the medical facilities. If farmers were in need of surgery, they had to go to general hospitals outside of the village and risked having to spend more than half their annual income for the whole household on the visit.

7.3.3 Saku Hospital and Dr. Toshikazu Wakatsuki

In 1943, Usuda village built a general hospital named "Saku Hospital." It was the first hospital in the area with proper medical facilities. The hospital was needed to improve the health of people living in the village, but was also part of a national program to produce healthy soldiers. While the Japanese government may have had military motivations, ultimately Saku Hospital had a mission to improve the health of farmers in the community.

In 1945, a year and a half after being established, Saku Hospital welcomed a surgeon from Tokyo named Dr. Toshikazu Wakatsuki (Fig. 7.2). Before his arrival, the hospital had not taken on any patients for hospitalization, serving only outpatients. This medical treatment structure reflected the gap in the medical services available at the hospital as well as the limited awareness of medicine within the community. Wakatsuki decided to dedicate his work to not only providing modern medicine but also to expanding the functions of the hospital and improving health literacy among farmers.

Under his leadership, Saku Hospital carried out many surgical operations—including breast cancer treatments—and started to accept in-patients for hospitalization. Furthermore, Wakatsuki (1971) encouraged the families of patients to observe surgical operations to improve the transparency of the hospital and its medical care. These new approaches led to greater trust between the community and the hospital.

Fig. 7.2 Home visits by Wakatsuki (Saku General Hospital n.d.)

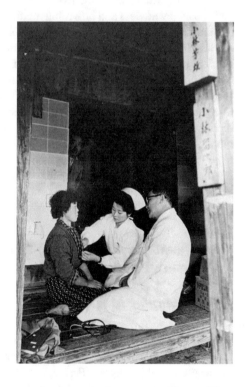

7.3.4   Health Promotion for Saving Lives

In 1957, while Saku Hospital was improving its health services to the rural population, the Japanese government was trying to achieve universal health coverage and
established a new payment system for such coverage. With the new system, patients
were asked to pay at medical hospitals/clinics immediately after their medical treatments. Before the new system had been introduced, all farmers' medical expenses
were paid upfront by a town hall and farmers paid it back to the town hall later on,
so that farmers could defer payments until they had the finances to cover it. However,
with the new payment system, the mayor of Yachiho village (one of the villages
served by Saku Hospital) and staff at Saku Hospital shared concerns that farmers
would be demotivated from going to the hospital due to the expected financial
burdens.

   Initially, the village decided not to follow the new system; however, their anti-
government action lasted no more than a year before the mayor of Yachiho village
and the people running Saku Hospital had to change their approach. If the community members they served were too poor to pay medical fees, the best solution might
be to avoid getting sick in the first place. They created two strategies: raising people's health awareness and providing medical checkups for villagers. To raise health
awareness, a theater group from Saku Hospital implemented health promotion more
actively in pieces of community theater and film. The second strategy of providing
medical checkups was initially not welcomed by villagers, since they had no real
concept of disease prevention, so the hospital provided medical education sessions
and distributed a medical handbook to each villager. The villagers were accustomed
to maintaining good health in their livestock by giving them vaccinations and
recording health checks in notebooks. For them, livestock was almost equivalent to
money, and they needed a stock of money to survive. However, they had never used
these notebooks for themselves or their families. To guide the villagers in prioritizing their health and to encourage them to use a notebook for their own health, it was
necessary to raise awareness and promote changes in behavior.

7.4   Wakatsuki's Strategy of Theater-Based Health Promotion

7.4.1   Planning Medical Drama

Wakatsuki's strategy to make use of medical drama began to develop when Saku
Hospital was invited to perform at a festival in Usuda village in 1946. Inspired by
Miyazawa's philosophy of "Farmer's Arts," Wakatsuki took this as an opportunity
to bond with local community members and to provide drama as a means of promoting health education.

In those days, the main problems in the Saku community were misunderstandings about medical care and a low awareness of the importance of healthy living. Wakatsuki was concerned by the extremely low health literacy within the community, and he realized that the existence of Saku Hospital by itself did not provide good community health care. Through pieces of drama conveying health care messages, Wakatsuki and Saku Hospital became health promoters in the community to improve access to and utilization of health care services. The goals of their medical drama pieces were set as: (1) promoting a better understanding of medical care, and (2) initiating community building through medical drama.

7.4.2 Scripts Using Jargon and Everyday Words with Local Dialogue

In 1950, the unadjusted primary school enrollment rate was 61% in Japan (Sumi 2014), and Japanese people in general were able to read and write everyday words. This held true for people living in Nagano prefecture. However, medical terminologies were difficult to understand for villagers. To improve their understanding of the role of medicine, every drama script was carefully written to mix jargon with everyday vocabulary from the region. During their visits to clinics, physicians from the Tokyo area had difficulty understanding the local dialect of the Saku community. Understanding the local dialect was critical to connect medical staff from outside of Saku with the local community, so Wakatsuki included local dialect as the key component to bridge Saku Hospital staff with the Saku community.

7.4.3 The Wider Impact of Theater-Based Interventions

Dramatic work is globally recognized as having the potential to motivate social change. During the Taisho democracy, many theater practitioners had also worked on theater-related practices like that of Kenji Miyazawa. Bertolt Brecht (1898–1956) was the one of them. A theater practitioner and theorist born in Germany in 1898, Brecht's concepts saw theater as a practice that "reveals truths, exposes contradictions, and proposes transformations" (Boal 1985). His plays contained messages of politics and social norms, and he imbued his characters with authenticity. By doing so, he encouraged audiences to think and to be critical of the messages actors conveyed in order to change audiences' mindsets and bring political changes (Gordon 2017).

Brecht's work also sowed the seeds for the work of Augusto Boal (1931–2009), who developed the "Theater of the Oppressed." Boal was a Brazilian theater practitioner who used theater to empower peasants who were oppressed by society. Theater of the Oppressed encouraged audiences to participate in theater, making

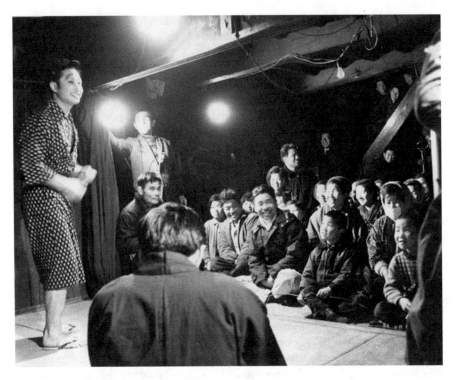

Fig. 7.3 Theater work "Haraita" (Saku General Hospital 1953)

them reactors to the drama rather than just observers. The emphasis of his work was on active participation, in that he encouraged participants to utilize their bodies on the stage (Fig. 7.3). Based on this philosophy and strategy, Boal implemented his own theater work in community settings, which led to various social movements (Boal 1985).

Both Brecht's and Boal's theater styles aimed to generate social changes by encouraging audiences to think and act based on messages conveyed by actors on the stage. One of the fundamental problems in the Saku community was the persistence of feudalistic mindsets. Wakatsuki used medical drama to promote liberation from old ideas prevalent in the village. Wakatsuki's ideas aimed to replace "naïve awareness" with "critical awareness," bringing back autonomy over one's own health to the community (Werner and Bower 1982). To empower the community, medical dramas addressed both medical problems and solutions to train the audience's ability to think and make decisions on their own.

The work of Brecht and Boal shared commonality with Miyazawa's philosophy and Wakatsuki's medical drama work, encouraging people to think and take action to overcome the problematic norms faced by their communities. During this period of time, theater transformed from a tool of entertainment into a tool for social change.

7.4.4 Involving Medical Professionals in Dramas

Starting with Wakatsuki himself, many medical staff at Saku Hospital were involved in the medical dramas. This was not just due to limited human resources; it also helped toward the goal of increasing their communication with farmers as well as boosting cohesion among the medical staff. Wakatsuki believed in the importance of getting closer to the local community to communicate with farmers. Art and culture were ways of expanding the minds of both the local community and the health care staff. One drama after another, the Saku community began to trust hospital staff. Wakatsuki stated his fundamental philosophy in his book, explaining: "…changing the farmer's health literacy must be the first and the final goal among all healthcare professionals" (Fujii 1999b, p. 215, translated by the author).

Theater-based health promotion created new connections between medical professionals and community members. Back in those days, medical professionals—especially medical doctors—were distant from other members of the community, as medical doctors were historically seen as people with a higher social status (Wakatsuki 1971). One of the intentions behind Wakatsuki's drama work was literally working with community people, and through this Wakatsuki revolutionized the hierarchy of doctor and community by letting doctors act in front of people in the community. Farmers began to recognize doctors as community members who made efforts to conquer the health challenges of the village together.

7.5 Results and the Development of Community Health

The first medical drama, titled "People with white coats," was performed in 1945. There was limited entertainment besides the drama in those days, so people in the Saku community welcomed it, and there were large audiences for every performance. It became the main event for the community and had considerable influence. The community farmers became aware of the role of hospitals and a variety of health services.

This theater-based health promotion activity was successfully conducted, and Saku Hospital combined medical drama and home visits as a community health intervention "package" provided free of charge. The intervention was carried out initially only on Sundays and national holidays, and was considered additional work for the hospital staff. However, once they saw the positive impact on the community, Wakatsuki and his colleagues decided to increase the frequency of offerings. Accordingly, in 1959, this increase in activity allowed Saku Hospital to set up a village health checkup system in Yachiho village.

7.5.1 The Work of Saku Hospital's Theater Group

Saku Hospital established a drama group whose mission was promoting health in the community by providing it with medical theater, as initiated by Wakatsuki in 1945. Wakatsuki and other doctors in Saku Hospital wrote a script for each drama. Examples of drama themes are listed in Table 7.1.

Table 7.1 Examples of drama themes extracted from Fujii 1999a, Fujii1999b, p. 324, translated by the author

Theme	Title	Summary	Year of the first performance
Role of Medicine	People in white coats (Hakuino-hitobito)	Describing the work of hospital staff in 1945	1945
Role of Medicine	A village song (Murano uta)	The need for a contagious disease unit in the hospital	1950
Role of Medicine	After the rain (Ame harete)	The hopes and challenges of a doctor in a famers' village	1956
Role of Medicine	At Ranbaneket (Ranbarene nite)	The life of Schweitzer in Africa	1974
Disease Prevention	Darkness (Kurayami)	The tragedy of a girl who develops coxotuberculosis from taking a therapy based on superstition	1946
Disease Prevention	Livetrap (Ikedori)	Ascariasis and Santonin therapy	1948
Universal Health Coverage	Health insurance card (Hoken-syou)	Seeking help from a local fortune teller due to financial difficulties	1947
Universal Health Coverage	Stomachache (Haraita)	A comedy about Ascariasis and universal health coverage	1953
Environmental Health	From the small window (Chiisaki mado yori)	The problems caused by agricultural chemicals containing mercury	1982
Social Norm	Hope (Kibou)	A soldier inspired by the democracy of the hospital union after World War II	1946
Social Norm	New departure (Atarashiki shuppatsu)	A movement to build a nursery school for widows	1948
Social Norm	Scream of liberation (Jiyu no oakebi)	A man's fight for democracy	1952
Social Norm	Medical laboratory (Igaku- dai kyoushitsu)	A message of anti-war sentiments and hope for the next generation through depictions of a medical laboratory and a doctor from China during World War I	1954

(continued)

Table 7.1 (continued)

Theme	Title	Summary	Year of the first performance
Social Norm	An old lady's death at dawn (Rouba akatsukini shisu)	The story of aging problems in a farmers' village	1986
Philosophy	Crime and punishment	Describing the mental anguish and moral dilemmas of Rodion Raskolnikov	1950 (original story written by Dostoevsky 1866, adapted for the stage by Dr. Wakatski)

The dramas had several themes such as the role of medicine, advocacy of universal health coverage, environmental health, the introduction of social norms, and life philosophy. They had a role in promoting well-being as well as health, and the drama group successfully wove both components into its work. As a result of the series of dramas, farmers in the community integrated medicine into their lifestyle and the community's health literacy increased (Sugiyama 1999). Consequently, the Saku community welcomed new medical facilities, such as new hospitals in distant areas, as well as their first nursery school. In addition, the dramas motivated hospital staff in their village health checkup work. Importantly, the medical dramas provided a source of knowledge for the village farmers (Wakatsuki 1971; Fujii1999a, Fujii1999b).

7.5.2 Development of Health Promotion with New Media

The medical dramas became annual events for community members in the Saku community. Farmers were delighted to watch the dramas. Gradually, however, farmers' interests shifted to new media such as TV and radio when the Japanese economic boom arrived in 1955. Day by day, fewer farmers showed up at community stages to watch medical dramas. As technology developed, media that could connect people and the hospital changed. Audience numbers decreased, and this led to the exploration of new media for health promotion (Sugiyama 1999). Wakatsuki forecasted this transition of the media in the community, and he and the drama group formed a new group to make films for medical educational purposes in 1952. The filmmaking group advocated health beyond the community. As a result, one national newspaper company—"Mainichi Shinbun sya"—brought attention to Saku Hospital's health promotion work, and the work was featured on a TV show and in the newspaper. After all of the drama work in health promotion initiated by Wakatsuki and his colleagues at Saku Hospital, the importance of a healthy lifestyle became ingrained in the communities of Saku and Sakuho villages (The name of the village was changed from Yachiho to Sakuho in 2005). As a result, Nagano prefecture became one of the healthiest prefectures in Japan (Nagano prefecture 2015).

7.6 Conclusion

Drama had not been used previously for health promotion in Japan when first implemented by Saku Hospital in 1945. However, to date, many health promoters implement works of theater as part of health promotion campaigns in community settings (Danbara and Morita 2010; Kaneko et al. 1991; Yokota et al. 2006), combined with health checkups and health education lectures in Japan. A main benefit of utilizing drama work for health promotion is its adaptability. In the 1940s, the Saku community was classified as a middle- to low-income community and had limited resources. In that context, community theater was financially efficient to provide medical education for all villagers. The impact of medical theater on the community served by Saku Hospital suggests that implementing theater-based health promotion can be an efficient intervention in other resource-limited settings. One example of this is "Theater for Change Ghana," a non-profit organization established in 2003 and based in Ghana. Theater for Change Ghana provides works of theater to tackle problems related to health, human rights, education, capacity building, and livelihood (Theater for Change Ghana 2019).

Wakatsuki's main purpose was not just to educate communities about medicine and the importance of healthy lifestyles, but also to change people's mindsets. He strongly recommended integrating cultural components from people's lives in the community. The arts and our lives have a close relationship; consequently, utilizing arts can be a springboard to address what communities need to know (see also Chap. 21).

It has been 75 years since the first medical drama was performed in the Saku community in Nagano prefecture. As people's health literacy increased, technology also developed. Presently, in the field of health promotion, many online-based educational opportunities are accessible. At the same time, medical drama is still used in the field of health promotion despite its non-digital quality. This is because—as Brecht, Miyazawa, Boal, and Wakatsuki proved—drama is an enduring and powerful intervention for changing people's mindsets. In particular, drama has unique characteristics whereby the relationship between the audience and the characters creates empathy. Empathy brings us the emotional experiences of the characters on stage as if the action of the play were happening to us (Boal 1985), triggering self-awareness and new mindsets, as was Wakatsuki's goal. Therefore, dramatic works can be a powerful intervention for health promotion regardless of a community's resources. Because of the reputation these dramatic works created, theater for health promotion has been now implemented for several decades (Mbizvo 2006).

Despite the positive impact of theater-based health promotion, research on theater for health promotion is limited. This may be due to low awareness of the importance of evidence-based practice among arts-based health care providers (Jahan

2012). In the case of health promotion, Inman et al. (2011) argue about the importance of evidence-based health promotion resources to enhance the effectiveness of these programs. Despite this, arts for health promotion interventions often prioritize the actual play and leave out evaluation of outcomes and related research (Richard 2002). Especially in Japan, research evaluation of arts-based interventions has been neglected, because theaters are not yet counted as important resources for improved health and quality of life. In order to codify theater-based health promotion interventions, it is important to increase research on their practice and potential.

Theater-based health promotion might not convey messages as fast as the Internet can, but it creates human connection that cannot be provided by apps or websites. The successful past intervention of theater works gives all health promoters a new strategy for addressing communities' problems, and challenges them to transform those problems into a performance that can be observed and discussed. History gives a strong argument for the power of theater-based health promotion to lead us to answers we could not find in existing non-theater-based approaches.

References

Aikawa, Y. (2003). Thoughts and its changing process of theatrical movement in rural area: A case study of Kenji Miyazawa's view of art and the activities of young men's circles and association in NAGATORO village. *Journal of Agricultural Policy Research, 4*, 27–51.

Aoki, M. (2008). Challenges of anti-tuberculosis measures in Japan. *Japanese Journal of Public Health, 55*(9), 667–670. (in Japanese).

Boal, A. (1985). *Theater of the oppressed.* New York: Theatre Communication Group.

Danbara, M., & Morita, T. (2010). Support to health promotion volunteers' activity by public health nurses—Structure and pattern of health promotion volunteers' role explanation by public health nurses. *Japanese Journal of Health Education and Promotion, 18*(2), 81–91.

Davies, C., Knuiman, M., & Rosenberg, M. (2016). The art of being mentally healthy: A study to quantify the relationship between recreational arts engagement and mental well-being in the general population. *BMC Public Health, 16*, 15.

Frishkopf, M., Hamze, H., Alhassan, M., Zukpeni, A. I., Abu, S., & Zakus, D. (2016). Performing arts as a social technology for community health promotion in northern Ghana. *Family Medicine and Community Health, 4*(1), 22–36.

Fujii, H. (1999a). Community health pre and post war (in Japanese). In T. Wakatsuki (Ed.), *History of Saku Hospital* (pp. 1–29). Tokyo: Keiso Shobou.

Fujii, H. (1999b). Toshikazu Wakatsuki's philosophy and practice (in Japanese). In T. Wakatsuki (Ed.), *History of Saku Hospital* (pp. 187–240). Tokyo: Keiso Shobou.

Funabashi, Y. (1992). Japan and the new world order. *Foreign Affairs, 70*(5), 58–74. https://www.foreignaffairs.com/articles/asia/1991-12-01/japan-and-new-world-order. Accessed 22 Apr 2019.

Gordon, R. (2017). Brecht, interruptions and epic theatre. https://www.bl.uk/20th-century-literature/articles/brecht-interruptions-and-epic-theatre. Accessed 15 May 2019.

Hamilton, C., Hinks, S., & Petticrew, M. (2003). Arts for health: Still searching for the holy grail. *Journal of Epidemiology Community Health, 57*, 501–402.

Inman, D. D., Van Bakergem, M. K., LaRosa, C. A., & Garr, R. D. (2011). Evidence-based health promotion programs for schools and communities. *American Journal of Preventive Medicine, 40*(2), 207–219.

Ito, Y. (2003). The influence of historical experiences on the Japanese political communication research (in Japanese). *Keio Communication Review, 25*, 3–17.

Jahan, S. (2012). Health promotion: Opportunities and challenges. *Journal of Biosafety Health Education, 1*(2). Japan.

Kaneko, M., Ogawa, M., Kitayama, M., Yamaisi, H., & Hirayama, A. (1991). Effect of public health nurses' activities on promotion stomach cancer screening test in a community (in Japanese). Chiba University School of Nursing Departmental Bulletin, Paper, 13, 19–27.

Konishi, S. (2015). The science of symbiosis and linguistic democracy in early twentieth-century Japan (in Japanese). *Interdisciplinary Description of Complex Systems, 13*(2), 299–317.

Massar, K., Sialubanje, C., Maltagliati, I., & Ruiter, R. (2018). Exploring the perceived effectiveness of applied theater as a maternal health promotion tool in rural Zambia. *Qualitative Health Research, 28*(12), 1933–1943.

Mbizvo, E. (2006). Essay: Theatre—A force for health promotion. *The Lancet, 368*, S30–S31.

Michalos, C. A. (2005). Arts and quality of life: An explanatory study. *Social Indicators Research, 71*, 11–59.

Ministry of Labor, Health, Labor, and Welfare. (2014). Annual report (in Japanese). Retrieved from https://www.mhlw.go.jp/wp/hakusyo/kousei/14/dl/1-01.pdf. Accessed 22 Apr 2019.

Miyazawa, K. (1957). *Kenji Miyazawa completion,* Vol. 11 (in Japanese). Tokyo: Chikuma Shobou.

Miyazawa, K. (1991). *Night of the Milky Way Railway* (trans: Strong, M. S.). London: An East Gate Book. (Original work published in 1934).

Miyazawa, K. (1994). *Gauche the cellist,* Little J Books (trans: Bester, J.). http://www.littlejbooks.com/publications.html. Accessed 22 Apr 2019. (Original work published in 1934).

Moriyama, S. (1963). The theory of popular arts (in Japanese). *Japanese Literature Association, 12*(7), 505–520.

Nagano Prefecture. (2015). Healthy life expectancy of people in Nagano prefecture (in Japanese). https://www.pref.nagano.lg.jp/kenko-choju/kensei/soshiki/soshiki/kencho/choju/documents/naganokenkochoju261117.pdf. Accessed 22 Apr 2019.

National Organization for Arts in Health. (2017). *Arts, health, and well-being in America.* https://thenoah.net/. Accessed 22 Apr 2019.

Nishirai, T. (1983). *For the sake of the people: The health revolution led by Saku Central Hospital* (JOICEP document series 9). Tokyo: Japanese Organization for International Cooperation in Family Planning.

Nomura Research Institute, & Agency for Cultural Affairs. (2015). Report of cultural and arts-based activities for solving social challenges (in Japanese). http://www.bunka.go.jp/tokei_hakusho_shuppan/tokeichosa/bunka_gyosei/pdf/h26katsudo_jirei.pdf. Accessed 22 Apr 2019.

Ren, G. (2015). The usage of theatre workshop in the field of medical and nursing education, Communication-Design (in Japanese). *Osaka University Knowledge Archive, 13*, 57–61.

Richard, S. (2002). Spend (slightly) less on health and more on the arts. *British Medical Journal, 325*(7378), 1432–1433.

Rinpoo Corporation. (n.d.). *Kenji Miyazawa sitting [Photograph].* Hanamaki: Rinpoo Corporation.

Saku General Hospital. (1953). *Theater work "Haraita"* [Photograph]. Saku: Saku General Hospital.

Saku General Hospital. (n.d.). *Home visits by Wakatsuki* [Photograph]. Saku: Saku General Hospital.

Stuckey, L. H., & Nobel, J. (2010). The connection between arts, healing, and public health: A review of current literature. *American Journal of Public Health, 100*(2), 254–263.

Sugiyama, A. (1999). Medical service in community (in Japanese). In T. Wakatsuki (Ed.), *History of Saku Hospital* (pp. 141–186). Tokyo: Keisou Shobou.

Sumi, T. (2014). Has the enrolment ratio of Japan lead the world? *Journal of Research Office for Human Rights, 17*, 19–31. (in Japanese).

Suzuki, A., Nakase, T., Yoshioka, S., & Sasaki, M. (2010). The enlightenment of action on stroke patients to the local populace and the pre-hospital emergency medical system (in Japanese). *Japan Journal of Stroke, 32*, 680–683.

Theater for Change Ghana. (2019). Retrieved from http://www.tfscghana.org/. Accessed 22 Apr 2019.

Wakatsuki, T. (1971). *Fighting for diseases in village* (in Japanese). Tokyo: Iwanami Syoten, Publishers.

Werner, D., & Bower, B. (1982). Looking at human relations affect health. In *Helping health workers learn: A book of methods, aids, and ideas for instructors at the village level* (pp. 546–584). https://archive.org/details/HelpingHealthWorkersLearn-DavidWerner. Accessed 22 Apr 2019.

White, M. (2009a). The preference of the wave: Case examples from Western Australia. In *Arts development in community health: Social tonic* (pp. 131–154). London: Radcliff Publishing.

White, M. (2009b). I am because we are: Case examples from South Africa. In *Arts development in community health: Social tonic* (pp. 155–176). London: Radcliff Publishing.

Woodson, E. S., Quiroga, S. S., Underiner, T., & Karimi, F. R. (2017). Of models and mechanisms: Towards an understanding of how theatre-making works as an 'intervention' in individual health and wellness. *Research in Drama Education: The Journal of Applied Theatre and Performance, 22*(4), 465–481.

World Health Organization. (1986). The Ottawa Charter for Health Promotion. https://www.who.int/healthpromotion/conferences/previous/ottawa/en/. Accessed 22 Apr 2019.

Yokota, K., Harada, M., Wakabayashi, Y., Inagawa, M., Ohima, M., Toriumi, S., Hirose, K., Shina, Y., Yamagishi, K., Cui, R., Ikeda, A., Yao, M., Noda, H., Tanigawa, T., Tanaka, S., Kurokawa, M., Imano, H., Kiyama, M., Kitamura, A., Sato, S., Shimamoto, T., & Iso, H. (2006). Evaluation of a community-based health education program for salt reduction through media campaigns. *Japanese Journal of Public Health, 53*(8), 543–553. (in Japanese).

Part III
Arts and Health Promotion: Tools and Bridges for Research

Chapter 8
Lights, Camera, (Youth Participatory) Action! Lessons from Filming a Documentary with Trans and Gender Non-conforming Youth in the USA

Robert A. Marx and Page Valentine Regan

> *With other people of color that were in the documentary,*
> *I wanted them to talk and I wanted them to speak their truth*
> *because I'm not gonna, I'm not gonna sugarcoat it. I don't want*
> *anyone else to sugarcoat it. I don't want them to whitewash*
> *it.* – Autumn (a pseudonym), age 17, Black genderqueer person

8.1 Introduction

Fifty years ago, Americans scarcely had the language to describe the uprising that queer people—specifically trans and gender non-conforming (TGNC) people of color—led at the Stonewall Inn in New York. When accounts of the riots were entered into the official record, journalists made clear their disdain and disgust for the lesbian, gay, bisexual, trans, and queer (LGBTQ) patrons involved: they were called slurs, were misgendered, and were described in terms that minimized their concerns and experiences (Eastmond 2017). On the rare occasions that their voices were included, they were mediated through straight authors' judgmental gaze—for example, in the cruelly titled *"Homo Nest Raided, Queen Bees Are Stinging Mad."* Even when the *New York Daily News* quotes participants directly, the straight, cisgender newsperson editorializes in an attempt to make them seem frivolous, misgenders them in an attempt at humor, and feigns confusion in an attempt to make queer people seem un-knowable and inherently perplexing (Lisker 1969).

R. A. Marx (✉)
Department of Child and Adolescent Development, San José State University,
San Jose, CA, USA
e-mail: robert.marx@sjsu.edu

P. V. Regan
Educational Foundations, Policy, and Practice, University of Colorado, Boulder, CO, USA
e-mail: page.regan@colorado.edu

© The Author(s) 2021

J. H. Corbin et al. (eds.), *Arts and Health Promotion*,
https://doi.org/10.1007/978-3-030-56417-9_8

In the 50 years that have followed, our culture has developed a vocabulary that enables more meaningful discourse around the experiences of those marginalized for their sexual orientation, gender identity, and gender expression. Mainstream media coverage of the riots, protests, and celebrations of the fiftieth anniversary of the Stonewall Rising, for example, demonstrates more nuance in their reporting. *The New York Daily News'* many stories in June 2019 offer less homophobic and antagonistic criticism of participants, and instead report the events in a more neutral, less judgmental tone, being careful to use appropriate terminology. Even more telling, though, is the companion piece written by Anthony Coron, who reflects on the experience of being at the Stonewall Inn on the first night of the riots (Coron 2019). By including his unmediated, first-person account of the events, the newspaper—potentially inadvertently—offers a corrective for its coverage 50 years ago: it implicitly acknowledges that marginalized people should express their own stories without being filtered through the gaze of judgmental outsiders.

Much in the same way, the current research project aimed to contribute to the discourse on TGNC youth of color by presenting their stories with as little mediation and involvement of outsiders as possible. The youth participatory action research (YPAR) project involved 12 youth and three adult advisors, with the youth responsible for the design and implementation of the research project. The young people worked together to film a documentary about the experiences of TGNC youth in a mid-sized southeastern city with the goal of authentically representing the challenges, triumphs, struggles, and resilience in their community. Moreover, the selection of art as the primary modality for the research enabled the young people to authentically and completely communicate their experiences in a compelling, effective way. This chapter begins with a brief background on the experience of TGNC youth in the USA with special attention to the health inequities and disparities they face, and then discusses the research process, culminating in critical reflections on the possibilities, challenges, and logistical needs of such a project.

8.2 The Experiences of TGNC Youth

Much of the research on trans and gender non-conforming (TGNC) youth folds the population under the umbrella of sexual and gender minority (SGM) youth, providing insight into the experiences of lesbian, gay, bisexual, transgender, queer, or gender non-conforming (LGBTQ+) young people. LGBTQ+ youth are at an elevated risk for victimization (Berlan et al. 2014; Dempsey 1994; Schneider et al. 2012). This victimization can negatively impact the healthy development of LGBTQ+ youth, as it has been associated with depression (Poteat and Espelage 2007; Russell et al. 2011; Toomey et al. 2010), substance use (Bontempo and D'Augelli 2002; Espelage et al. 2008; Goldbach et al. 2014), and suicidality (Bontempo and D'Augelli 2002; Friedman et al. 2006; Russell et al. 2011).

Although much of the research on queer young people simply groups LGBTQ+ youth together, TGNC students may be at even greater risk for negative outcomes.

TGNC youth report higher levels of depression (Bazargan and Galvan 2012; Budge et al. 2013), attempted suicide (Goldblum et al. 2012; Grossman and D'Augelli 2007; Haas et al. 2014; Toomcy et al. 2018), and problematic drug use (Klein and Golub 2016; Reisner et al. 2015) than their peers. They also report a lack of resources, support, and safety in their environments as a result of being TGNC (Grossman and D'Augelli 2007). The majority of TGNC youth report feeling unsafe at school (McGuire et al. 2010). Further, potentially due to the higher rates of victimization and lower feelings of support, being a TGNC student is associated with lower academic achievement, increased fear-based truancy, and lower academic goals (Greytak et al. 2009). When compared with their victimized gay, lesbian, and bisexual (GLB) peers, TGNC students experience higher levels of victimization, harassment, school disengagement, and absence of resources for support (Greytak et al. 2009).

It is important to note that although this research may present a bleak picture of TGNC youth's experiences, recent research demonstrates TGNC youth's resilience, especially when supported by parents, school systems, and communities that acknowledge their needs and treat them with respect. When asked about what supports are important for their healthy development, TGNC students note that access to education systems that acknowledge and affirm their identities are important sources of resilience (Hatchel et al. 2018; Singh et al. 2014). Further research demonstrates the importance of a supportive school environment: TGNC students at schools with appropriate resources and supports (e.g., Gay-Straight or Gender Sexuality Alliances, anti-harassment policies, or information about LGBTQ+ people in the school library) indicate that their school is safer and are less likely to skip school (Greytak et al. 2009). School belonging is also associated with lower rates of suicidality and depression for trans adolescents (Hatchel et al. 2018), and it may protect TGNC young people from drug use (Hatchel and Marx 2018) and poor mental health outcomes (Hatchel et al. 2018). Family support is also associated with resilience, as TGNC youth who report supportive families also report decreased distress, improved mental health, and self-acceptance (Budge et al. 2013; Pflum et al. 2015; Sánchez and Vilain 2009). For TGNC adults, a supportive family is associated with fewer suicide attempts (Haas et al. 2014; Mustanski and Liu 2013) and depressive symptoms and a greater quality of life (Austin 2016; Mustanski and Liu 2013).

It is clear, then, that the experiences of TGNC youth are more complicated than traditional research methods may be able to capture; there is a tension between the health disparities that impact their well-being and healthy development and the strength and resilience they derive from environments that acknowledge and affirm their identities. Beyond resilience and health disparities, another tension that exists in representing the experiences of TGNC lies in the unique experiences of TGNC youth of color. In addition to a sense of belonging, family supports, and school-based resources, TGNC young people of color express the need for affinity spaces based on race, as well as access to representation of other LGBTQ-identified people of color (Singh 2012). While access to social media might be a vehicle for expanding community and increasing access to knowledge around the experiences of

TGNC people of color, the absence of empirical research at the intersection of race and gender speaks to the added pressures on this population of young people.

Indeed, community-based participatory research and youth participatory action research (Cammarota and Fine 2010; Kemmis et al. 2013; Kidd and Kral 2005) offer researchers the opportunity to include the voices of marginalized groups directly and with limited external mediation, capturing the many nuances of their experiences. In line with the values espoused in health promotion (see Chap. 1, this volume), by including young people as experts and giving them the opportunity to determine what research products best represent their own experiences, we offer them the space to control the conversation and thereby harness the power to shape their own narratives.

The complexity of TGNC youth's experiences may be best captured through arts-based research, as it inherently allows for—and potentially encourages—the intricacies and contradictions of their experiences in environments that at turns may result in increased mental and physical health concerns but may also be supportive and health-promotive. Prior work with documentary film as a medium for research notes that the creation of a documentary film engenders a necessarily rich text that can capture and document data that may be otherwise difficult to access, especially with marginalized groups (Parr 2007). Moreover, the practice of collaborative documentary filmmaking may allow for participants to accurately represent themselves in ways that sidestep the hierarchical nature of traditional research, opening new avenues for embedded and embodied knowledges (Kindon 2003) and potential resulting in increased synergy (see Chap. 21, this volume, for theoretical background on synergy). For these reasons, this research project aimed to leverage the power of participatory documentary film to amplify the voices and share the unique and specific experiences of TGNC youth in ways that more traditional research methodologies may have silenced, flattened, or rendered untenable.

8.3   The Untitled Trans Youth Film Project

In December of 2017, the 14- to 18-year-old members of "Just Us," a program for LGBTQ+ youth at a local non-profit community center in a mid-sized southeastern city, sat down to watch *The Trans List*, an HBO-produced documentary film that profiled 11 trans and gender non-conforming US celebrities, activists, athletes, and figures of note. Page Regan—then the program coordinator of Just Us, now a doctoral researcher and co-author of this chapter—selected the film to connect with the young people's experiences and to offer visions of potential futures for TGNC youth, who were so often shown only limited options. Robert Marx, who was at the time an adult advisor for the youth group and is now a researcher and co-author of this chapter, was eager to see the young people's responses to the video. As they watched, the youth were clearly interested; side conversations stopped, and they snapped their fingers to indicate support and agreement as figures on the screen shared experiences that resonated with their own. At the conclusion of the film, Page facilitated a talk-back session that invited the young people to consider the strengths of the movie. Although the feedback was overwhelmingly positive, many young people offered that the stories depicted on screen did not conform to their own experiences: those interviewed seemed wealthier, older, and more binary in terms of their gender identity (i.e., they tended to identify as either a trans man or a trans woman, rather than as non-binary or genderqueer).

During that conversation, one young person suggested that they could make their own film—sort of a *Youth Trans List*—that more accurately captured their narratives. Several other students expressed interest, and the idea gained buzz and critical traction. Following the meeting, Robert and Page met to determine ways forward. Robert had previous experience with a youth participatory action research (YPAR) project that focused on marginalized youth's experiences of discrimination and saw an opportunity to bring that framework to the documentary film project. Because both Page and Robert wanted the young people to be able to create a product that they would be proud of and that would accurately capture their experiences, they saw YPAR as a way of ensuring that the young people adopted a systematic approach that yielded meaningful findings. We then approached the young people with the more formal procedures of a YPAR project, and they were very open to it. Because their vision of the documentary film already included key aspects of research such as participant recruitment, interview design, and thematic analysis, the young people adopted the YPAR framework naturally and saw the benefit of approaching the project with systematicity and an eye toward research.

In line with the tenets of YPAR, the young people determined the research design, the participants, and the procedure, and they conducted the research and analysis themselves. Robert and Page served as adult advisors for the project, securing meeting space and other resources, ensuring that the young people respected each other and allowed all voices to be heard, and assumed liability, as the young people were under 18. Importantly, Robert and Page also provided research training for the young people, instructing them on best practices for recruiting participants, designing interview protocols, conducting interviews, and engaging in thematic analysis.

In the sections that follow, we outline the process from idea to execution, noting the successes and difficulties we encountered along the way following the Bergen Model of Collaborative Functioning (see Chap. 21, this volume). Throughout the research process, both the adult advisors and the youth participants remained singularly focused on sharing the stories of TGNC youth. We aimed to capture the complexity and variety of TGNC experiences in the hopes that audiences would have a better understanding of the realities of TGNC youth's lives.

8.3.1 Inputs: Mission, Participants, Partners, and Funding

From its inception, the documentary film project had a clear and direct mission: the young people wanted to share their worlds, their experiences, and their hearts with a broader audience. In creating the film, the young people hoped to document the aspects of their lives that were most difficult, as well as their triumphs and goals for the future. In describing why a documentary film was the medium of choice for the project, one participant said, "The documentary literally allows you to see…because [in other situations] you see people, but you don't see them. You don't necessarily consider them, or you don't consider what they like to do… You don't consider what their favorite color is. You don't consider how difficult it is for them to walk down the street, whether or not they've been walking on the street and feel secure, and whether they're going to be sexually assaulted. You don't consider any of that…You don't consider them, and you don't see them; and so, I think that the ... I do like the idea of the documentary being, like, you see them, and then, you *see* them."

In our first meeting as a research team, we opened the group to any young person who was interested in creating a documentary film, and we recruited from among the youth who came to the community center for LGBTQ+ programming, as well as from other youth in the area who might be interested. Twelve young people, aged 14–19, attended our first meeting, representing a variety of gender identities and expressions. Most young people identified as TGNC, but two young people identified as cisgender allies. In that first meeting, the young people determined that the film would focus specifically on the most marginalized among TGNC youth: TGNC youth of color. Research team members cited the high rates of violence and murder that TGNC youth of color experience, as well as the fact that mainstream accounts of TGNC youth often omit or exclude youth of color, neglecting to consider the ways that racism impacts the experience of transphobia. For many of the research team members, this was also a personal project—more than half of the young people identified as youth of color, and their desire to illuminate their experiences came from a sense of not being heard in other forums.

To support the research endeavors, we relied on several key partnerships that proved invaluable. Because Page was a full-time employee of the community center, we could use the space as needed for meetings and, eventually, for filming. We could also recruit participants for the film and advertise through the community center, which made finding interview participants easier. Robert, who was then a doctoral student in the area, leveraged connections with his university and with the local library to help the project come to fruition. Robert received a small grant from the Community Engaged Research Core that provided both funding for the research project and guidance in managing the many moving pieces that go along with YPAR projects; this money funded everything from pizza at research team meetings to external hard drives to server access for uploading video segments. Robert also reached out to the local library, which fortuitously ran a studio and maker space for teenagers. The library provided editing equipment and space, which allowed young people to collaboratively edit the project, and it also had trained professionals who could offer guidance. An additional partnership proved important: the parent of one of the research team members was a professional filmmaker and had considerable camera and lighting equipment, as well as expertise with filming.

8.3.2 Throughputs: Implementation, Execution, and Analysis

As clear as the mission was and as natural as the partnerships came to be, other aspects of the research process were more nebulous. The young people had varying experience and interest in some aspects of making a documentary film, and so we split into two groups: one group focused on the specifics and aesthetics of the filming, and the other focused on the content of the documentary. This meant that one group focused on determining which cameras would be used, what the set-up would be, where and when we would film, and what the overall aesthetic vision was. The other group determined who would conduct the interviews, who would be interviewed, what questions would be asked, and what the overall emotional tenor of the film would be. This division enabled those with more interest in or knowledge about filmmaking to deepen their commitment to the technical aspects of the film, while allowing those who were more concerned with the recruitment of participants and the storytelling to focus on that aspect of the research. The research team met once a week for 5 months; we would begin as a full group and then split into the two teams, with one adult advisor going with each group, and then return to a large group meeting to share progress. Approximately a month into the project, a third adult advisor who also worked full time at the community center and who has considerable experience with digital media and filmmaking, joined the group and served as a technical advisor to ensure that the project was feasible and appropriate.

Over the course of these meetings, the research team determined the particulars of all aspects of the film, making most decisions by consensus and working to hear all voices. Each subgroup elected a leader who was responsible for the deliverables and for ensuring that all necessary work was completed. The young people put together dioramas of the filming day, wrote out interview questions, contacted young people to be interviewed, determined the schedule for filming, and even arranged for a local photographer—the parent of one of the research team members—to take photographs of the interview participants. Over the course of the meetings, the young people maintained unwavering focus on including the stories of TGNC youth of color and allowing them to be as complicated and complete as possible. Nonetheless, the young people engaged in vigorous debate concerning the specifics of achieving their vision; in particular, the youth had a bit of difficulty deciding on the scope of the interview questions, the participants to include, and who would conduct the interviews. This was the result, mainly, of thoughtful and judicious consideration of how to best meet their goals—they determined that young people of color might respond best to an interviewer of color, and they also struggled to balance their desire to focus only on youth of color with their concern that not enough young people would want to be interviewed. Similarly, their debate over interview questions centered on their desire to avoid leading participants into sharing overly sanitized, happy versions of their lives, but also wanting to avoid setting their participants up to only speak about damage and sadness. In the end, the research team reached a compromise by designing open-ended questions that allowed participants to respond in a variety of ways, but also by asking a set of specific questions, some of which included:

- How does your gender identity affect your daily life?
- What aspects of your identity are you comfortable with?
- Are there aspects of your identity that you hope to change?
- When do you feel the safest or most acknowledged?
- What would you like to tell other LGBTQ+ people?
- What has it been like to deal with living in a society that is often hostile to your existence?
- Where do you see yourself in 10 years?
- What are you excited about?

They also created a schedule and rotated through interviewers so that everyone who wanted to participate as an interviewer could.

Over the course of the planning meetings, the young people engaged in all stages of the arts-based research project design. They finalized interview protocols through piloting and practicing questions with group members, determining which questions were too broad, which were too closed off, and which worked effectively. They also drafted a list of potential participants from their own network of TGNC youth of color, created recruitment material, and recruited participants. Additionally, the technical team created specifications for all aspects of the day of filming, including mocking up filming plans; determining the lighting plan; and designating who would set up, run cameras A and B, and get extra footage of the participants to intercut with their interviews.

The planning meetings culminated in a day-long filming session during which all interviewees were photographed, interviewed on camera, and filmed in informal interactions with the camera to capture their personalities. The research team set up all camera equipment and lighting the day before, then spent 12 hours filming eight interviews with TGNC youth. The interviews varied in length, but all were between 25 and 75 minutes. Following the filming of the interviews, three members of the research team worked at the local library to edit the film down. They began by removing verbal tics and fillers, and then brought transcripts of the interviews to the whole research team.

The research team spent a month reading each transcript, watching raw footage, and determining what aspects of each interview to highlight. They also engaged in thematic coding, surfacing key ideas across interviews to divide the film into units. The editing team then cut together the footage thematically, creating a 15-minute rough cut of the final documentary. The research team was trained in thematic analysis and engaged in a modified constant-comparative method that involved the reading and re-reading of transcripts, the identification of codes and themes, and the re-examination of transcripts to ensure that the identified themes still fit as the analysis continued. Because the YPAR team determined that their main product would be the documentary film (and not, for example, an academic article or a blog post), all research and analysis were conducted with the documentary film in mind.

That is, the transcripts were analyzed with an eye toward the documentary, and the themes that were surfaced were those that would be present in the film. The transcripts were coded and analyzed systematically, but only in terms of which aspects of the interviews provided salient material for the documentary. As the major themes coalesced, the research team then read through each transcript to find the clearest and most captivating examples. One salient theme, for example, was the racial divide within the LBGTQ+ community—the research team deeply resonated with the respondents' experiences of racism and isolation within nominally inclusive spaces or histories. The research team then selected moments from interviews that highlighted the lack of representation of queer people of color in LGBTQ+ history-telling and spoke to the isolation experienced in spaces for LGBTQ+ youth that were predominantly white. Another example of the research process centered on familial tensions. For example, after the team surfaced a theme concerning the complicated dynamic between trans youth and their parents—who could be both supportive and closed-minded—they re-read all transcripts for the voices and moments that best captured this idea. In this way, although the research team engaged in a systematic analysis of the data they had collected, their sole focus was the creation of the documentary film and the sharing of their findings in that way.

8.3.3 Output: The In-Progress Film

Although the research team worked cohesively to design, implement, film, and initially edit the documentary film, progress flagged in the months following filming. As other priorities came to the forefront—our research team was all students, after all—and as the required work became more technically demanding, weeks went by without progress. As of this publication, the film is still in progress. The research team has functionally disbanded; although they remain committed to having a completed documentary, we lack the traction and time to bring the project to completion. The third adult advisor, who has more technical experience, has recently taken on the task of beginning to edit together the rough cut into a final documentary film, but progress remains slow.

Although the film is not yet in its final form, both authors have shared clips of the film in trainings, classes, and educational settings. The response has been overwhelmingly positive, and viewers have reflected on how much they have deepened their understanding of TGNC youth of color's experiences. Specifically, audiences have noted the terminology they have learned and the additional insight into both the strength that TGNC youth of color have as well as the many challenges they face in their daily lives. One tangible impact of the film is that viewers at a center for sexual assault survivors have changed their intake forms and their trainings around gender and sexuality. These preliminary results, of course, must be taken lightly, as the film has not yet been finalized.

In addition to assisting with advising the research team, Robert also conducted interviews with many of the research team members in the hopes of better understanding the impact of working on the documentary film. The young people offered clear examples of the ways in which their participation had deepened their commitment to social justice and their belief in the power of documentary film. Additionally, though, the young people reflected on some of the challenges in the research project. In the discussion section, we include some of these reflections alongside our own thoughts. For the most part, the research team members' thoughts resonated with our own interpretations of the events of the project.

8.4 Discussion

Engaging in this arts-based YPAR project has contributed to the dialogue and discourse surrounding TGNC youth of color. Despite the very limited release of the documentary film in its current form, it nonetheless contains important data about the lives of a group of people who are too rarely discussed. Moreover, the film contains the voices of the young people themselves and is deeply and rigorously informed by TGNC youth of color in every stage of the research project. In the following section, we discuss the possibilities that such a project offers, as well as the challenges that we faced in its execution. We finish with lessons we have learned through the process.

8.4.1 Possibilities and Promise

In many ways, this project represents a fulfilment of the promise of YPAR and documentary film. It represents a valuable source of data that would otherwise not be available—a rich text that captures TGNC youth's experiences unmediated, direct from the source. In many respects, this was possible only because the project was participatory in nature and organized and completed by the youth themselves; their own connection to the material and to the art form enabled the project's success. Moreover, the young people who pioneered this project were familiar with each other because of their shared attendance at after-school, queer-centered programming, meaning that they were also connected to one another. The project also afforded students an opportunity to connect more deeply around a shared purpose. Many of the research team participants reported that a defining characteristic of the group was their shared commitment to a goal, and they credited this shared commitment to the success of the project.

Importantly, the project represented great diversity among participants. The research team represented different ethnic and racial groups, different schools, and different embodied identities related to trans and queer life; this rich diversity propelled the project forward in immeasurable ways. The young people were able to provide a more complete, accurate, and thorough depiction of TGNC youth's lives because they lived those lives and knew which questions would elicit the richest discussion. They knew which misconceptions and half-truths needed to be corrected and which words would be most useful to dispel the myths that surrounded them. Further, they knew which aspects of TGNC life would most impact their audience, and they skillfully chose to share certain portions of their world to improve outcomes. Moreover, the young people represented diversity in skill and interest around making a documentary film: some students were adept with camera and lighting, others had experience interviewing, and others were merely willing to learn. The diversity of talent also meant that the young people were able to learn from each other and teach one another, and by the end of the project, all participants had additional research skills. Because the team was trained in basic research methods to complete the project, they all gained skills around recruiting participants, crafting interview protocols and conducting interviews, and performing thematic analysis of qualitative data.

One of the chief sources of success of the project was thoughtfully chosen partnerships. Although the adult advisors had considerable experience working with youth and running YPAR projects, they had very limited experience with documentary filmmaking. Partnering with the local library, which was able to provide both equipment and expertise, and the parent of a research team member, who was a filmmaker, supplemented the gaps in our experience and made the project possible. Similarly, the partnership with the Community Engaged Research Core provided financial support for the project and made all aspects of it easier. Our ultimate partnership with the third adult advisor also helped the project along, and it is our hope that with her guidance, we will have a completed film soon. Finally, the project represents a partnership between the university—of which Robert was a representative—and the community, in which Page worked. This partnership enabled the leveraging of important resources and expertise, as Page could draw on past program participants and their connection to youth, while Robert could address research concerns such as Institutional Review Board approval and incentives for participation.

Although the rough cut of the film has only preliminarily been released, we hope that it is fulfilling the promise that the young people have and making their community safer, stronger, and more supportive. As family support and school support are two key drivers of TGNC resilience, we hope that showing this film—albeit to only a few dozen people—has improved their interactions with TGNC youth and has created a healthier environment for sexual and gender minorities. Even if the project only served to touch the young people involved in the creation of the film, it was certainly a success: the research team shared time and again how valuable the experience was and how important it was for them to be a part of it. The young people came to see themselves as agents of change and shapers of knowledge—two key aspects of resilient, healthy youth.

8.4.2 Challenges

Although the project delivered on much of its promise, it was hindered by a number of challenges, both foreseen and unforeseen. A foreseen, consistent challenge was continuity. All students involved in the project attended school full time and were responsible for familial and work commitments that could not be compromised by their participation in the documentary project. Sometimes the students were able to meet every week, completing large aspects of the planning process and even devoting extra time to the work, while at other times sessions became few and far between. We found that without a clear set of expectations for the editing process, and without a stable person to help support this process, film editing was slowed almost completely to a halt. We did not expect that students' interest, availability, and productivity would drop off so suddenly after filming was completed; students were committed to the designated weekly meetings, the planning of the filming and interviewing, and the events leading up to and including the day of filming. Following that, though, the project slowed considerably, and many research team members spoke of the film as if it were complete and finished, even though it was not. Moreover, because only one or two team members could edit at a time, it was difficult to maintain continuity or interest once all participants had read the transcripts and selected key parts.

Another foreseen challenge that nonetheless hindered the progress of the documentary film was the tension in our roles as adult advisors of a YPAR project. We found it difficult to know when we should step in and intervene, and when we should allow the young people to solve the problems for themselves. For example, at times the young people worked together as a perfectly functional group, allowing each other to speak and contribute ideas equally. At other times, though, we felt compelled to intervene to ensure that all voices were heard. Similarly, we were unsure how much of a hands-on role to take in the planning and scheduling of meetings, especially after filming. Leading up to the filming day, the young people took considerable initiative and scheduled extra meetings, but after filming, they were less available. As adult advisors, we did not know how much we should push the issue or force the students to have meetings or to complete deliverables. This is an ongoing challenge, as we still work to complete the film and are unsure how much external guidance and structure we can impose on the young people.

An unforeseen challenge in this work was the labor that the narrative involved. In the filming process, several participants became deeply emotional as they were invited to unveil past trauma around their identities. Given the emotional and immersive nature of qualitative data collection and the potential burdens borne of eliciting and transmitting truth through narrative, we should have been more cognizant of the environment that was created. Many of our research team members became involved in the emotional care and support of our interview participants, and we had not prepared sufficiently for this. We were fortunate to have access to exemplary mental health services and guidance for young people through our partnership with the community organization.

Another unforeseen challenge was the gap between young people's desires to participate and the skills they needed to complete tasks. Many of the students expressed interest in joining the research team so that they could develop skills with camerawork, lighting, and editing. As adult advisors for the project, we were excited to have young people who wanted to learn, and we hoped that our partnership with the library would help bring them the needed skills. Unfortunately, we did not realize just how much training is required to become a competent video editor, and our research team members lacked the time to devote to learning these new skills. At times, it was easier for our partners to complete tasks rather than train our team members to complete them, which frustrated those who wanted to learn. For example, on the day of the shoot, the filmmaker parent of one of the research team members found that it was more expedient to set up the lights himself, and therefore did not train a team member to set them up. This frustrated the team members and made the experience less valuable for them. Nonetheless, when shooting on a deadline, it is understandable that the lights needed to be set up quickly. Resolving this challenge, therefore, is difficult.

8.4.3 Lessons Learned

Over the 2 years of this project, we have learned a number of lessons that would make the completion of an arts-based YPAR project with marginalized youth more successful. Drawing on the many strengths of our project, we have learned the importance of assembling a diverse team that has partnerships across equipment, skill level, financial support abilities, and life experiences. Moreover, involving the population of interest directly in all aspects of the process leads to a richer, more important final product. Additionally, creating a university-community partnership alleviates many of the sticking points of traditional YPAR; we were able to rely on each other for recruitment, finding space, obtaining Institutional Review Board approval, and moving through the phases of the research project.

From our many challenges, we also derived several recommendations for similar projects moving forward. Creating a firm but flexible timeline from the outset that runs throughout the entirety of the project would have made our project run more smoothly and would have ensured timelier completion. Although timelines are rarely strictly adhered to, having a more specific sense of when the editing process should begin and be finished would have enabled us to set more appropriate goals and deadlines. Additionally, allowing for the ramping up of skills, especially around the editing process, would help the project move to completion; had we selected several students and had them learn about editing techniques from the beginning of the project, they would have been up to speed by the time editing was needed. Finally, expecting the drop off in engagement and participation following the completion of filming would have potentially allowed us to build in additional events, activities, or workshops that would have continued interest and sustained the project's momentum.

In sum, our main lessons learned were the importance of strong partnerships and the need for key planning for multiple deadlines to ensure that interest and engagement did not flag throughout the process.

8.5 Conclusion

This arts-based research project that culminated in the filming of a documentary about the lives and experiences of trans and gender non-conforming youth of color offers many possibilities for deeper understanding and for the creation of health-promoting families, schools, and communities. Importantly, this documentary film project aligns itself with tenets of critical race theory in research, especially as it engages in counter-storytelling that draws on, centers, and highlights the experiences and knowledges of TGNC youth of color (Solórzano and Yosso 2002). Although the research team may not have employed the language of critical race methodology, their work actively sought to address the intersecting forms of subjugation across race, class, gender, and sexual identities, giving voice to the complexities of experiences shaped not only by their gender identities but also by their racialized and classed identities (Solórzano and Yosso 2002). Further, their work speaks back to the traditional, deficit-focused narrative of TGNC youth, acknowledging both their sources of strength and their hopes for the future. In these ways, the documentary film project offered participants the opportunity to engage in counter-storytelling, adding multivocal accounts that push back against majoritarian, privileged stories and accounts (Solórzano and Yosso 2002).

Although we encountered many challenges and are still in the process of finalizing the film, this research project makes clear the importance of using art as a medium to capture what traditional research methods might leave unexplored and unexpressed. Documentary film—and art, more broadly—may offer new inroads into work that aims to offer a more complete and complex understanding of people's lived experiences. These methods may offer "new ways to see" (Leavy 2015, p. 291) and new ways to understand what is seen. More traditional research methods may omit certain aspects of TGNC youth's experiences and may render salient moments invisible (Hesse-Biber and Leavy 2008); the documentary film may function as a source of data that highlights and celebrates these salient moments (Parr 2007). The sharp intake of breath before a participant shares a story of familial rejection, the broad smile as a participant talks about her future as an aesthetician, the cautious look to the ground as a participant offers advice to their former self—these subtle nuances and quiet moments are often obscured in the written word. Documentary film relies on these moments as text and as data, capturing the nuance and subtlety that often goes unspoken and unacknowledged in other work. Further, documentary film as a medium welcomes a broader audience than more traditional academic research products do (Leavy 2015); although the film has only had very limited release, its audience has included more diverse thinkers and viewers than a journal article would. The research team aimed to appeal to a wide audience that included TGNC youth, their parents and teachers, and those who had no prior knowledge of gender theory, and documentary film as a medium offered them that opportunity.

Moreover, by including the population of interest in every step of the research process, we were able to create a richer, more meaningful text that ultimately offers many ways forward for the health of trans and gender non-conforming youth. By engaging in participatory video that enabled TGNC youth to share their experiences and thoughts directly with the audience, the research team created a final product that harnessed the transformative potential of documentary film (Kindon 2003). As many scholars have argued, participatory video offers an important and natural means of making manifest complicated concepts and realities, especially unearthing aspects of experience that may be harder to access through more traditional, hierarchical, researcher-centered projects (Braden and Mayo 1999; Kidd 1994; Mitchell et al. 2012). Traditional researchers may not think to ask questions that the TGNC youth did, may not recognize the answers in the way that the research team did, or may not put forward the often-messy and still-forming conversation as the youth did. The research team focused on sharing their truths with the audience, rather than representing themselves in ways that a traditional researcher could acknowledge and incorporate into the researcher's work. This necessarily has implications for the knowledge produced and the research product. This participatory video may also open space for societal transformation as it offers a way of allowing research subjects to direct the audience's gaze and control the audience's understanding of the subjects' experiences (Kindon 2003). This radical restructuring of the research process not only transfers power to those who may otherwise be powerless within a traditional research paradigm, but it also enables the types of discussions that may give rise to material changes in the lives of TGNC youth.

As the documentary film continues post-production and is eventually released to the public, the research team will further its goal of providing a platform for individuals who are often overlooked or unheard to control their own audiovisual reality and representation. For all of its shortcomings and challenges, the research team set out to create a document that offers nuance and insight into lives that are often rendered flat and two-dimensional, and the collaborative, arts-based method they chose allowed them the power to turn those dreams into a reality.

Acknowledgements The authors would like to acknowledge the many people who came together in order to make this larger project possible. First and foremost, we are greatly indebted to the young people who worked so diligently to create the documentary project. We also partnered with a local community center and a local library, without which we would not have been able to complete the project. Additionally, the project received funding from the Meharry-Vanderbilt Community Engaged Research Core.

References

Austin, A. (2016). "There I am": A grounded theory study of young adults navigating a transgender or gender nonconforming identity within a context of oppression and invisibility. *Sex Roles, 75*(5–6), 215–230. https://doi.org/10.1007/s11199-016-0600-7.

Bazargan, M., & Galvan, F. (2012). Perceived discrimination and depression among low-income Latina male-to-female transgender women. *BMC Public Health, 12*(1). https://doi.org/10.1186/1471-2458-12-663.

Berlan, E. D., Corliss, H. L., Field, A. E., Goodman, E., & Austin, S. B. (2014). Sexual orientation and bullying among adolescents in the Growing Up Today study. *Journal of Adolescent Health, 46*, 366–371.

Bontempo, D. E., & D'Augelli, A. R. (2002). Effects of at-school victimization and sexual orientation on lesbian, gay, or bisexual youths' health risk behavior. *Journal of Adolescent Health, 30*(5), 364–374. https://doi.org/10.1016/S1054-139X(01)00415-3.

Braden, S., & Mayo, M. (1999). Culture, community development, and representation. *Community Development Journal, 34*(3), 191–204.

Budge, S. L., Adelson, J. L., & Howard, K. A. S. (2013). Anxiety and depression in transgender individuals: The roles of transition status, loss, social support, and coping. *Journal of Consulting and Clinical Psychology, 81*(3), 545–557. https://doi.org/10.1037/a0031774.

Cammarota, J., & Fine, M. (2010). *Revolutionizing education: Youth participatory action research in motion*. New York: Routledge.

Coron, A. (2019, June 28). 'Quite a scene': New Yorker inside Stonewall Inn 50 years ago recalls police raid that sparked a rebellion. *The New York Daily News*. https://www.nydailynews.com/new-york/ny-witness-to-stonewall-history-20190628-adglogadpbh5vhfmkkcexkxvpm-story.html. Accessed 22 Sept 2019.

Dempsey, C. L. (1994). Health and social issues of gay, lesbian, and bisexual adolescents. *Families in Society: The Journal of Contemporary Social Services, 75*(3), 160–167. https://doi.org/10.1177/104438949407500304.

Eastmond, D. (2017, February 6). LGBT+ history month: how the press reported the stonewall riots in 1969. *HISKIND Magazine*. https://hiskind.com/lgbt-history-month-how-the-press-reported-the-stonewall-riots-in-1969/. Accessed 22 Sept 2019.

Espelage, D. L., Aragon, S. R., Birkett, M., & Koenig, B. W. (2008). Homophobic teasing, psychological outcomes, and sexual orientation among high school students: What influence do parents and schools have? *School Psychology Review, 37*(2), 15.

Friedman, M. S., Koeske, G. F., Silvestre, A. J., Korr, W. S., & Sites, E. W. (2006). The impact of gender-role nonconforming behavior, bullying, and social support on suicidality among gay male youth. *Journal of Adolescent Health, 38*(5), 621–623. https://doi.org/10.1016/j.jadohealth.2005.04.014.

Goldbach, J. T., Tanner-Smith, E. E., Bagwell, M., & Dunlap, S. (2014). Minority stress and substance use in sexual minority adolescents: A meta-analysis. *Prevention Science, 15*(3), 350–363. https://doi.org/10.1007/s11121-013-0393-7.

Goldblum, P., Testa, R. J., Pflum, S., Hendricks, M. L., Bradford, J., & Bongar, B. (2012). The relationship between gender-based victimization and suicide attempts in transgender people. *Professional Psychology: Research and Practice, 43*(5), 468–475. https://doi.org/10.1037/a0029605.

Greytak, E. A., Kosciw, J. G., & Diaz, E. M. (2009). Harsh realities: The experiences of transgender youth in our nation's schools. Retrieved from GLSEN website: https://files.eric.ed.gov/fulltext/ED505687.pdf.

Grossman, A. H., & D'Augelli, A. R. (2007). Transgender youth and life-threatening behaviors. *Suicide and Life-threatening Behavior, 37*(5), 527–537. https://doi.org/10.1521/suli.2007.37.5.527.

Haas, A. P., Rodgers, P. L., & Herman, J. L. (2014). *Suicide attempts among transgender and gender non-conforming adults* (p. 18). Los Angeles: The Williams Institute.

Hatchel, T., & Marx, R. (2018). Understanding intersectionality and resiliency among transgender adolescents: Exploring pathways among peer victimization, school belonging, and drug use. *International Journal of Environmental Research and Public Health, 15*(6). https://doi.org/10.3390/ijerph15061289.

Hatchel, T., Valido, A., De Pedro, K. T., Huang, Y., & Espelage, D. L. (2018). Minority stress among transgender adolescents: The role of peer victimization, school belonging, and ethnicity. *Journal of Child and Family Studies, 28*, 2467–2476. https://doi.org/10.1007/s10826-018-1168-3.

Hesse-Biber, S. N., & Leavy, P. (2008). Pushing on the methodological boundaries: The growing need for emergent methods within and across the disciplines. In S. N. Hesse-Biber & P. Leavy (Eds.), *Handbook of emergent methods* (pp. 1–15). New York: Guilford Press.

Kemmis, S., McTaggart, R., & Nixon, R. (2013). *The action research planner: Doing critical participatory action research*. Singapore: Springer Science and Business Media.

Kidd, D. (1994). Shards of remembrance: One woman's archaeology of community video. In P. Riaño (Ed.), *Women in grassroots communication: Furthering social change* (pp. 179–191). Thousand Oaks: Sage Publications.

Kidd, S. A., & Kral, M. J. (2005). Practicing participatory action research. *Journal of Counseling Psychology, 52*(2), 187–195.

Kindon, S. (2003). Participatory video in geographic research: A feminist practice of looking? *Area, 35*(2), 142–153. https://doi.org/10.1111/1475-4762.00236.

Klein, A., & Golub, S. A. (2016). Family rejection as a predictor of suicide attempts and substance misuse among transgender and gender nonconforming adults. *LGBT Health, 3*(3), 193–199. https://doi.org/10.1089/lgbt.2015.0111.

Leavy, P. (2015). *Method meets art: Arts-based research practice*. New York: Guilford Press.

Lisker, J. (1969, July 6). Queen bees are stinging mad | American Experience | PBS. https://www.pbs.org/wgbh/americanexperience/features/stonewall-queen-bees/. Accessed 22 Sept 2019.

McGuire, J. K., Anderson, C. R., Toomey, R. B., & Russell, S. T. (2010). School climate for transgender youth: A mixed method investigation of student experiences and school responses. *Journal of Youth and Adolescence, 39*(10), 1175–1188. https://doi.org/10.1007/s10964-010-9540-7.

Mitchell, C., Milne, E.-J., & de Lange, N. (2012). Introduction to *Handbook of participatory video*. In E.-J. Milne, C. Mitchell, & N. de Lange (Eds.), *Handbook of participatory video* (pp. 1–18). Lanham: AltaMira Press.

Mustanski, B., & Liu, R. T. (2013). A longitudinal study of predictors of suicide attempts among lesbian, gay, bisexual, and transgender youth. *Archives of Sexual Behavior, 42*(3), 437–448. https://doi.org/10.1007/s10508-012-0013-9.

Parr, H. (2007). Collaborative film-making as process, method and text in mental health research. *Cultural Geographies, 14*(1), 114–138. https://doi.org/10.1177/1474474007072822.

Pflum, S. R., Testa, R. J., Balsam, K. F., Goldblum, P. B., & Bongar, B. (2015). Social support, trans community connectedness, and mental health symptoms among transgender and gender nonconforming adults. *Psychology of Sexual Orientation and Gender Diversity, 2*(3), 281–286. https://doi.org/10.1037/sgd0000122.

Poteat, V. P., & Espelage, D. L. (2007). Predicting psychosocial consequences of homophobic victimization in middle school students. *The Journal of Early Adolescence, 27*(2), 175–191. https://doi.org/10.1177/0272431606294839.

Reisner, S. L., Greytak, E. A., Parsons, J. T., & Ybarra, M. L. (2015). Gender minority social stress in adolescence: Disparities in adolescent bullying and substance use by gender identity. *The Journal of Sex Research, 52*(3), 243–256. https://doi.org/10.1080/00224499.2014.886321.

Russell, S. T., Ryan, C., Toomey, R. B., Diaz, R. M., & Sanchez, J. (2011). Lesbian, gay, bisexual, and transgender adolescent school victimization: Implications for young adult health and adjustment. *Journal of School Health, 81*(5), 223–230. https://doi.org/10.1111/j.1746-1561.2011.00583.x.

Sánchez, F. J., & Vilain, E. (2009). Collective self-esteem as a coping resource for male-to-female transsexuals. *Journal of Counseling Psychology, 56*(1), 202–209. https://doi.org/10.1037/a0014573.

Schneider, S. K., O'Donnell, L., Stueve, A., & Coulter, R. W. S. (2012). Cyberbullying, school bullying, and psychological distress: A regional census of high school students. *American Journal of Public Health, 102*(1), 171–177. https://doi.org/10.2105/AJPH.2011.300308.

Singh, A. (2012). Transgender youth of color and resilience: Negotiating oppression and finding support. *Sex Roles, 68*(12), 690–702.

Singh, A. A., Meng, S. E., & Hansen, A. W. (2014). "I am my own gender": Resilience strategies of trans youth. *Journal of Counseling & Development, 92*(2), 208–218. https://doi.org/10.1002/j.1556-6676.2014.00150.x.

Solórzano, D. G., & Yosso, T. J. (2002). Critical race methodology: Counter-storytelling as an analytical framework for education research. *Qualitative Inquiry, 8*(1), 23–44.

Toomey, R. B., Ryan, C., Diaz, R. M., Card, N. A., & Russell, S. T. (2010). Gender-nonconforming lesbian, gay, bisexual, and transgender youth: School victimization and young adult psychosocial adjustment. *Developmental Psychology, 46*(6), 1580–1589. https://doi.org/10.1037/a0020705.

Toomey, R. B., Syvertsen, A. K., & Shramko, M. (2018). Transgender adolescent suicide behavior. *Pediatrics, 142*(4), 10.

Chapter 9
From Arts to Action: Project SHINE as a Case Study of Engaging Youth in Efforts to Develop Sustainable Water, Sanitation, and Hygiene Strategies in Rural Tanzania and India

Anise Gold-Watts, Marte Hovdenak, Aruna Ganesan, and Sheri Bastien

9.1 Arts-Based Engagement in Research: Project SHINE

Through creative and collaborative processes, arts-based methods have been used to varying degrees within health promotion research and evidence-based public health interventions (Delgado 2015; Israel et al. 2005; Leavy 2015; Chap. 1, this volume). Art is fundamentally communicative and expressive (Barone and Eisner 2012), thus capable of inciting collaboration, perspective, emotion, dialogue, and/or action. Studies have demonstrated that arts-based methods, when applied to research approaches, can be used to develop community partnerships, to manage sensitive issues, to involve community members in the interpretation of data, and as a dissemination tool to communicate knowledge and empower participants to catalyze change in their communities (Delgado 2015; Lambert and Hessler 2018; Lohan et al. 2015; McEwan et al. 2013; Vindrola-Padros et al. 2016). Additionally, arts-based methods hold the potential to promote communication beyond language and

A. Gold-Watts (✉)
Department of Public Health Science, Faculty of Landscape and Society, Norwegian University of Life Sciences, Ås, Norway
e-mail: anise.gold-watts@nmbu.no

M. Hovdenak
Department of Health Promotion and Development, University of Bergen, Bergen, Norway

A. Ganesan
Sri Narayani Vidyalaya School, Vellore, India

S. Bastien
Department of Public Health Science, Faculty of Landscape and Society, Norwegian University of Life Sciences, Ås, Norway

Department of Community Health Sciences, Cumming School of Medicine, University of Calgary, Calgary, AB, Canada

© The Author(s) 2021
J. H. Corbin et al. (eds.), *Arts and Health Promotion*,
https://doi.org/10.1007/978-3-030-56417-9_9

encourage close collaboration between academic researchers and community participants throughout the research process.

There are several different art forms often used in arts-based research, including the performing arts such as music, spoken word, and drama; visual arts such as painting, drawing, design, and crafts; community and cultural affairs such as festivals, fairs, and events; literature, poetry, and creative writing; and online, digital, or electronic arts (Cahnmann-Taylor and Siegesmund 2018; Delgado 2015; Lambert and Hessler 2018). These arts-based methods can be applied to research approaches in various ways (Coemans and Hannes 2017; Wang et al. 2017), thus reflections on the application and effects of arts-based methods are key in continuing to develop this field of research. The arts-based methods discussed in this chapter were used as tools of inquiry, awareness raising, adaptation, and knowledge translation. Knowledge translation is a process of contextualization and application (Campbell 2012; Graham et al. 2006), which according to the Canadian Institutes of Health Research promotes the "synthesis, dissemination, exchange, and ethically-sound application of knowledge" to improve health outcomes (Straus et al. 2009). Throughout this chapter, we will reflect on several distinct features of arts-based methods as (1) a tool for awareness raising, knowledge translation, and action and (2) a process of promoting meaningful and equitable partnerships in community-based participatory research (CBPR) within the frame of Project SHINE (Sanitation and Hygiene INnovation in Education) in India and Tanzania.

Implemented in two countries, Project SHINE is a school-based intervention that aims to improve water, sanitation, and hygiene (WASH)-related knowledge, attitudes, and behaviors among students, teachers, and local communities. In addition to supporting participatory approaches in the classroom, SHINE encourages youth to become health promoters and change-makers within their communities through the development of life and leadership skills. Unlike other WASH interventions that may employ techniques that promote "shame" or "social stigma" as a means for behavior change (Bartram et al. 2012; Kar and Chambers 2008; Pattanayak et al. 2009), Project SHINE uses an assets-based approach that incorporates CBPR and various arts-based methods throughout all phases of the research as a tool for awareness raising, knowledge translation, and action to promote meaningful engagement for participants and community members to result in synergy (for further background on the concept of synergy, see Chap. 21).

Throughout the intervention in Tanzania, art was used as a means to facilitate dialogue and promote knowledge-sharing and meaningful participant engagement. Arts-based health promotion activities such as open defecation mapping, a sanitation mural, a sanitation time capsule, digital stories, songs, and a sanitation science fair were incorporated throughout the intervention. These activities were used in formative research, implementation, and knowledge translation phases of the intervention and promoted participant inquiry and reflection, youth mobilization, and leadership focused on water, sanitation, and hygiene in the community.

During our adaptation to the southern Indian cultural context, the medium of photography was incorporated into the formative research phase through the CBPR process of photovoice. Here, we sought to develop a supportive research environment in which participants were positioned as experts and photography was used to stimulate knowledge production, participation, and co-learning (Wang and Burris 1997). This arts-based method enabled student participants to identify and represent (Wang et al. 1998) their communities and lived experiences in order to help us understand WASH-related contextual factors and facilitate the interpretation, adaption, and translation of Project SHINE to the local cultural context.

9.2 SHINE Tanzania: An Application of the Arts to Create a Broad Platform for Youth Expression and Engagement

SHINE Tanzania was developed and implemented in 2014 (see Fig. 9.1) as a pilot study to engage students in two secondary schools and the wider community in the development and evaluation of strategies to improve water, sanitation, and hygiene. The focus of the intervention was grounded in community concerns regarding the impact of parasitic infection on child health and from local hospital records, which indicated that fecal-oral transmitted diseases including helminth infections and protozoa are prevalent in the region. SHINE Tanzania was first implemented in a Maasai pastoralist community in the Ngorongoro Conservation Area (NCA) in rural and remote Tanzania. It was a collaboration between academic researchers and students from the University of Calgary, Canada, and the Catholic University of Health and Allied Sciences, Tanzania, as well as through a long-term partnership with communities of Maasai pastoralists in the NCA. The transdisciplinary research team included members with expertise in diverse fields—ranging from education, psychology, and anthropology to global health, veterinary medicine, and bioengineering—who work within a One Health paradigm (Zinsstag et al. 2011), which focuses on the interrelationships between humans, animals, and the environment. The study design has been described in full elsewhere (Bastien et al. 2016), as has the process and outcome evaluation of the intervention (Hetherington et al. 2017). In the intervention, a sequenced suite of participatory arts-based methods were used, including: open defecation mapping (9.2.1), a sanitation mural (9.2.3.1), a time capsule (9.2.3.2), songs, the capstone event of the sanitation science fair (9.2.2), and subsequent digital stories (9.2.3.3) to engage youth in reflecting on their experience with SHINE.

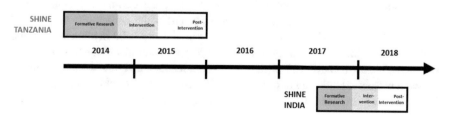

Fig. 9.1 Project SHINE timelines

9.2.1 Open Defecation Mapping

During the formative research phase, which involved qualitative research both in schools and in the wider community (see for instance Henderson et al. 2016), we wanted to engage youth in an icebreaker activity that would raise the potentially sensitive issue of open defecation in a non-threatening way. We refrained from asking about individual practices and instead asked about how the community and physical environment were structured and what common WASH practices were. This approach simultaneously contributed to our understanding of the broader community context and of WASH behaviors. Using poster paper and markers, we invited the students to draw a map of their village, indicating *bomas* (houses) where people and animals sleep, water sources, and places where animals and people commonly defecate. We then asked them a series of questions, such as what different water bodies are used for (washing clothes, drinking water for humans and livestock), what happens when it rains, if flies are common in the area, how they understand contamination, and what they perceive to be "safe" water. This led to a reflective discussion on health and how participants understand the causes of diarrheal disease. This exercise also provoked laughter among the students, who were at first tentative to draw on the paper but once they understood the purpose became animated and engaged.

9.2.2 Sanitation Science Fair—Culturally Relevant Knowledge Translation Strategies

The development and evaluation of the sanitation science fair has been described in detail elsewhere (Bastien et al. 2017); however, in brief, it was designed to engage and empower youth and communities in the development and evaluation of locally relevant and sustainable health promotion strategies to improve sanitation and hygiene. Student teams were separated into three broad categories (e.g., water, sanitation, and hygiene) and with the guidance of biology teachers and the research team developed sanitation science fair projects, which were showcased at a One Health sanitation science fair in November 2014. Approximately 400 Form 3 students participated from two secondary schools. Then, an evaluation team consisting of a broad cross-section of community members was tasked with identifying promising projects that were particularly relevant given the community context and which held potential for social entrepreneurship. The wider community was invited to attend the science fair, and there were between 500 and 1000 in attendance at the two schools, which included representatives of the Pastoralist Council (local government), local education authorities, traditional leaders, and out-of-school youth.

Each project included a knowledge translation component, which focused on the public health implications of the science fair project findings for the wider community. Through discussions with our local community partners regarding what would be culturally relevant techniques to transmit knowledge in the local Maasai context, students used approaches such as songs, which were an engaging means to involve students actively and reflexively in applying and translating what they had learned throughout the SHINE intervention to the wider community. One such example is a team of students that developed an experiment to test how many folds in a cloth were needed in order to filter water. Based on their findings, they developed a song to teach to women that could be sung while collecting water.

9.2.3 SHINE Arts-Based School and Community Event

As part of the knowledge translation activities post-intervention, a one-day event was organized at the school to engage youth and community members in a series of arts-based approaches to elicit perspectives on what participating in Project SHINE meant to them. The day was organized around a series of facilitated stations whereby youth, teachers, and community stakeholders—including the evaluation team from the sanitation science fair—circulated to each station to participate in an activity and contribute to broadening our understanding of the impact of the study from their perspective. The stations included: (1) posters with visuals developed by the Bachelor of Health Sciences students from the University of Calgary to depict the main findings of the study and to gather perspectives to help interpret the findings; (2) a sanitation mural whereby participants were invited to paint what their experience with SHINE meant to them; (3) a Foldscope station that provided another opportunity to prepare and look at locally collected samples of water, soil, and plants collected from the schoolyard; and (4) a digital storytelling station. Highlights from the selected facilitated stations are elaborated on below.

9.2.3.1 Sanitation Mural

The sanitation mural was used as a visual method through the project to elicit student perspectives on what participating in Project SHINE meant to them. We provided a white sheet and a selection of paints and brushes on a table and asked participants to illustrate by any means what their SHINE experience meant to them (Figs. 9.2 and 9.3). The canvas was ceremoniously initiated by a traditional leader and member of the SHINE evaluation team giving a speech and painting the first stroke. Students and the wider community used words, phrases, and pictures to highlight the essence of the project, and it was later showcased in the school and formed part of the time capsule. In discussion with students and teachers, it became clear that painting was not an activity they had engaged in previously, but one which they enjoyed tremendously.

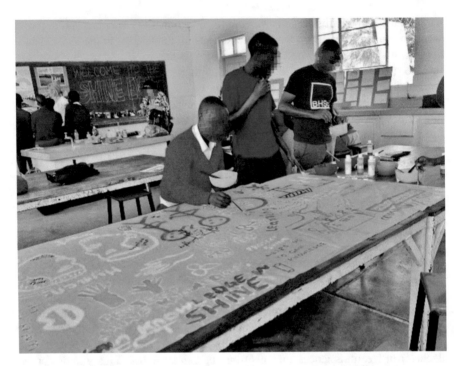

Fig. 9.2 Students and teachers collaborating on the development of a sanitation mural

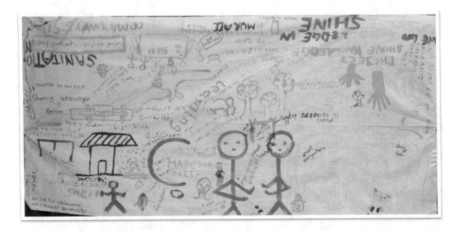

Fig. 9.3 Sanitation mural from SHINE Tanzania

9.2.3.2 Time Capsule

A time capsule is a historic cache of information or items that can be used both as a memory that participants can look back and reflect on at a later date and as a method of communicating with people in the future, to share perspectives, hopes, and dreams from an earlier time period. Within Project SHINE, this assignment was given in a civics class and framed as a means to get students to think about what they envision in the future for their community and the changes they might like to see in the next 5 years. The assignments consisted of a worksheet with a series of questions, including what their vision for a healthy Maasai community consisted of and what they perceived their role in achieving this to be. Prompts to guide the reflection included: access to clean water and toilets/latrines; food; access to a doctor/hospital/healer; and physical, social, and spiritual health. The worksheet also included a section where they could use the arts and draw their vision. The sheets were completed by SHINE participants and, together with the sanitation mural and science fair posters, were put into a container that was buried under the ground at the school. After 5 years have passed, the intention is that the Project SHINE time capsule will be opened, and the students and community will be able to discuss and reflect on the changes that have taken place.

9.2.3.3 Digital Stories

Storytelling is deeply engrained in Maasai culture, and in order to tap into this mode of expression to capture and convey what it meant to participants to be involved in the project, digital stories were created in partnership between the research team and participants. Digital storytelling permits participants to build narratives about their experiences through different mediums such as video, audio, imagery, music, or text (Lambert and Hessler 2018). It was explained to participants that we wanted to use a technique that was culturally relevant to the Maasai to share the SHINE story to the wider world, and that using visual means and digital stories might be a useful tool for reflecting and sharing participant experiences.

The photos that were taken of the sanitation science fair by students with disposable cameras were printed and shared with students. In addition, photos taken by the research team were included among the options students could select from for the digital stories, so that there was a wide range of photographs to choose from to represent participant memories and experiences. Storyboarding sessions were facilitated by members of the University of Calgary team with guiding questions to help students organize the sequence of photos and develop captions for the digital stories.

When this activity was completed, those who wished their experiences and reflections to be captured on film were taken to an adjacent room for filming. Upon their return to Canada, the University of Calgary students, with the assistance of a filmmaker, finalized the digital stories and stored and shared them on USB devices

with all participants and with the school as a token of appreciation for their participation in the study and to serve as a memory of the project. Although not all or even
most students are likely to have a computer on which they can view the photos, they
do have access to computers on the school premises, and the digital stories can be
shared with parents at school meetings.

9.3   Formative Research: Application of Photovoice in the Adaption of Project SHINE to an Indian Community

Throughout India, poor sanitation and hygiene is a widespread public health challenge. Indians account for one-third of the 2.3 billion people worldwide who do not
have access to improved sanitation in their home (World Health Organization and
UNICEF 2017), and this is a leading contributor to the diarrheal disease burden of
children under age five (Boschi-Pinto et al. 2008). Given India's vulnerability to
diarrheal disease and other sanitation-related challenges, solutions that incorporate
the country's social, cultural, and environmental context are in great demand.
Project SHINE was a relevant health promotion intervention that contributed to the
country's existing efforts to improve WASH-related health outcomes for communities. However, given India's rich cultural heritage and distinct historical legacy, a
rigorous adaptation and translation process from the Tanzanian context was needed.

SHINE India evolved from mutual interests in water, sanitation, and hygiene
conveyed by leadership from the locally based Sri Narayani Hospital and Research
Centre in Sripuram, Thirumalaikodi, and Dr. Bastien facilitated the partnership.
Once a partnership was formally established, an academic research team was
formed including doctoral and master students from Norwegian academic institutions (Norwegian University of Life Sciences and University of Bergen), local
schools, community stakeholders, and spiritual leadership. Implemented from June
2017–July 2018 in the rural community of Sripuram, Thirumalaikodi within the
Vellore District of Tamil Nadu (see Fig. 9.1 for timeline), in SHINE India, arts-
based research methods were incorporated into the study design as a critical component of the formative research phase and adaptation framework. The study protocol
was approved by the Norwegian Centre for Data Research (reference number:
53162) in Norway and the Institutional Ethics Committee/Institutional Review
Board at the Sri Narayani Hospital and Research Centre (reference number:
30/25/02/17) in India. As an initial step, a month-long photovoice sub-study was
conducted at a local school, which aimed to engage adolescent students in a group
process of critical reflection and dialogue to assist in the adaptation and translation
of the intervention to the local cultural context. Rooted in the tradition of documentary photography, photovoice provided adolescent students with cameras so that
they could accurately capture and share their community's assets, challenges, and
needs in relation to issues concerning water, sanitation, and hygiene (Wang and
Burris 1997). These photographs, accompanied by critical discussion and reflection,

helped inform changes to the SHINE India adaptation that was subsequently implemented in their school.

Artistic expression when applied to CBPR approaches can trigger discussions that facilitate the co-creation of knowledge between researcher and participant. Although there are several approaches that can develop a researcher's understanding of the cultural context, we felt that using an arts-based method not only could help co-create knowledge, but could also encourage and promote genuine partnerships, participation, and engagement through discussion and intimate sharing. In order to embark on this process, we needed to understand students' everyday lives. Figure 9.4 demonstrates how photovoice was utilized in the formative research and adaptation processes to help increase the cultural relevance, appropriateness, and appeal to student participants (Viswanathan et al. 2004).

9.3.1 Photovoice: An Effective and Engaging Tool for Adapting the SHINE Intervention

In the photovoice sub-study, a purposive sampling strategy was used to recruit participants. Here, the school principal and teachers recruited ten students (three boys and seven girls) aged 13–15 through classroom announcements and the distribution of project brochures. The research team, school principal, and a local project coordinator worked closely with participants throughout the sub-study. The project coordinator was a local schoolteacher and attended school with the students daily. She was also available to discuss any issues about the project if students were uncomfortable or unsure how to communicate with the principal investigator. The project coordinator was not present in photo discussion sessions (PDS) so that

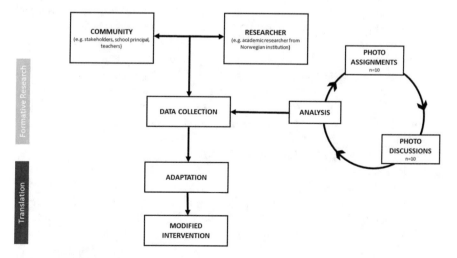

Fig. 9.4 Adaptation framework for Project SHINE India using arts-based method: Photovoice. (Adapted from McKleroy et al. 2006)

students would not associate the photo discussions with a school assignment and would be able to communicate freely. Additionally, the project coordinator had regular meetings with the school principal to provide updates on the photovoice substudy progress and student feedback.

Participants attended one information meeting, seven PDS, and one wrap-up meeting over a three-week period. They were formally introduced to the photovoice sub-study in the initial information meeting, which the local project coordinator cofacilitated with the principal investigator. The main purposes of this information meeting were (1) for participants to become acquainted with the photovoice process and method, and (2) to build rapport between the participants and the principal investigator prior to in-depth PDS. Participants were also taught about photography ethics (see Box 9.1), how data and identities would be protected throughout research activities, and how to obtain informed written consent when taking photographs of people. They also had the opportunity to ask questions in English or in their native language, Tamil.

Box 9.1 Photography Ethics: Implications and Procedures

Susan Sontag discusses ethical implications embedded within the artistic medium of photography when she describes the camera as "a tool of power" (Sontag 2001); therefore, the first photovoice training included a discussion on photography and ethics. The technical processes involved when taking photos can offer a "permanent record" (Price 1994) or an "authentic" visual representation of the photographer's reality (Ball and Smith 1992; Collier and Collier 1986). However, when viewing a photograph, an individual may interpret it or react to it differently than the photographer intended (Killion 2001). Consequently, it is important that both researchers and participants discuss and reflect upon the power of taking pictures before they mutually decide to engage in a photovoice project. Since visual content can be easily objectified when revealed without context (Cooper and Yarbrough 2010; Frosh 2001), SHINE India participants were encouraged to take photos and narrate experiences from their own everyday lives (Cooper and Yarbrough 2010). Also, in this project, we discussed the importance of "storytelling" or providing context when sharing photographs. Guided by a handout and a short exercise in which students went through an example, the photovoice facilitator (PI) modeled how contextual descriptions can complement a photograph (such as descriptions of what the picture conveys and why the photographer chose to take this photo) to prevent misunderstandings and/or other misconceptions (Frosh 2001; Sontag 2001). Additionally, participants were carefully instructed that informed written consent must be obtained anytime they took a photograph of a person's face or any other identifiable feature because visible identifiers can easily connect individuals to an image, which has several other ethical implications in research. These consent processes were established to protect both the individuals in photographs and the photographers themselves (student participants) from harm, thus preventing issues such as unwanted attention, involuntary participation, marginalization, embarrassment, or shame.

In this information meeting, participants were trained on how to use digital cameras. The group talked about their prior understanding of photography. Discussing the group's prior knowledge about the medium was an important step before distributing cameras, and it helped the facilitator structure the rest of the meeting based on the students' experience levels. Students expressed a major concern: is sanitation photogenic? The group had little to no experience using a camera, so we showed the group examples related to different research questions to help them conceptualize future assignments. During an explanation on the photovoice method, students browsed *Visual Voices: 100 Photographs of Village China by the Women of Yunnan Province* (Wu 1996) to see examples of photos from another photovoice project in China. After flipping through the book and seeing the different ways that these women photographed their community, students felt reassured and excited for the first photo assignment. It is important to consider that many students will reference advertisements or portraiture as the types of photographs that are customary in their environment. Here, it was crucial to bring examples of other ways to take photographs that illustrate reality or everyday life (e.g., newspaper clippings, postcards, books) so that students could see examples of different types of photography. We also discussed how to take photographs and photo aesthetics such as lighting, focus, and composition.

Once participants indicated that they understood the process, the first PDS were scheduled, and participants separated into single-sex groups to ensure that they were comfortable when talking about sensitive topics in front of their peers. After each photo assignment, each group would come together to share their photographs. All PDS followed the same procedure in both male and female groups; however, since the groups were conducted separately, the photo assignments generated differed. It is also important to note that participants were included and involved in the research question development processes, helping to ensure that the study genuinely addressed community-identified needs and interests.

Prior to each PDS, participants would select one or two photographs that they had taken for that day's photo assignment that they would like to share with the group. When the session started, each participant would share their selected photographs with the group. After all participants had shared their photographs, the entire group would vote on one photograph to discuss in depth.

To facilitate these in-depth discussions, we used an inductive mneumonic questioning technique known as the SHOWED method (questions include: what do you **See**; what is **Happening**; how does this relate to **Our** lives; **Why** does this situation/ strength exist; how can we become **Empowered** by our new understanding; what can we **Do**?) (Shaffer 1985). This method is based on Freirean processes of listening, dialogue, and action (Freire 1973, 2000) that were used to "trigger" critical dialogue and reflection (Wallerstein 1994). During discussions, the initial questions elicited critical dialogue first through description (See, Happening), then personalization (Our), while subsequent questions probed further critical analysis (Why), problem-posing (Empowered), and action (Do) (Wallerstein 1994).

It can be argued that the central focus of these discussions was not the photographs themselves, but the critical dialogue that ensued. For example, in one PDS a

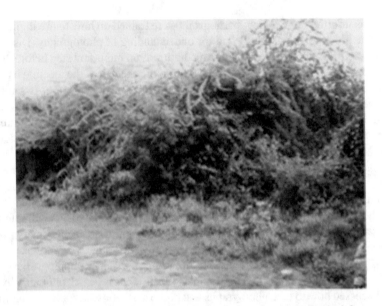

Fig. 9.5 Photovoice assignment 4: What habits do people have that are not hygienic?

participant shared a photograph (see Fig. 9.5) of a bush plant which generated an in-depth discussion about hygiene habits such as waste disposal and traditional health practices. Participants explained how this bush plant was not beneficial for their community because it grew thorns, produced no food, and did not have any medicinal value; therefore, people would dump waste on or around it. Then students began to discuss strategies for improving the community. For example, they spoke about how they could cut down the bush to prepare the land for planting medicinal herbs. This would perhaps sway people's attitudes about dumping their waste there.

9.3.2 Shared Power: From Critical Dialogue to Action

From the PDS, the academic research team identified key themes and applied them to a blend of adaptation frameworks traditionally used to translate evidence-based health promotion interventions such as Intervention Mapping (Bartholomew et al. 1998) and the Map of Adaptation Process (McKleroy et al. 2006). Using the photovoice data, these frameworks guided the intervention adaptation and knowledge translation of the SHINE school curriculum from Tanzania to the Indian cultural context. For example, students' photographs and discussions often revealed the cultural importance and sacredness of the natural/ecological environment, environmental sanitation, and waste management, which helped inform the translation of specific lessons in the SHINE Tanzania curriculum to have a more explicit focus on environmental sanitation and the natural environment for SHINE India. The adapted curriculum with the input from the photovoice sub-study was disseminated to over

300 students in two schools in the SHINE India intervention in the local community of Sripuram, Thirumalaikodi.

9.3.2.1 Project SHINE India Adaptation

The main outcome of the photovoice project was to make changes in the SHINE India curriculum. Throughout India, many people do not use toilets and instead defecate out in the open because toilets are considered dirty and it is seen as defiling to clean an impure space (Lüthi 2010) such as a toilet. Students suggested in the PDS that they could help with cleaning and other household chores, therefore transforming social norms. According to social cognitive theory, social modeling is a powerful method of health behavior change (Bandura 1998; Glanz et al. 2008). Inspired by photovoice student participants, we decided to include a lesson in the intervention that included proper hygienic practices such as cleaning toilets and reusing waste.

9.3.2.2 Photovoice Photograph Exhibition

Similar to SHINE Tanzania, as part of the main intervention, students and teachers held a sanitation science fair where they came up with projects related to water, sanitation, and hygiene. Many students constructed models and performed demonstrations for their science fair projects. Parents, community members, and students from other classes were invited to tour the projects. In addition to the science fair, photovoice students decided that they would like to include their photographs in a display. This small photo exhibition was suggested by the local project coordinator and discussed during the final group meeting. Students saw an exhibition as an opportunity to display their work to their peers and community as well as promote awareness about key issues discussed during the project. The gallery of photographs and captions was displayed outside the sanitation science fair so that all attendees could view it before they entered the main exhibition.

9.4 Reflections, Considerations, and Lessons Learned

As arts-based research methods gain momentum, academic researchers and practitioners must also engage in continuous processes of self-reflection and self-evaluation (Minkler 2005; Minkler and Wallerstein 2003). Although these methods exhibit the potential to communicate and elicit discussion beyond traditional research praxis through various data collection and knowledge translation methods, we must also reflect on further methodological and epistemological limitations. Each SHINE intervention was implemented within distinct social, cultural, and environmental settings and populations. The following reflections illustrate the similarities and differences across these contexts while simultaneously unpacking the methodological dilemmas and experiences in practice concerning participant engagement, community partnerships, power, and empowerment.

9.4.1 Meaningful Processes of Participant Engagement in Participatory Arts-Based Research

Ensuring meaningful participant engagement was essential throughout both the formative research and implementation phases of both SHINE interventions. The inclusion of arts-based methods within SHINE contributed to broader and more authentic engagement of participants and community members because of the methods' capacity for equitable participation that encourages personal expression and sharing of one's lived experiences (Finley 2008). Often, this type of engagement contributed to critical reflection processes that addressed sensitive or stigmatized concerns (Switzer et al. 2015) and acted as an entry point for participants to engage in discussions concerning potentially sensitive health issues, such as open defecation and its effects on community health. Additionally, in the SHINE photovoice, students shared photographs of their everyday lives and spoke openly about their personal experiences with hygiene-related illnesses and disease in their community, thus contributing to the depth and richness of our understanding of the contextual setting. Moreover, in many instances, arts-based methods such as the sanitation mural in Tanzania facilitated an open dialogue and ensured that participant experiences and expertise remained at the center of the inquiry, while also helping balance power dynamics by providing opportunities for participants to share their perspectives in a way that resonates and is most relevant to their culture and context. However, engaging with arts-based methods is not without challenges, and upon reflection of our own positionalities and experiences, it is important to acknowledge and deconstruct the complexities of employing arts-based methods in health promotion research.

In both settings, a foundational component of the project was the collaborative efforts put forth by academic researcher-community partnerships; therefore, stakeholder inclusion in all phases of research was fundamental to the SHINE approach. While participatory arts-based methods were incorporated throughout the project to encourage authentic participation and equitable partnerships, we also collaborated with students, teachers, and the wider community beyond these methods in various forums such as think tanks, workshops, and focus groups in which participants, stakeholders, and researchers met and exchanged knowledge. In Tanzania, a think tank approach to engaging community stakeholders at the local hospital, schools, and wider community included traditional leaders, traditional birth attendants, out-of-school youth, and parents in all phases of the piloting of SHINE, which supported equitable participation and community ownership of the intervention. While think tanks generated a space for community participants to articulate potential concerns about the intervention at each stage, the platform also encouraged the development of community-driven mitigation strategies, thus exemplifying co-learning processes between academic researchers and community collaborators in which local knowledge and skill helped navigate challenges and structures that the research team might lack. Additionally, the evaluation teams for the sanitation science fairs, which consisted of a broad spectrum of community stakeholders, were highly engaged in the process of selecting culturally relevant strategies for improving WASH and subsequently served as an advisory board for the project. Their participation constitutes another means whereby the project incorporated a diverse cross-section of stakeholders with an aim to contribute to the overall sustainability of the project.

Although Project SHINE was deeply committed to developing equitable partnerships, it is also important to consider that systems of oppression, structural hierarchies, and power imbalances exist at the local community level, which may influence community-researcher partnerships. In India, although we held regular meetings with community stakeholders/gatekeepers who were involved with the local community-based organizations, hospitals, schools, and spiritual leadership, it is important to acknowledge that while diverse in their position and expertise, our collaborating partners do not represent all voices within the community. Although we may envision comprehensive community participation and representativeness, it may not be feasible within a complex community structure. Stakeholders can represent and communicate many concerns; however, we must not assume they are able to represent the entire community (Wallerstein and Duran 2006). The community is composed of a multitude of voices, and stakeholders/gatekeepers may not adequately represent certain segments of a community, such as the elderly and other hard-to-reach groups. Although we hoped to include the community in shaping the research project in order to ensure that the project addressed community-identified needs, it is important to recognize and reflect upon how each community has dynamic and complex historical, political, and cultural forces that shape knowledge and power. In SHINE India, community members such as parents and local elders were not directly involved in our formal stakeholder engagement process, though we did attempt to ameliorate this with informal interactions throughout our daily activities in the community. Sripuram, Thirumalaikodi is a community with a strong spiritual legacy, and engaging in this aspect of community life was central to our own investment in the partnership. This included daily participation in *puja* and regular participation in *seva* activities. We also chose to wear locally appropriate clothing and follow cultural norms and rituals regarding traditional activities. Participation in these activities was essential to showing our commitment and engagement in the community. However, formalized stakeholder meetings were especially important arenas of knowledge exchange, allowing us to report on current project activities and receive feedback on our progress. As these formal processes failed to reach certain segments of the community, such as the elderly or parents, we felt it was essential for the research team to build relationships outside of formalized space. To do so, we attended temple daily, attended school-based and religious or cultural celebrations, and greeted parents in the schoolyard to foster further engagement, trust, and mutual respect with community members.

9.4.2 The Potential for Arts-Based Methods as a Tool for Empowerment and Catalyst for Social Change

One of the main aims of Project SHINE has been to encourage youth through the development of life and leadership skills. Powerlessness is a social determinant of health, and thus empowerment is essential to improving health outcomes. The World Health Organization (WHO) distinguishes between individual and community empowerment, defining individual empowerment in terms of an ability to make decisions and control one's personal life, while community empowerment is defined as collective action to "gain influence and control over the determinants of health and the quality of life in their community" (World Health Organization 1998). The goals of Project SHINE are both to aid in the participants developing life skills that lead to greater autonomy over their own health, and also to help them develop leadership skills that allow them to take part in leadership and civic engagement activities in the long term. With arts-based methods such as photovoice, time capsules, and murals, SHINE aimed to create a participatory platform that would foster engagement, ownership, and self-determination among the participants, which in turn would encourage the development of various life skills as well as self-confidence in their role as change makers in their communities (Wilson et al. 2007).

Project SHINE was developed as a CBPR project that creates a platform for data collection, art, and youth empowerment. Nevertheless, we should not assume that participation is inevitably empowering for the participants or co-collaborators, especially given the social structures surrounding youth participants. Action is a foundational component of CBPR, with participants engaging with stakeholders, gatekeepers, and policymakers to create social change. However, Strack et al. (2004) state that it is important to bear in mind that arts-based methods such as photovoice are a "process," and empowerment may not be completely realized by participants by the conclusion of a project or research study. Empowerment is a personal journey and likely a lifelong project for most people, and thus cannot be reduced to a simple measurable outcome of participation in a year-long study. Therefore, it is important to understand the value of processes of reflection and dialogue as crucial first steps in personal growth processes that lead to mobilization and empowerment, especially when working with youth who are undergoing intense experiences of personal growth and change (Strack et al. 2004).

While photovoice and other CBPR methods encourage participants to make contact with policymakers to create change in their communities, this may not always be a realistic goal, and a singular focus on this can be discouraging for the long-term success of a project (Johnston 2016). Both SHINE interventions were implemented in settings that had distinct social structures. In India, hierarchical social structures that value seniority shape systems and cultural norms that influence how youth are perceived, seen, and heard. In this context, social structures may also prevent students from having access to power within society. This leads to a question: to what extent can youth participants share their "voice"? In many countries around the world, youth are unable to vote or participate in civic organizations without consent from an adult. Even to participate in Project SHINE, all students needed to obtain parental consent. As we managed goals and expectations of the project, we also acknowledged that adolescents often must act through proxy and reflected upon local systems of power and processes of empowerment. However, this is not to suggest that empowerment cannot be achieved through skills development and feelings of self-confidence and self-worth; rather, it is to remind us that researchers must acknowledge potential benefits and limitations of methods in order to effectively facilitate and support project participants. Additionally, researchers engaged in arts-based CBPR research should be cautious when raising expectations of project participants. In the SHINE PDS, participants brainstormed solutions for identified challenges without limitations, such as a discussion on potential sanitation enforcement strategies that are punishable by fines, or imprisonment for individuals who are seen dumping waste in the community's water sources. However, society, power structures, corruption, and resources may limit participant control of everyday life and their abilities to implement such strategies.

9.4.3   Tapping the Potential of Arts-Based Methods for Unlocking the Creativity and Curiosity of Youth in Health Promotion Interventions

Arts-based methods were also integrated into SHINE to provide a platform for youth as social actors, future educators, scientists, and leaders and to enable them to express themselves in diverse ways that would resonate with their culture and context. The linguistic complexity of the setting was one factor in adopting a participatory arts-based method within the project. Although English is the language of instruction at secondary schools in Tanzania, as well as in our partner schools in India, it is not the participants' first language in either setting. Moreover, given the strong community focus within the project, the predominately oral culture among Maasai pastoralists, and potentially low literacy levels, including a more diverse spectrum of possibilities for expression within the project was important in terms of inclusion of diverse perspectives and modes of expression, as well as ensuring a broader reach and overall sustainability of the project.

We found students to be positively engaged in this component of the project, and it was frequently mentioned that they lacked a similar creative outlet within their school setting. Community members reflected that it was important that the knowledge created as part of the project be shared beyond the walls of the classroom and spread to the wider community, speaking to the potential of arts-based methods in health promotion to span the divide that often exists between schools and communities. Teachers similarly expressed appreciation for the inclusion of arts-based methods in the project, yet discussion indicated that within the national curriculum there is insufficient focus and space devoted to the arts. Similarly, the inclusion of arts such as dance and theater in SHINE India's knowledge translation and dissemination activities resonated with the local culture, where such performing arts are a common part of community life. After the photovoice sub-study, three students wrote and directed a short skit about the importance of water (a key takeaway from the photo discussion sessions and a community-identified health concern), while other students choreographed a dance about handwashing (see Fig. 9.6). Participants expressed that they felt happy sharing their knowledge and experiences with their peers through art.

9.4.4 Can Arts-Based Methods Alleviate Power Imbalances?

Power imbalances can exist within community-researcher, young-elder, and other superior-subordinate relationships that are replicated and reinforced by history, politics, culture, and tradition (Muhammad et al. 2015). In many ways, the inclusion of arts-based methods in Project SHINE was intended to mitigate power differentials in the research process. As mentioned above, the SHINE Tanzania intervention was implemented in a context of considerable linguistic complexity. The incorporation of arts-based methods was crucial to giving a broad and diverse platform for youth expression. Additionally, literacy levels among both students and community members could not be assured; therefore, providing a medium that nurtured personal expression and sharing was essential for equitable engagement.

However, despite efforts to minimize power differentials, we acknowledge several difficulties of establishing truly equitable partnerships. In the SHINE India project, the photovoice process aims to overcome imbalances in power in the relationship between participant and researcher; however, this is especially difficult when working with youth in a setting where distinct social structures are prominent. To overcome this, we tried to develop a supportive environment where we could learn together, with participants and their experiences as the focal point of all interactions. Although we had certain time constraints, we focused on building rapport and allowing space in all our conversations with participants for questions and debate. We discussed the participants' roles as co-researchers and the instrumentality of

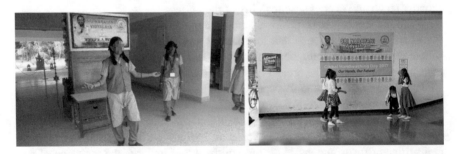

Fig. 9.6 Students in SHINE India engage in performing arts to teach peers about the importance of water (left) and handwashing (right)

their experiences and concerns to the development of the research project. Through looking at the photographs and discussing the various issues they identified within their community, we started to develop new knowledge and understanding of the local context together. The cultural significance of the natural environment quickly emerged as important to the participants, alongside concerns about generational divides regarding the importance of ecological preservation. Exploring these ideas and concerns was essential to the adaptation of the SHINE curriculum to the Indian context. We continuously tried to communicate the implications and impact of the research and the importance of the participants' involvement. However, power imbalances between participants also posed a challenge to the equitability of the PDS experience. Janes (2016) discusses how in some ways CBPR can preserve power differentials in community-researcher partnerships despite the approach's claims to prevent and/or mitigate oppressive research practices. As only one photo is selected and discussed, dominant members of the group can end up controlling the direction of the discussion, and certain participants may not have their voices heard, potentially resulting in antagony (for background on this issue, see Chap. 21, this volume). To prevent this, we selected the photo for discussion through an anonymous vote and developed group norms aimed at creating an open, inclusive, and supportive environment in which everyone felt comfortable expressing their opinions during the initial photovoice meeting.

Through the application of a CBPR approach, the research project brought academic researchers, communities, and students together to exchange knowledge and disseminate findings. However, a research project developed with the intention to encourage equitable partnerships can also contribute to the very power dynamics it seeks to disrupt (Janes 2016). We hope to expose additional tensions related to power within this type of work to encourage a push toward more reflexive and transparent research praxis. As we build meaningful partnerships with community collaborators, it is crucial that we try to understand how research skills are applied in the local context, so these skills and capacity can be leveraged outside the research project to ensure that the project is mutually beneficial throughout the entirety of the research process. In Project SHINE, although participants were excited about the intervention itself, we experienced difficulties recruiting community collaborators to contribute to the academic writing processes (i.e., we have not been able to reach a teacher who was deeply involved in implementing SHINE Tanzania to co-author this chapter). Mindful of the potential threat of tokenism (Arnstein 1969)—which would consist of merely including names to give the appearance that we engaged the community—we used this opportunity to reflect and learn more about local ways of communicating and disseminating information, which often included visual and performing arts such as theater, song, and dance (described in previous sections). As collaborative partners, we should also explore alternative methods of dissemination, since academic publications may not represent "currency" to local counterparts or be accessible to collaborating communities. By limiting knowledge translation to the confines of academic tradition, we sustain the power and privilege of academics and diminish inclusive and equitable practices of the CBPR approach. Therefore, it is necessary to critically reflect on such challenges and limitations in an attempt to build the academic researcher's capacity to become more adept in understanding alternative communication methods and knowledge translation.

9.5 Conclusion

In Project SHINE, arts-based methods were used at various stages of the intervention to engage youth, teachers, and the wider community not only in the development of culturally relevant and sustainable strategies to improve water, sanitation, and hygiene, but also more broadly to promote youth leadership and to provide an additional avenue or platform for expression within the project. This demonstrates how arts-based methods can be integrated into health promotion interventions to increase authentic engagement, encourage empowerment processes, increase understanding, translate knowledge, and aid in knowledge translation to the wider community. However, from a methodological standpoint, systematic and thoughtful inclusion of arts-based methods at all phases of the research—alongside more traditional methods such as in-depth interviews, focus group discussions, and surveys—is a promising strategy for meaningfully engaging youth and communities and enhancing triangulation within a study. The use of arts-based methods also allowed the researchers to gain a deeper understanding of the cultural contexts we were working in through engaging with personal and communal forms of artistic expression and encouraging active listening and continuing reflection throughout the process. In many ways, the incorporation of the arts was a continuous organic process which made it challenging to evaluate their effect and impact. Therefore, we recommend that similar interventions aiming to reach youth should systematically plan and sequence the incorporation of arts-based methods into an evaluation. This would help further strengthen legitimacy of methods and allow for effective and systematic evaluation of processes and outcomes.

Although each SHINE intervention incorporated different arts-based research methods during different phases of research to help achieve research project objectives under a CBPR frame, future iterations would need to develop meaningful indicators and apply systematic evaluation frameworks in order to realize the full potential of arts-based methods when applied to research. However, throughout these two interventions, we witnessed participants sharing their personal insights, reflections, and experiences through creative expression, which—despite criticisms of voice, power, and empowerment—did inspire a sense of responsibility to the community and improve our understanding of the health issues that were important to the community. Moreover, the inclusion of arts-based methods has fostered alternative methods of knowledge translation that markedly challenge us as academic researchers to disrupt and critique traditional academic praxis and work toward more equitable and creative approaches in future projects. Although the use of methods differed, their inclusion led to unique partnership engagement, knowledge sharing, and learning, demonstrating how these methods can be utilized in health interventions as a tool for education, knowledge translation, and action.

Acknowledgements Grand Challenges Canada (Tanzania) and CINIM (India) funded this project.

We would like to thank all the schools, teachers, students, and community stakeholders in the Tanzanian and Indian communities who participated and contributed to this research project. In addition, we would like to acknowledge the contributions and support of Erika Laurel Friebe and "Godwin" Saningo Olemshumba (SHINE Tanzania) and Ramesh Shanmugasundaram, Nathalie Latham, Balaji Nandagopal, Sri Sakthi Amma, and photovoice participants (SHINE India).

References

Arnstein, S. R. (1969). A ladder of citizen participation. *Journal of the American Institute of Planners, 35*(4), 216–224.

Ball, M. S., & Smith, G. W. (1992). *Analyzing visual data*. Thousand Oaks: Sage Publications.

Bandura, A. (1998). Health promotion from the perspective of social cognitive theory. *Psychology and Health, 13*(4), 623–649.

Barone, T., & Eisner, E. W. (2012). *Arts based research*. Thousand Oaks: Sage Publications.

Bartholomew, L. K., Parcel, G. S., & Kok, G. (1998). Intervention mapping: A process for developing theory and evidence-based health education programs. *Health Education & Behavior, 25*(5), 545–563.

Bartram, J., Charles, K., Evans, B., O'hanlon, L., & Pedley, S. (2012). Commentary on community-led total sanitation and human rights: Should the right to community-wide health be won at the cost of individual rights? *Journal of Water and Health, 10*(4), 499–503.

Bastien, S., Hetherington, E., Hatfield, J., Kutz, S., & Manyama, M. (2016). Youth-driven innovation in sanitation solutions for Maasai pastoralists in Tanzania: Conceptual framework and study design. *Global Journal of Health Education and Promotion, 17*(1).

Bastien, S., Hetherington, E., Williams, K., Hatfield, J., & Manyama, M. (2017). The development of an innovative one health sanitation science fair to cultivate change agent capacity among pastoralist youth in rural Tanzania. In S. Bastien & H. Holmarsdottir (Eds.), *Youth as architects of social change* (pp. 77–95). Cham: Palgrave Macmillan.

Boschi-Pinto, C., Velebit, L., & Shibuya, K. (2008). Estimating child mortality due to diarrhoea in developing countries. *Bulletin of the World Health Organization, 86*, 710–717.

Cahnmann-Taylor, M., & Siegesmund, R. (Eds.). (2018). *Arts-based research in education: Foundations for practice*. New York: Routledge.

Campbell, S. (2012). *Knowledge translation curriculum*. Ottawa: Canadian Coalition for Global Health Research.

Coemans, S., & Hannes, K. (2017). Researchers under the spell of the arts: Two decades of using arts-based methods in community-based inquiry with vulnerable populations. *Educational Research Review, 22*, 34–49. https://doi.org/10.1016/j.edurev.2017.08.003.

Collier, J., & Collier, M. (1986). *Visual anthropology: Photography as a research method*. Albuquerque: University of New Mexico Press.

Cooper, C. M., & Yarbrough, S. P. (2010). Tell me—Show me: Using combined focus group and photovoice methods to gain understanding of health issues in rural Guatemala. *Qualitative Health Research, 20*(5), 644–653.

Delgado, M. (2015). *Urban youth and photovoice: Visual ethnography in action*. New York: Oxford University Press.

Finley, S. (2008). Arts-based research. In *Handbook of the arts in qualitative research: Perspectives, methodologies, examples, and issues* (pp. 71–81). Thousand Oaks, CA: SAGE Publications.

Freire, P. (1973). *Education for critical consciousness*. London: Bloomsbury.

Freire, P. (2000). *Pedagogy of the oppressed*. New York: Continuum.

Frosh, P. (2001). The public eye and the citizen-voyeur: Photography as a performance of power. *Social Semiotics, 11*(1), 43–59.

Glanz, K., Rimer, B. K., & Viswanath, K. (2008). *Health behavior and health education: Theory, research, and practice*. San Francisco: Jossey-Bass.

Graham, I. D., Logan, J., Harrison, M. B., Straus, S. E., Tetroe, J., Caswell, W., et al. (2006). Lost in knowledge translation: Time for a map? *Journal of Continuing Education in the Health Professions, 26*(1), 13–24.

Henderson, R. I., Hatfield, J., Kutz, S., Olemshumba, S., Van Der Meer, F., Manyama, M., et al. (2016). 'We can't get worms from cow dung': Reported knowledge of parasitism among pastoralist youth attending secondary school in the Ngorongoro Conservation Area, Tanzania. *Journal of Biosocial Science, 48*(6), 746–766.

Hetherington, E., Eggers, M., Wamoyi, J., Hatfield, J., Manyama, M., Kutz, S., et al. (2017). Participatory science and innovation for improved sanitation and hygiene: Process and outcome evaluation of project SHINE, a school-based intervention in rural Tanzania. *BMC Public Health, 17*(1), 172.

Israel, B., Eng, E., Schultz, A., & Parker, E. (2005). *Methods in community-based participatory research for health*. San Francisco: Jossey-Bass.

Janes, J. E. (2016). Democratic encounters? Epistemic privilege, power, and community-based participatory action research. *Action Research, 14*(1), 72–87.

Johnston, G. (2016). Champions for social change: Photovoice ethics in practice and 'false hopes' for policy and social change. *Global Public Health, 11*(5–6), 799–811.

Kar, K., & Chambers, R. (2008). *Handbook on community-led total sanitation*. Brighton: Institute of Development Studies, University of Sussex; http://www.communityledtotalsanitation.org/resource/handbook-community-led-total-sanitation. Accessed 10 June 2020.

Killion, C. M. (2001). Understanding cultural aspects of health through photography. *Nursing Outlook, 49*(1), 50–54.

Lambert, J., & Hessler, H. B. (2018). *Digital storytelling: Capturing lives, creating community*. New York: Routledge.

Leavy, P. (2015). *Method meets art: Arts-based research practice*. New York: Guilford Publications.

Lohan, M., Aventin, Á., Oliffe, J. L., Han, C. S., & Bottorff, J. L. (2015). Knowledge translation in men's health research: Development and delivery of content for use online. *Journal of Medical Internet Research, 17*(1).

Lüthi, D. (2010). Private cleanliness, public mess: Purity, pollution and space in Kottar, South India. In E. Dürr & R. Jaffe (Eds.), *Urban pollution: Cultural meanings, social practices* (pp. 57–85). New York: Berghahn Books.

McEwan, A., Crouch, A., Robertson, H., & Fagan, P. (2013). The Torres indigenous hip hop project: Evaluating the use of performing arts as a medium for sexual health promotion. *Health Promotion Journal of Australia, 24*(2), 132–136.

McKleroy, V. S., Galbraith, J. S., Cummings, B., Jones, P., Harshbarger, C., Collins, C., et al. (2006). Adapting evidence-based behavioral interventions for new settings and target populations. *AIDS Education and Prevention, 18*(4), 59–73. https://doi.org/10.1521/aeap.2006.18.supp.59.

Minkler, M. (2005). Community-based research partnerships: Challenges and opportunities. *Journal of Urban Health, 82*(2), ii3–ii12.

Minkler, M., & Wallerstein, N. (Eds.). (2003). *Community based participatory research for health*. San Francisco: Jossey-Bass.

Muhammad, M., Wallerstein, N., Sussman, A. L., Avila, M., Belone, L., & Duran, B. J. C. S. (2015). Reflections on researcher identity and power: The impact of positionality on community based participatory research (CBPR) processes and outcomes. *Critical Sociology, 41*(7–8), 1045–1063. https://doi.org/10.1177/0896920513516025.

Pattanayak, S. K., Yang, J.-C., Dickinson, K. L., Poulos, C., Patil, S. R., Mallick, R. K., et al. (2009). Shame or subsidy revisited: Social mobilization for sanitation in Orissa, India. *Bulletin of the World Health Organization, 87*(8), 580–587.

Price, M. (1994). *The photograph: A strange confined space*. Palo Alto: Stanford University Press.

Shaffer, R. (1985). *Beyond the dispensary*. Nairobi: African Medical and Research Foundation.

Sontag, S. (2001). *On photography*. New York: Macmillan.

Strack, R. W., Magill, C., & McDonagh, K. (2004). Engaging youth through photovoice. *Health Promotion Practice, 5*(1), 49–58.

Straus, S. E., Tetroe, J., & Graham, I. (2009). Defining knowledge translation. *CMAJ, 181*(3–4), 165–168.

Switzer, S., Guta, A., de Prinse, K., Carusone, S. C., & Strike, C. (2015). Visualizing harm reduction: Methodological and ethical considerations. *Social Science & Medicine, 133*(SI), 77–84.

Vindrola-Padros, C., Martins, A., Coyne, I., Bryan, G., & Gibson, F. (2016). From informed consent to dissemination: Using participatory visual methods with young people with long-term conditions at different stages of research. *Global Public Health, 11*(5–6), 636–650.

Viswanathan, M., Ammerman, A., Eng, E., Gartlehner, G., Lohr, K. N., Griffith, D., et al. (2004). *Community-based participatory research: Assessing the evidence: Summary. AHRQ evidence report summaries* (pp. 1–8). Rockville: Agency for Healthcare Research and Quality.

Wallerstein, N. (1994). Empowerment education applied to youth. *Multicultural Challenge in Health Education*, 161–162.

Wallerstein, N., & Duran, B. (2006). Using community-based participatory research to address health disparities. *Health Promotion Practice, 7*(3), 312–323.

Wang, C., & Burris, M. A. (1997). Photovoice: Concept, methodology, and use for participatory needs assessment. *Health Education & Behavior, 24*(3), 369–387.

Wang, C., Yi, W. K., Tao, Z. W., & Carovano, K. (1998). Photovoice as a participatory health promotion strategy. *Health Promotion International, 13*(1), 75–86.

Wang, Q., Coemans, S., Siegesmund, R., & Hannes, K. (2017). Arts-based methods in socially engaged research practice: A classification framework. *Art/Research International: A Transdisciplinary Journal, 2*(2), 5–39.

Wilson, N., Dasho, S., Martin, A. C., Wallerstein, N., Wang, C. C., & Minkler, M. (2007). Engaging young adolescents in social action through Photovoice—The youth empowerment strategies (YES!) project. *Journal of Early Adolescence, 27*(2), 241–261. https://doi.org/10.1177/0272431606294834.

World Health Organization. (1998). *Health promotion glossary*. https://www.who.int/healthpromotion/about/HPR%20Glossary%201998.pdf?ua=1. Accessed 10 June 2020.

World Health Organization, & UNICEF. (2017). *Progress on sanitation and drinking water: 2017 update and SDG baselines*.

Wu, K. (1996). *Visual voices: 100 photographs of village China by the women of Yunnan Province*. Yunnan: Yunnan People's Publishing House.

Zinsstag, J., Schelling, E., Waltner-Toews, D., & Tanner, M. (2011). From "one medicine" to "one health" and systemic approaches to health and well-being. *Preventive Veterinary Medicine, 101*(3–4), 148–156.

Chapter 10
Photovoice for Health Promotion Research, Empowerment, and Advocacy: Young Refugee Stories from Turkey

Ozge Karadag Caman

10.1 Introduction

Forced migration is one of the most significant consequences of man-made and natural disasters throughout history. Today, millions of people are forced from their homes by war, persecution, and poverty, driving a global migration crisis (UN 2018). Factors such as poverty, unhealthy living conditions, and lack of nutritious food—in addition to poor access to health care, social care, education, and employment opportunities—cause forced migrants (e.g., refugees and asylum seekers) to be among the most vulnerable groups with respect to health (Karadag Caman and Altintas 2010).

The United Nations Convention Relating to the Status of Refugees (1951) defines a refugee as "a person who owing to a well-founded fear of being persecuted for reasons of race, religion, nationality, membership of a particular social group or political opinion, is outside the country of his nationality and is unable or, owing to such fear, is unwilling to avail himself of the protection of that country; or who, not having a nationality and being outside the country of his former habitual residence as a result of such events, is unable or, owing to such fear, is unwilling to return to it" (UNHCR 1951). The United Nations High Commission for Refugees (UNHCR) has called the Syrian emergency "the biggest humanitarian and refugee crisis of our time." Since the start of the conflict in Syria, an estimated 6.6 million persons have been displaced inside the country and an additional 5.6 million persons have fled to other countries. More than 90% of people fleeing Syria have sought asylum in three countries: Turkey, Lebanon, and Jordan (UNHCR 2019). According to the World Migration Report (2018) of the International Organization for Migration (IOM), Turkey has the highest number of refugees in the world (3.6 million), with the

O. Karadag Caman (✉)
Center for Sustainable Development, Earth Institute, Columbia University, New York, NY, USA
e-mail: ok2267@columbia.edu

© The Author(s) 2021
J. H. Corbin et al. (eds.), *Arts and Health Promotion*, https://doi.org/10.1007/978-3-030-56417-9_10

majority being Syrian. Latest national statistics indicate that over 95% of the refugees live in urban areas, and young people constitute the majority of the refugee population in Turkey, where more than 70% of the refugees are below 30 years old (Turkish Ministry of Interior 2019).

Young refugees are among the most vulnerable population groups with respect to physical, mental, and social health problems; sexual and gender-based violence; trafficking; and early and forced marriage (Karadag Caman and Bahar Ozvaris 2010; Women's Refugee Commission 2016). Refugee youth also face numerous challenges including barriers to accessing quality learning, education, and employment opportunities, as well as youth-friendly health care and social care (Norwegian Refugee Council 2018; UNHCR 2017). In Turkey, although health care is freely available for registered refugees, use of health services—especially the uptake of preventive services—remains low due to factors such as health literacy problems, lack of awareness about available services, language problems, and cultural barriers including gender inequalities (Karadag Caman 2015; Kaya and Kiraç 2016). However, little research to date has examined how to bridge this gap. Qualitative research may be useful in this regard, as it is known to be effective in learning more about different values, perspectives, attitudes, behaviors, and social contexts of specific population groups. Using qualitative methods can sometimes be more helpful than quantitative research when working with vulnerable and/or disadvantaged groups because these methods encourage learning about a given phenomenon from individuals themselves, rather than driven solely by researchers' framing of the issue. As a result, qualitative research can help both researchers and policy makers to better understand the complex reality of a given context and can also complement quantitative research (Mack et al. 2005). One qualitative approach is Community-Based Participatory Action Research (CBPAR), which has been recognized as a unique approach to conducting research with—rather than on—communities. CBPAR involves researchers, community members, and decision makers and aims to combine research with advocacy and action for achieving change (Holkup et al. 2004). CBPAR differs from traditional research in many ways. Instead of creating knowledge for the advancement of a field or for knowledge's sake, CBPAR is an iterative process, integrating research, reflection, and action in a cyclical process (Holkup et al. 2004).

In the early 1990s, Dr. Caroline Wang, a professor and researcher with the University of Michigan, developed photovoice, a creative approach to participatory action research. According to Wang, photovoice has three main goals: (1) to enable people to record and reflect their community's strengths and concerns, (2) to promote critical dialogue and knowledge about important issues through group discussion of photographs, and (3) to reach decision makers to change policies and programs (Wang and Burris 1997). Among CBPAR methods, photovoice is designed to empower members of vulnerable or disadvantaged groups by giving them an opportunity to tell their own stories and have their voices heard (Budig et al. (2018). Photovoice enables researchers, community members, and policy/decision makers to work in a collaborative manner to achieve social change through photography. By documenting their own worlds and critically discussing with policy makers the images they produce, communities can initiate social change (Wang et al. 2004). Using cameras, participants may focus on a wide range of individual, family, and community assets and needs. By sharing and talking about their photographs, participants may also use the power of visual images to communicate their life experiences, expertise, and knowledge (Wang et al. 1998). Therefore, photovoice can be used more widely in health promotion research, especially among more vulnerable/disadvantaged groups such as refugees and youth, as an empowerment and advocacy tool and as a social bridge. Within this framework, the project described in this chapter aimed to involve young people in health promotion research and advocacy through the use of photovoice to assess and increase awareness on the most pressing public health problems they faced.

10.2 The Photovoice Process

10.2.1 Setting

The present study was conducted with young refugee and local youth aged 18 to 30 years in Hatay, which is one of the provinces with the highest per capita concentration of refugees in Turkey. The study was conducted as part of a larger project between December 2015 and April 2016 with the collaboration of a national NGO (Community Volunteers Foundation), United Nations Population Fund (UNFPA) Country Office, and Hacettepe University in Turkey.

Photovoice was selected as part of a mixed-methods study to complement quantitative data collection in the field. The quantitative needs assessment study was conducted with 251 young refugees (aged 18–30 years). The quantitative data collection aimed to assess the current situation of young refugees in order to plan evidence-based interventions with respect to health, education, employment, and gender issues. The main motivation to complement this quantitative survey with a photovoice approach was to select a research method that enables active participation of young refugees in identifying their own problems and finding solutions, as well as to increase social cohesion and mutual understanding between refugee and local youth. Creation of visual materials that could attract more attention of stakeholders than written materials was another strong motive in choosing this specific photography-based approach.

10.2.2 Participants

Young people experiencing forced migration were recruited during the quantitative survey portion of the larger project in Hatay, in which the survey participants were asked about their willingness to participate in another study that used photography and group discussions. After the quantitative data collection was completed, the young people who had volunteered to take part in the photovoice study were contacted via e-mail or mobile phone and were invited to an introductory meeting with the research team (principal investigator, OC, and two local facilitators). In addition, local youth within the same age group were contacted by local NGOs using snowball sampling and were invited to take part in the same study. The study was conducted with a group of 12 young people (nine refugee and three local youth) who gathered in meetings before, during, and after data collection in the field. The country of origin for refugee youth was Syria and they had "temporary protection status," which is a legal status giving forced migrants access to certain services and employment opportunities in Turkey. The main goals in bringing together refugee and local youth were to increase interaction and to improve mutual understanding between the two groups of young people, who were living in the same urban area in *physical* terms but in mostly different environments in *social* terms.

10.2.3 Study Timeline and Steps

Taking into consideration the proposed stages of photovoice by Dr. Wang et al. (1998), the following study steps were taken as shown in Fig. 10.1.

The methodology involved an introductory half-day meeting with the participants to: (1) introduce the photovoice approach with its participatory nature; (2) discuss, get input, and agree on the overall aim of the study; (3) receive written informed consent of participants; (4) introduce specific features of the distributed

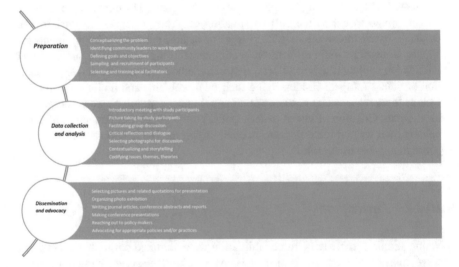

Fig. 10.1 Photovoice study steps of the present project. (Reproduced with permission from the author. Copyright © 2021 Ozge Karadag Caman. All rights reserved)

cameras; (5) discuss data collection procedures; and (6) discuss ethical issues regarding taking photos in the field.

This first meeting lasted around three and a half hours in total (two sessions with a half-hour coffee break in between). The meeting was mainly led by two local and bilingual facilitators, who were trained by the principal investigator on the study methodology. The local facilitators were members of local NGOs and were leading several other projects in the study area. Therefore, they were already knowledgeable about the local context and had previous contact with some of the study participants, which made it easier for young people to participate and devote time to this photo-voice project on a voluntary basis. After the introduction to the project, there was a general discussion about the major individual and environmental health concerns for young refugees, as well as the potential barriers that they may face in accessing health care. Thereafter, the main aim of the study was discussed and agreed upon with the participants—namely, that the study should aim to reflect the main challenges that young refugees face with respect to healthy living conditions and access to health care services in Turkey. The facilitators delivered information about the photo-taking process, including important features of the distributed digital cameras and how and where to use the cameras. During this time, several ethical issues were also discussed in the group, such as the importance of getting permission when taking photos of other people and the rules for taking photos of minors. Finally, potential participants provided written consent to participate, and the group agreed to meet in the same place two weeks later.

The first part of the data collection process lasted two weeks and involved reflection of refugees' individual- and environmental-level health issues/problems through photographs taken by both refugee and local youth. After the two-week data collection period was over, all participants were invited to meet again for a general group discussion and reflection on their experience in this photovoice study.

The second meeting with the same participants was a two-hour focus group meeting in which all photographs taken by the participants were discussed. This group meeting was led by the principal investigator and included one facilitator helping in Arabic-Turkish translation and facilitating discussion while the other facilitator took written notes about the discussion. The discussion was guided by the following series of questions adapted from the SHOWeD guide (Wang 1999):

General discussion with the group:

1. In your opinion, what kind of factors affect the health of young people experiencing forced migration?
2. In your opinion, what kind of barriers do young people experiencing forced migration face when trying to access health care services in Turkey?

Individual reflections for each photo taken:

3. What would you like to share with the group about this photo?
4. What was the main reason why you took this photo?
5. What kind of barriers does this photo show regarding young people's health promotion and/or accessing health care?
6. Do you have any recommendations to solve this problem or to overcome this barrier?

General discussion with the group:

7. Do you have any other opinions or recommendation to promote the health of young people experiencing forced migration?
8. How can young people's access to health services be improved?

Upon participants' request to continue taking photos for two more weeks, the same cycle of data collection and group discussion was repeated once more. All group discussions were voice-recorded (after obtaining written consent of participants) and were then transcribed and translated verbatim. The qualitative data from the study were analyzed using thematic content analysis. The initial analysis was performed by the principal investigator with input from the two facilitators; the initial set of themes were shared with youth for their feedback, which was incorporated in an iterative process continuously throughout project discussions.

10.3   Project Findings and Impact

The photos and the group discussions about those photos demonstrated that although health care services in the public sector were widely available for registered refugees, social determinants of young refugees' health at the individual and environmental levels were mostly unfavorable. Refugees faced language, financial, social, cultural, and educational barriers, as well as gender and stigma-related barriers, to accessing health care services and healthy environments in urban areas. Some of the main themes that emerged during data analysis included: (1) *unhealthy living conditions* (crowded households, rental costs, unsafe buildings, and problems with access to clean water and heating; see Fig. 10.2a); (2) *nutrition and hygiene problems* (vitamin and mineral deficiencies, lack of access to healthy food and cooking facilities, and hygiene-related problems—especially by female participants, who were traditionally more involved with this topic; see Fig. 10.2b); (3) *barriers to accessing education* (financial and language problems, the need to work and earn money to sustain living conditions, inability to find a secure job, low-paying jobs, occupational hazards, and the need for vocational trainings); (4) *child labor* (unhealthy working conditions, unregistered employment, and lack of access to primary education for children, especially for those living out of camps; see Fig. 10.2c); (5) *early marriage and adolescent pregnancies* (polygamy, unregistered marriages, unregistered children, human trafficking issues, gender inequalities, low health literacy, language and cultural barriers to accessing health care, lack of awareness on available health services, problems in access to reliable health information, and low uptake of preventive services); and (6) *high mobility and uncertainty* (unregistered refugees, dreams to return to home country or to move to another country, adaptation problems, problems arising with moving from one city to another including limited access to services without an updated registration, continuous uncertainty in

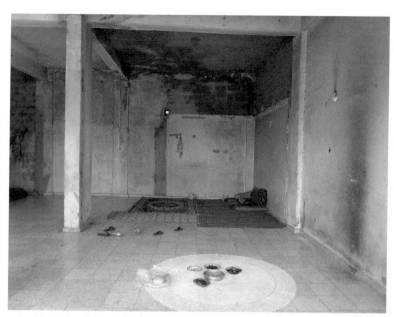

10 çocuklu ailenin yaşadığı yer. Aile kâğıt toplayıcılığı yapıyor.
A family with 10 kids live here. Family is earning their living by collecting paper for recycling.

هذا مكان يعيش فيه عائلة لديهم 10 أطفال. العائلة تعمل في لم الورق (خرده)

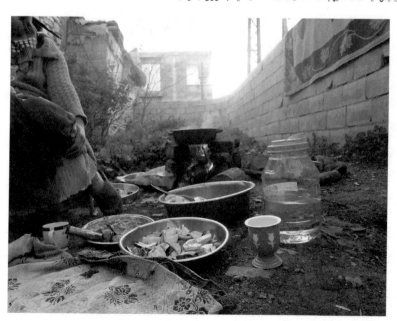

Dışarıda yakılan ateşte pişen yemekler…
Foods cooked on bonfire.

طبخات تطبخ على نار....

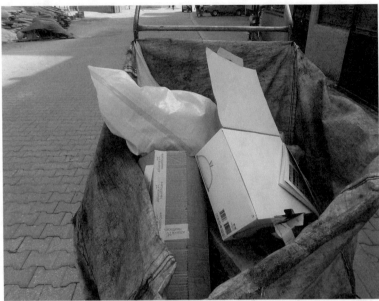

Kağıt toplayan iki çocuğun arabası.``Okul kıyafetimiz olsa bizi de çekerdin ama böyle utanırız`` dediler.
Cart of two children collecting paper. They said: "We would allow you to take our photo if we were on
our school outfits, but we are ashamed like this"

هذه العربة للطفلين الذين يلمون كراتين و ورق .

- هذه طفلين يقولون إن كانت لدينا ملابس المدرسة كنت تصورينا أن تصويرينا في الوقت الحالي لانريد أن نتصور بهذه الملابس الوسخة إننا نخجل.

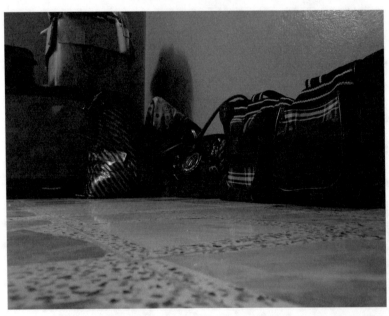

Eşyalar, bavullar, kutular hep toplu... Sürekli bir taşınma hali, istikrar yok. Sürekli bir gitme hali...
Stuff, luggages, boxes always packed... Always in a state of moving, no stability. Constant state of departure...

أعراضهم دائما في حقائب لم يستقرو في مكان دائماً يرحلون من منطقة إلى آخره لأنهم لم يحسون أن هذا المكان تابع لهم.

Fig. 10.2 (**a–d**) Example photos taken by youth and used in analysis, reporting, and dissemination of research findings. (Reproduced with permission from the author. Copyright © 2016 Ozge Karadag Caman. All rights reserved)

life, acceptance problems including stigma and discrimination toward refugees, and mental health problems; see Fig. 10.2d).

The findings above were the main themes that emerged—with mutual agreement among the study participants—during the two group discussion meetings. Several other issues were also brought up by some of the participants; however, after discussing those issues in the larger group, they were found to be very rare, individual-level experiences that were not shared or experienced by most of the participants, and hence were not included among the major themes that emerged. There were also several ethical concerns that arose during the group discussions and during selection of the photos for wider dissemination in the photo exhibitions and publications. Although all photos were either taken with permission or did not show people's faces for privacy reasons, there were still some concerns about potential identification of some people, including some minors. Therefore, photos that were not found suitable for wider dissemination were extracted from the database and were not shared in any electronic or printed medium.

10.3.1 Advocacy Through Dissemination

In the study, data analysis with feedback and contribution of participants was followed by the production of short reports, conference papers, and other publications for disseminating findings to different stakeholders, such as academics, civil society members, and policy makers at the national and international level. These written documents for dissemination were written by the primary investigator with input from the youth throughout the process. The youth also selected which photos would be used in the dissemination efforts and co-wrote the quotes to use with the photos. The publications were coupled with advocacy activities, such as photo exhibitions that brought together policy makers, health service providers, civil society organizations, host communities, and young people to achieve positive change through joint action. The photo exhibition—which was organized on World Refugee Day (June 20, 2016) with the joint efforts of the Community Volunteers Foundation, UNFPA, and a municipality in Ankara—attracted a large number of visitors from different sectors and resulted in high media coverage of the different young refugee stories. In the exhibitions, each photo was displayed with the name of the participant, the name of the photographer, and a short excerpt from the participant's own words, hence combining photos with voices. Youth participants also attended the photo exhibitions and interacted with policy makers and other stakeholders, and some of them were interviewed by journalists, later appearing in newspapers with their photos and stories. Although the project team did not use a specific evaluation method for these exhibits, verbal reflections of the exhibition participants indicated that both the photos and the young people's physical presence in the exhibitions were the major contributors to raising awareness and increasing observers' perception of the reality of problems faced by young people.

10.4 Discussion

The present qualitative study aimed to use a CBPAR approach to assess public health problems faced by young refugees in Turkey. The study also aimed to advocate for their health rights, as well as to involve young refugees in health promotion research and have their voices heard by policy makers. The findings of this photovoice study indicated that refugees living in urban areas faced serious problems regarding shelter, education, employment, income, and access to health services, in addition to language barriers, cultural differences, stigma, and discrimination. There was a significant gender-based difference between the challenges faced by young refugees, indicating a need to tailor unique approaches based on gender.

The overall experience of young people with the photovoice approach was found to be very positive. This particular approach enabled the researchers to involve participants actively throughout the research process, while helping the research team to compare their experience with different research methods and question their own roles and limitations in the research processes. The team agreed that active involvement of study participants contributed to the research process in many different ways and increased the validity of findings and the quality of research in general. These positive outcomes can mainly be attributed to the continuous feedback that was received from the participants. In traditional research, there is usually a one-way flow of data, where all data are analyzed and then interpreted by the researchers. On the other hand, when properly facilitated, participatory approaches like photovoice enrich the data analysis and interpretation process by enabling the flow of data, information, ideas, and suggestions in two directions throughout the whole process (from participants to researchers and vice versa).

Community involvement is usually described as the involvement of communities in the planning, implementation, and evaluation of policies and practices. In disaster or humanitarian settings, many programs implemented by governments and non-governmental organizations have been found to be successful during the initial phase of responses but to effect decreasing success as time passes. There can be many reasons for this phenomenon; however, lack of participation and capacity building of the affected communities remains a major factor in inadequate sustainability (Rajeev 2014). Literature shows that in the past, important decisions were made by higher authorities based on their perception of the communities' needs, where the affected communities served as passive receivers of aid. This approach was typically ineffective because it failed to meet the real needs of communities (Pandey and Okazaki 2012). Previous experience indicated that community members need to be involved from the initial phase of responses and should continue to be involved in later stages, including long-term development efforts. Equitable partnerships require sharing power, resources, credit, results, knowledge, and skills at each stage of the research project, including problem definition, research design, data collection, data analysis, results interpretation, and determination of how the results should be used for action (Minkler and Wallerstein 2008). Unless people are involved in research-related decisions—and, therefore, included as research partners, or (co-)researchers—it is not participatory research, but rather an example of pseudo-participation (Bergold and Thomas 2012). In truly participatory research, community members have control (shared leadership) over the research, and they are more likely to accept the legitimacy of the research and pay attention to its findings if they know it was conducted by people like themselves. Participatory research also trains citizen researchers, who can turn their skills to other community-level problems. Skills learned by researchers in the course of participatory research are also carried over into other areas of researchers' lives (University of Kansas 2018). However, when working with youth, we found that several adaptations to a traditional CBPAR approach were necessary to achieve project goals within study constraints.

First, due to organizational and financial reasons, the preparation stage of our photovoice study was comparatively less participatory than later stages; however, the data collection, analysis, and dissemination stages were very dynamic with continuous communication between all project stakeholders. In an ideal participatory research setting, the preparation stage should be as participatory as the following stages, but this was not an option in our study. Despite the initial phase, our overall experience showed that when compared to other research approaches, participatory action research was more effective in developing concrete plans for disseminating findings and driving advocacy to create a change. In our own experience, the high motivation of the research team and the participants was kept alive throughout the process due to the collaborative and iterative nature of the study. This approach provided an opportunity to discuss study findings, revisit data for further analysis, and prepare dissemination and advocacy materials with the continuous contribution of the participants. The photovoice approach also helped to improve social cohesion and social ties between refugee and local youth, in addition to building partnerships among different stakeholders for more comprehensive youth health promotion efforts—covering potential changes at the individual, social, and environmental levels. Overall, research-related costs were not high, and outputs (visual findings and stories) were more attractive for, and easy to grasp by, the target audience.

Second, the language barrier between the principal investigator and the refugees might have affected some of the group interactions as well as the interpretation of some of the findings, although this limitation was thought to be minimal since the facilitators that translated all group discussions and the local participants that contributed to the translation process during group discussions were bilingual. In contrast to studies using qualitative interviews, photovoice studies are less affected by language barriers, since photos, which are taken by the participants, either complement or speak more strongly than words. In addition to these issues, it was challenging to build and sustain collaboration and to share decision-making between all partners, especially when the partners are youth who have important lived experiences but are typically less experienced in political and financial processes to make sustained change. Considering these challenges, this study aimed to bring together youth who has local wisdom with stakeholders who have expertise in research, advocacy, and policy making for all partners to learn from each other and to plan more concrete actions for social change.

Although this qualitative study was conducted with a rather small sample size in one city, the findings still point to an urgent need for developing multidimensional and multi-sectoral interventions on health, education, employment, and gender issues regarding young refugees in Turkey. Within this framework, potential interventions that were brought up during group discussions were: (1) increasing health literacy and awareness on available health care services; (2) improving social determinants of health, including the promotion of healthy living and working conditions; (3) increasing awareness of policy makers and service providers on gender inequities and how to tackle them; (4) decreasing refugee-related stigma among local communities; and (5) empowering young refugees and promoting their social and mental health. In this regard, it was agreed that community involvement should be an integral part of these interventions in order for the health promotion responses to be successful and linked to sustainable development efforts in the long term, because effective participation and capacity building of the affected communities are critical factors for sustainability.

In the present study, social cohesion of refugee and host communities—as well as increased motivation of local young people (host communities) to think about problems faced by their refugee peers—were additional gains, since working in mixed groups can strengthen social ties and values to build a shared environment between refugee and local youth. Thus, while photovoice can be a strong "tool" for health promotion research and advocacy, our experience demonstrates that the photovoice approach has a strong potential to act as a "bridge" to create synergy (See Chaps. 1 and 21, this volume for further background on these concepts). In the context of our study, photovoice methodology created social bridges in many different ways. First, photovoice was often a language bridge for young people, who experienced forced migration from a neighboring country with a different language and a different alphabet. Depending upon their experiences getting to and living in the host country, photovoice might also have helped to create a channel for young people to talk about their migration-related traumas or challenges. This participatory methodology and the mixed nature of the study group created a bridge between refugee and local youth, building connections and feelings of belonging and mutual understanding. Photovoice also acted as a bridge to policy makers and other stakeholders, who had the power to create system-level changes. By seeing the photos and reading the quotations, they might have felt something viscerally that moved them, through empathy, to change certain policies and/or practices.

10.5 Conclusion

The number of studies using CBPAR methodology with refugees/migrants is still scarce. Therefore, despite some of its limitations, the project described in this chapter may potentially motivate health promotion researchers and professionals to involve vulnerable or disadvantaged populations in future health promotion research and practice. In particular, photovoice might be very helpful in understanding real-life problems of minority populations, as well as in supporting them with tools and bridges to identify and advocate for their own solutions. This experience indicated that photovoice, as one of the CBPAR approaches, can be used more widely with vulnerable or disadvantaged groups to promote health and decrease inequalities. In forced migration settings, photovoice can also facilitate social cohesion of refugee and local individuals, and photography can be a strong tool to engage refugees in health promotion work.

In conclusion, participation of refugees in refugee-related research, policy, and practice in host countries—as well as in the promotion of their own health—is essential for efficiently using available resources and planning culturally appropriate interventions in the short term, and for supporting sustainable development efforts of host countries in the long term.

Acknowledgements   The author is thankful to all the participants and facilitators of the photovoice study and acknowledges with appreciation the invaluable support provided by the Community Volunteers Foundation, the Yuva Association, and the UNFPA Country Office in Turkey during data collection and organization of the photo exhibition.

References

Bergold, J., & Thomas, S. (2012). Participatory research methods: A methodological approach in motion. *Historical Social Research, 37*(4), 191–222. https://doi.org/10.12759/hsr.37.2012.4.191-222.

Budig, K., Diez, J., Conde, P., Sastre, M., Hernán, M., & Franco, M. (2018). Photovoice and empowerment: Evaluating the transformative potential of a participatory action research project. *BMC Public Health, 18*(1), 432. https://doi.org/10.1186/s12889-018-5335-7.

Center for Community Health and Development, University of Kansas. *Community tool box, Section 2. Community-based participatory research.* https://ctb.ku.edu/en/table-of-contents/evaluate/evaluation/intervention-research/main. Accessed 24 Nov 2018.

Department General of Migration Management, Turkish Ministry of Interior. (2019). *Migration statistics: June, 2019.* https://www.goc.gov.tr/icerik6/gecici-koruma_363_378_4713_icerik. Accessed 14 June 2019.

Holkup, P. A., Tripp-Reimer, T., Salois, E. M., & Weinert, C. (2004). Community-based participatory research: An approach to intervention research with a native American community. *Advances in Nursing Science, 27*(3), 162–175.

International Organization for Migration (IOM). (2018). *World migration report.* https://www.iom.int/wmr/world-migration-report-2018. Accessed 26 Nov 2018.

Karadag Caman, O. (2015). *Needs assessment study among young Syrian refugees on health, education, employment and gender issues in Turkey: Final report.* Ankara: Community Volunteers Foundation, Yuva Association, UNFPA.

Karadag Caman, O., & Altintas, K. H. (2010). Refugees and health. *TAF Prev Med Bull, 9*(1), 55–62.

Karadag Caman, O., & Bahar Ozvaris, S. (2010). International migration and women's health. *Health and Society, 20*(4), 3–14.

Kaya, A., & Kiraç, A. (2016). *Vulnerability assessment of Syrian refugees in Istanbul.* Support to Life.

Mack, N., Woodsong, C., Macqueen, K., Guest, G., & Namey, E. (2005). *Qualitative research methods: A data collector's field guide.* USAID/Family Health International.

Minkler, M., & Wallerstein, N. (Eds.). (2008). *Community-based participatory research for health: From process to outcomes* (2nd ed.). San Francisco: Jossey-Bass.

Norwegian Refugee Council. (2018). *10 challenges of refugee youth*. https://www.nrc.no/news/2018/august/10-challenges-of-refugee-youth/. Accessed 18 Nov 2018.

Pandey, B., & Okazaki, K. (2012). *Community-based disaster management: Empowering communities to cope with disaster risks*. United Nations Centre for Regional Development, Japan.

Rajeev, M. M. (2014). Sustainability and community empowerment in disaster management. *International Journal of Social Work and Human Services Practice, 2*(6), 207–212.

UNHCR. (1951). *UN Convention relating to the status of refugees*. http://www.unhcr.org.tr/MEP/FTPRoot/HTMLEditor/File/anasayfa/sozles me.pdf. Accessed 10 Dec 2018.

UNHCR. (2017). 3RP progress report: regional refugee & resilience plan 2017–2018. https://data2.unhcr.org/en/documents/download/60340. Accessed 28 Nov 2018.

UNHCR. (2019). *Syria emergency*. http://www.unhcr.org/en-us/syria-emergency.html. Accessed 12 June 2019.

United Nations. (2018). *Refugees*. http://www.un.org/en/sections/issues-depth/refugees/. Accessed 12 Nov 2018.

Wang, C. (1999). Photovoice: A participatory action research strategy applied to women's health. *Journal of Women's Health, 8*, 185–192.

Wang, C., & Burris, M. A. (1997). Photovoice: Concept, methodology, and use for participatory needs assessment. *Health Education & Behavior, 24*(3), 369–387.

Wang, C. C., Yi, W. K., Tao, Z. W., & Carovano, K. (1998). Photovoice as a participatory health promotion strategy. *Health Promotion International, 13*(1), 75–86. https://doi.org/10.1093/heapro/13.1.75.

Wang, C. C., Morrel-Samuels, S., Hutchison, P. M., Bell, L., & Pestronk, R. M. (2004). Flint photovoice: Community building among youths, adults, and policymakers. *American Journal of Public Health, 94*(6), 911–913.

Women's Refugee Commission, United Nations Refugee Agency, United Nations Population Fund. (2016). *Initial assessment report: protection risks for women and girls in the European refugee and migrant crisis*. https://www.unhcr.org/en-us/protection/operations/569f8f419/initial-assessment-report-protection-risks-women-girls-european-refugee.html

Chapter 11
Reframing Health Promotion Research and Practice in Australia and the Pacific: The Value of Arts-Based Practices

Wendy Madsen, Michelle Redman-MacLaren, Vicki Saunders, Cathy O'Mullan, and Jenni Judd

11.1 Introduction

In health promotion research, the arts can take many forms: as the focus of the research or evaluation; as a tool of inquiry; as an avenue of dissemination; or as a combination of each of these. Each art form occurs within a place-based or social and spatial context, and it is the interdependence of form and context that gives rise to ethical and methodological tensions. In this chapter, we argue that arts-based research (ABR) is an aesthetic, iterative, and organic research process and health promotion practice that brings to the fore ethical and methodological tensions

---

W. Madsen
School of Health, Medical and Applied Sciences CQ University,
Rockhampton North 4702, QLD, Australia
e-mail: w.madsen@cqu.edu.au

M. Redman-MacLaren
College of Medicine and Dentistry James Cook University, Cairns 4870, QLD, Australia
e-mail: michelle.maclaren@jcu.edu.au

V. Saunders
First Peoples Health Unit, Queensland Conservatorium Research Centre, Griffith University,
Gold Coast Campus, Parklands Dr, Southport 4222, QLD, Australia
e-mail: v.saunders@griffith.edu.au

C. O'Mullan
School of Health, Medical and Applied Sciences, CQ University Bundaberg,
Bundaberg 4670, QLD, Australia
e-mail: c.omullan@cqu.edu.au

J. Judd (✉)
Centre for Indigenous Health Equity Research, Centre for Emotional Health and Wellbeing,
School of Health Medical and Applied Sciences, Central Queensland University,
Bundaberg 4670, QLD, Australia
e-mail: j.judd@cqu.edu.au

© The Author(s) 2021
J. H. Corbin et al. (eds.), *Arts and Health Promotion*,
https://doi.org/10.1007/978-3-030-56417-9_11

inherent in participatory research. The value of ABR lies in how it advances and enhances scientific practices and methodologies. However, there are also tensions inherent in designing studies that respond to community-led research priorities because ABR provides opportunities for ethical and methodological development/ advancement.

11.2   Framing and Reframing Arts and Health Promotion Research

Arts-based research (ABR) emerged from within qualitative research approaches of the 1990s (Capous-Desyllas and Morgaine 2018), although visual and audio data have been used in social anthropology and historical research for many decades (Banks 2007). Whereas anthropological and historical researchers used visual and audio data in association with other data such as documentary evidence or informant interviews, ABR's relationship with data is often more multifaceted and multidirectional. ABR disrupts more traditional understandings of what data are and can be. Data generated in ABR can take the form of visual, auditory, performance, or literary art; the art may pre-exist the research or be created as part of the research process. The art may also be used to generate meaning within the research process or as part of the knowledge translation process (Fraser and al Sayah 2011). Critically, ABR can "extend" what and how we understand by opening alternatives to propositional or conceptual ways of knowing to also include symbolic, expressive, experiential, and practical knowledge (Daykin and Stickley 2016). These primarily aesthetic extensions can disrupt, or challenge, established research traditions.

While the use of qualitative research methods is central to much health promotion research to better understand communities' needs (Salazar et al. 2015; see also Chap. 1, this volume), there are a number of challenges associated with using ABR practices and approaches. These challenges include ontological and epistemological (what is real and how it is known) differences, as well as ethical and methodological issues arising before, during, and after the research. Arts practitioners and researchers usually employ constructivist, critical, or participatory paradigms. In contrast, health promotion researchers and practitioners are not immune to broader narratives around evidence-based practice, and there are pressures to demonstrate effectiveness and use evidence that is not "too" subjective. Thus, it is not surprising that more positivist approaches, such as quantitative or mixed methods research, are increasingly being used to evaluate the impact of ABR approaches, resulting in fundamental differences in opinion as to whether or not it is possible to quantify the "unquantifiable" (Blomkamp 2015).

Related to these epistemological issues are pragmatic issues in how the arts have been co-opted to meet the agendas of other fields of study, such as personal well-being (Scott et al. 2018), social and economic development (Ashley 2015), and urban renewal (Pollock and Paddison 2014; Webb 2014). Health promotion researchers and practitioners are at risk of such instrumentalism when working in partnership with artists to undertake ABR projects in which the art emphasizes process over product or outcome over process (this can also lead to team antagony; see Chap. 21, this volume). Instrumentalism overlooks the broader aesthetics of the art process (aesthetics of experience) and product (aesthetics of beauty) (Graham 2005; Stroud 2014). Thus, it is helpful for health promotion practitioners and researchers to critically reflect upon their relationships with the artists they work with as well as how they view the role of art in their work. When ABR is undertaken by the researcher who is also the artist, such aesthetic tensions become less relevant.

There is potential for the arts to be used across the five action areas of the Ottawa Charter—develop personal skills, create supportive environments, strengthen community action, reorient health services, and build healthy public policy—to directly address the social determinants of health (World Health Organization 1986; see also Chap. 1, this volume). The four case studies outlined in this chapter focus on strengthening community action, developing personal skills, and creating supportive environments. Written as place-based narratives, each case study explores ethical and/or methodological challenges associated with ABR. Reflecting the strengths of ABR, it is in the telling of a place-based narrative that the learning is revealed.

11.3 Case Studies

11.3.1 Case Study 1: Evaluation of IT ALL BEGINS WITH LOVE

The first case study outlines a mixed methods evaluation of a theater production. In this case, there was methodological complexity and a few ethical complications. These complications relate to the diverse ways many health promotion practitioners have used the arts to tap into the public's cognitive and emotional understanding of difficult social topics.

IT ALL BEGINS WITH LOVE emerged out of a series of community consultations undertaken in 2012 by Creative Regions, a not-for-profit arts-production company in Bundaberg, Queensland, Australia. Domestic and family violence (DFV) was identified as a significant issue in the community that needed to be talked about to decrease the social stigma associated with it so more women would seek help. Rod Ainsworth, a renowned playwright, worked with local counseling, DFV support agencies, and local media to develop a verbatim theater production to raise social consciousness around the issue. Twelve women who had experienced DFV but who were then safe were interviewed, and excerpts from these transcripts were used to develop the script—a process that took three years as various drafts were distributed between Rod and the counselors.

Wendy Madsen (WM), one of the authors of this chapter, was asked to evaluate the production after it gained funding for a tour of Queensland in 2015. As a qualitative health promotion researcher committed to participatory research, WM could not countenance undertaking a pre-post survey of a stage production around such an emotional topic. Wendy also recognized the range of confounding factors that could influence any evaluation, such as: the venue was different for every performance, meaning the actors would need to adapt to each venue; the actors were professional, but their energy levels would vary between performances; the audience may or may not have insights into theater techniques of communication; and the relationship between the audience and their theater could condition them to expect entertainment, when this production was meant to challenge rather than entertain. Trying to undertake in-depth interviews was unrealistic, as the production was frequently moving. Wendy needed to find a participatory approach that provided depth as well as breadth around the following issues: (1) Could a socially engaged theater production raise social consciousness around such a sensitive topic? (2) What were some of the challenges of undertaking and touring such a production?

Luckily, Rod was not only the playwright but also the producer and was committed to working in a participatory manner. We formed a small group consisting of Rod, a representative from one of the counseling agencies who provided on-site counseling support, a representative from the funding body, one of the actors, and WM. Together we worked through the issues of how to evaluate this production in a way that was sensitive to the topic and context, but also practical. We decided to draw data from a range of sources. We offered audience members two online surveys (one was available immediately after each performance, and one was open for a month after the last performance to allow audience members to reflect on the production). Next, we provided audience members with paper and pens and allowed five minutes between the end of the performance and the beginning of the Question and Answer session for them to write down thoughts and questions (these pieces of paper were collected at the end of each event). Finally, we utilized ethnographic data consisting of in-depth interviews with various stakeholders, as well as field notes. Wendy was responsible for the analysis and write-up of the project and so was consistently in touch with the other members of the research team, seeking out their views and interpretations of these data.

This was WM's first time working with professional artists to evaluate an arts-based production that had health promotion implications. WM admits she was on a huge learning curve as she tried to understand issues of evaluation within the arts sector and how these issues related to health promotion. There have been many claims over the years that the arts contribute to the health and social well-being of communities; however, these claims have been frequently questioned by insufficient evidence. While not "gold standard," we were nevertheless able to demonstrate that this production contributed to raising the consciousness around DFV for many who saw the performance. The results suggested that many in the audience felt increased empathy for those caught in DFV situations, and some audience members reflected on the quality of their own relationships. We concluded that when undertaken as part of a broader shift in social conversations, the arts can and do play a significant role in tapping into the public's cognitive and emotional understanding of these difficult social topics (see Madsen 2018 for more on this project).

11.3.2   Case Study 2: IMPACT Community Choir

The second case study shifts the focus from evaluation of the arts to using the arts to generate data with members of the disability community—a group generally seen as difficult to research. Compared to the first case study, additional ethical complexities impacted the methodology of this second case. As such, this next case demonstrates how arts-based methods were used as a tool to elicit understanding and generate knowledge and well-being.

Once a week the halls of IMPACT, a community service organization in Bundaberg, are filled with the sweet sounds of the IMPACT Community Choir. The choir was established in 2011 for people with a disability and includes people with profound and multiple disabilities; it has also expanded to include community members from a diverse range of local community organizations who are experiencing mental health issues. There are now over 60 members. Volunteers support the choir, as do paid carers (i.e., caregivers) and support staff who assist with the musical accompaniment. Performances are in high demand, and the choir regularly travels throughout the region in the widely acclaimed "rock-bus." It is now well known that choir singing is associated with a range of health benefits; participating in a choir also provides the opportunity for members to access additional social support and may provide a new social identity (Hassan 2017). For people living with a disability or a mental health condition, being part of a choir presents an opportunity for meaningful activity and social connectedness. As part of an ongoing research partnership with IMPACT, we (Cathy O'Mullan and Jenni Judd, two of this chapter's authors) were asked to develop a creative way to showcase the impact of the choir for the participants—in particular, how participating in the choir contributes to improving their health and well-being.

Historically, people with a disability are an underrepresented group in research and in the evaluation of programs and services, and this is particularly true for people who have profound and multiple disabilities. Although we were keen to hear the perspectives of those in the IMPACT choir, we were also conscious that many members had limited cognitive abilities and would not be able to participate in more traditional research approaches such as focus groups or interviews. As such, if we used these methods, only the most able (a small number) would be able to participate, which presented us with a dilemma since we wanted to ensure that we could hear all choir members' points of view. We needed to find a participatory research approach that was inclusive and allowed individuals the autonomy of making their own decisions without further marginalizing people with a disability. Fortunately, IMPACT is committed to working in a participatory manner and was open to forming a working group to oversee the project. The group consisted of us (Cathy and Jenni), a paid support worker, and case managers with experience in working with these choir members. As part of this group, we brainstormed moral and ethical issues relating to the project and practical ideas for moving forward.

We chose to use photovoice—an arts-based method using photographs to provide insight into participant experiences—to engage and provide a "visual voice" to all choir members who chose to participate. Photovoice is a participatory action research methodology that uses photography as a tool to access other people's worlds (Wang and Burris 1997). By taking photographs, individuals are able to explore their experience of daily life and promote critical dialogue with respect to important community issues. While the methodology can be used flexibly (Seed 2016), individuals are typically encouraged to select a number of photographs for discussion either in a group setting or on a one-to-one basis. Over the past two decades, photovoice has been effectively used as a participatory research approach for engaging with marginalized and vulnerable populations (Dassah et al. 2017) and offers an empowering and creative tool to help gather rich, qualitative data. Participatory research methods such as photovoice have provided a much-needed research approach to capture the voices of those with a physical or intellectual disability. Indeed, a number of projects have used photovoice as an avenue for people with a disability to communicate their health priorities and actively contribute to health promotion planning and service delivery (Dassah et al. 2017). Although there is a dearth of literature involving those with profound and multiple learning disabilities, Cluley (2017, p. 42) argues that photovoice can be used flexibly to provide such individuals with an opportunity to "voice their words visually," thereby opening up this approach to include people of all cognitive abilities.

Based on discussions with the working group and through our communication with choir members, it was apparent that photovoice's "gold standard" approach, which typically includes interviews and focus groups to help analyze the photographs, was not going to work. To facilitate inclusion, we needed to be realistic and mindful about the contribution expected from choir members. Hence, photovoice was used flexibly and adapted to suit this project. While speaking for people with a disability is widely frowned upon, we included support workers across all stages of the project to facilitate the inclusion of members' voices. Each support worker, for example, partnered with a choir member to help them to identify photo opportunities and select appropriate photos. In partnership, they worked together to interpret the meaning of each photograph and to develop a caption. We then analyzed the photos and captions based on conversations with each choir member (when appropriate) and their support worker.

Our findings reveal how participation in the choir has made a positive impact on choir members' self-esteem, their sense of calm and well-being, and their growth as individuals. Furthermore, participation has also fostered a sense of belonging and social connectedness among members. At a community level, those who have been involved as volunteers, researchers, and as part of an audience have reported feeling elevated and deeply moved by the experience. Of note, the findings have also resulted in the publication of a community photo book (see Fig. 11.1), which is being used to raise awareness of the benefits of this type of program.

Although we had used photovoice before, we had never used this approach with people who have a disability. What we have learned is that we can include individuals with profound and multiple disabilities in participatory and emancipatory research projects. The IMPACT choir performances demonstrate the power of singing to bring people and communities together, to promote social inclusion, and

Fig. 11.1 Example of a photovoice photograph titled "Growth: The choir helps me learn and grow". (Reproduced with permission from the authors. Copyright © 2021 Wendy Madsen, Michelle Redman-MacLaren, Vicki Saunders, Cathy O'Mullan, and Jenni Judd. All rights reserved)

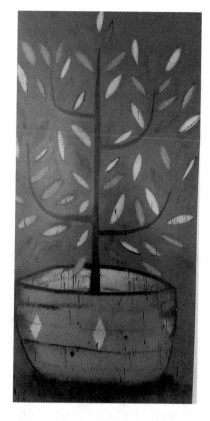

importantly to provide a collective voice for people with a disability and/or a mental health condition. This case study shows that ABR can provide a highly inclusive approach to research, allowing those who have traditionally been excluded from the data-generation process to be active participants.

11.3.3 Case Study 3: Implications of Male Circumcision for Women in Papua New Guinea, Including for HIV Prevention

The third case study again uses an arts-based method to generate data and to make meaning from the data, and takes into account some ethical and methodological challenges associated with researching cross-cultures, gender, language, and varied literacy levels.

For many women in Papua New Guinea (PNG), HIV is an ever-present risk. PNG is a hyper-diverse Pacific island nation experiencing a concentrated human immunodeficiency virus (HIV) epidemic that is largely heterosexually transmitted.

Addressing HIV in PNG is a challenge. The seven million people of PNG speak over 830 languages. The rural majority (85%) live a predominantly subsistence life-style, with limited educational opportunities for girls and women; approximately 50% of women in PNG are illiterate. Given that male circumcision reduces the risk of female-to-male HIV transmission and thus reduces HIV at a population level, it is currently being explored as an HIV-prevention option in PNG. Exploring the implications of male circumcision with women is essential to inform balanced, evidence-based health policy that will result in positive, intended consequences.

In 2013–2014, I (Michelle Redman-MacLaren, one of this chapter's authors) and Rachael Tommbe, a health researcher from Enga Province in PNG, worked with over 60 rural and urban women in seven interpretive focus groups at two sites to explore implications of male circumcision for the women as wives, partners, and/or mothers (Redman-MacLaren et al. 2017). Qualitative research methods often rely on individual or group interviews to co-generate stories that help the researcher/s understand the phenomenon being studied. These methods are consistent with the way information is shared in PNG, where knowledge, art, and lore are often trans-mitted orally. However, the highly accepted oral way of communicating in PNG is to rely upon a *big man* or *big meri* (literally, important man or important woman) to be a spokesperson for the group. In this study, we needed to understand the implica-tions of male circumcision for all women, not just for the spokeswomen/leaders. Thus, we used ABR to enhance participation and inclusivity in the research process. During the interpretive focus groups, whole-of-group discussions were initially held with women to contextualize the research. Women then worked in smaller story circles to discuss "chunks" of existing data from a previous male circumcision study. A final process involved storyboarding.

Storyboarding is a technique used in the visual arts and has recently been adapted for use in community development and participatory research (Pittaway and Bartolomei 2012). In this study, storyboarding was used to elicit different under-standings about male circumcision from a wide range of rural and urban women. Women self-organized into story circles of four to five participants, discussed the prompt questions, and drew their responses. The following were the four prompt questions used to elicit information: (1) What is happening (how, who, where, when)? (2) What is the outcome for men? (3) What is the outcome for women? (4) What needs to happen next? (See Fig. 11.2 for an example process of storyboarding.)

Women drew pictures on large sheets of paper using crayons, felt pens, high-lighter pens, and pencils (Fig. 11.3). Various-sized drawings emerged, and women organized information and drawings differently. Some women drew only pictures, while others drew a combination of pictures and words (Fig. 11.4). Some women started drawing immediately; other story circles took more time to discuss the ques-tions first and then draw considered responses. Although a spokeswoman from each story circle shared an explanation of the drawings with the whole group, the draw-ings often led to extended discussions with a wide range of women participating.

The visual method of storyboarding was well received by the women we worked with in PNG. Storyboarding stimulated succinct, targeted representations of

Storyboarding to understand implications of male circumcision for women

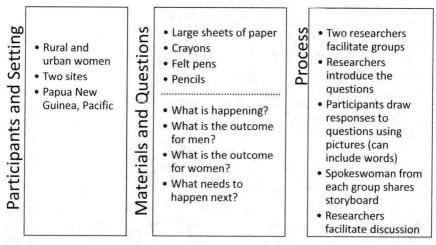

Participants and Setting
- Rural and urban women
- Two sites
- Papua New Guinea, Pacific

Materials and Questions
- Large sheets of paper
- Crayons
- Felt pens
- Pencils
....
- What is happening?
- What is the outcome for men?
- What is the outcome for women?
- What needs to happen next?

Process
- Two researchers facilitate groups
- Researchers introduce the questions
- Participants draw responses to questions using pictures (can include words)
- Spokeswoman from each group shares storyboard
- Researchers facilitate discussion

Fig. 11.2 Storyboarding to understand implications of male circumcision for women. (Reproduced with permission from the authors. Copyright © 2021 Wendy Madsen, Michelle Redman-MacLaren, Vicki Saunders, Cathy O'Mullan, and Jenni Judd. All rights reserved)

women's knowledge and experience of male circumcision, and it offered a different way of communicating about sensitive sexual health issues that encouraged high levels of participation in the research process. The kinesthetic experience of drawing appeared to elicit different types of information to that shared in interviews and focus groups. The storyboard artifacts were used to provide more detailed reporting of research findings in a way that transcended language and cultural barriers. The findings recorded have informed health promotion activities with men and women, guided advocacy with policy makers, and furthered other research projects.

In this case study, ABR provided an ethical means of including a diverse range of participants in the research process.

11.3.4 Case Study 4: Using Poetic Inquiry to Story Aboriginal Recovery in Mental Health Care

In the fourth and final case study, we describe ABR as a way of ethically and methodologically engaging with stories of well-being and recovery of Indigenous Australians experiencing mental health issues. However, this final case challenges us to consider our positionality as health promotion researchers.

In the texts that inscribe Indigenous peoples in mental health care statistics, stories of recovery or living life well with a diagnosis of mental illness are not usually included. In the reports that inscribe stories of well-being and recovery in mental health care service delivery, indicators to describe Indigenous peoples are not often

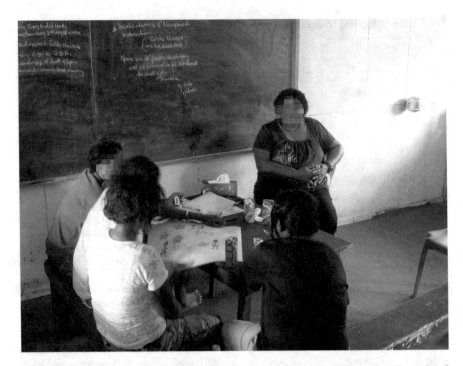

Fig. 11.3 Young women draw their storyboards, supported by Rachael Tommbe. (Reproduced with permission from the authors. Copyright © 2021 Wendy Madsen, Michelle Redman-MacLaren, Vicki Saunders, Cathy O'Mullan, and Jenni Judd. All rights reserved)

recovery-oriented. This research project began with the search for indicators of recovery among stories of Indigenous people living with a diagnosis of mental illness in Far North Queensland. To amplify Indigenous voice and modes of storytelling, and to engage with the silences and the ethical and moral imperatives that asking Indigenous questions about statistics and stories of Indigenous recovery foregrounded, the research methodology evolved into poetic inquiry.

Poetic inquiry is the transformation of ideas or words from research into poetry (Butler-Kisber and Stewart 2009). According to Monica Prendergast (2009), poetic inquiry as a process of seeing, caring, and understanding is all about voice, and there are three main types of voice used in poetic practices and methods of research: vox theoria, vox participare, and vox autoethnographia. Poetic inquiry can be performed using found poetry, where the actual words of participants are used (vox participare); or it can be performed using generated poetry, where researchers poetically reflect on their own subjectivities/responses in the work (vox autoethnographia); or it can be written from, or in response to, works of literature/theory in a discipline or field or poems written about poetry and/or inquiry itself (vox theoria) (Prendergast 2009). The results can be shared publicly or kept as a private interpretive tool (Butler-Kisber 2017) in which poems are approached as a source of data, a form of data, a way of representing complex or ineffable social dilemmas, or a

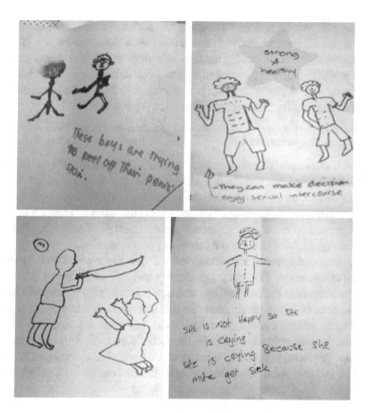

Fig. 11.4 Responses to questions considered by women in the story circles. (Reproduced with permission from the authors. Copyright © 2021 Wendy Madsen, Michelle Redman-MacLaren, Vicki Saunders, Cathy O'Mullan, and Jenni Judd. All rights reserved)

methodology or means through which to link research processes to research outcomes for transparent, powerful effect (Van Luyn et al. 2016). Poetics can be viewed as a discourse articulating "the relationship between the creative work and its critical inputs and outcomes" (Lyall 2014, p. 134, citing the work of Lasky 2013).

Indigenous poetics necessarily includes another dimension of representation or expression—it includes a way of listening that is active and deep and centers around a particular sense of place, belonging, and country. Miriam Rose has called this dimension of Indigenous listening *"Dadirri"* see Miriam Rose Foundation https://www.miriamrosefoundation.org.au/)—a way of listening that does not just involve the ears; that is not necessarily about sound; and that is sometimes about listening to the absence of sound, the absence of a story where there once was one, or where there perhaps should be one. It is also about storywork, or the work of stories. It is about the way stories embed multiple layers of meanings that interweave cultural signifiers as reference points between the reader/listener and the storyteller (Archibald 2008a, b; Bessarab and Ng'andu 2010; Kovach 2010).

A Gunggari woman and an Aboriginal researcher, Vicki Saunders, one of the authors of this chapter, works with and within what Sousain Abadian (2006) has called "culturally toxic stories." This term describes the way settler or colonizing stories do harm to Indigenous storytelling practices, cultural and community stories in an ongoing way. A key quote from one of the storytellers and co-researchers that shaped the direction for this research project captures it well:

> *It's about the way they tell their stories about us. It's about the way we then have to tell our stories within their stories. No wonder you go womba (mad/crazy)* (Saunders 2016, p.16).

All research at its core is about questioning, and it is the form and type of research question that drives methodological choice. The questions asked of VS as an Aboriginal researcher and woman required a more holistic methodological response and deliberation (and unlearning). The poem that concludes this section captures in poetic form some of the critical deliberations and findings of answering these questions. (See Fig. 11.5 for an example process of poetic inquiry).

As an Aboriginal researcher embedded within a place-based web of ancestral and social relationships that locate her identity and citizenship status, Vicki cannot *not* be a participant in the storytelling; that is, she is not quite nor can she be objective in this context. Underpinning her research standpoint is a foundational assumption that to do so could create harm and could also harm the precious stories that Indigenous peoples hold and share. Using poetic license, Vicki listened deeply for the absence of stories of recovery in contexts of Aboriginal mental health care. She listened to the way these absences revealed themselves through people's stories through the poetic—through verse rather than prose—disrupting the way the stories

Using poetic inquiry to story Aboriginal recovery in mental health care

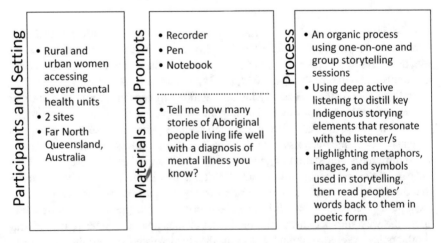

Fig. 11.5 Using poetic inquiry to story Aboriginal recovery in mental health care. (Reproduced with permission from the authors. Copyright © 2021 Wendy Madsen, Michelle Redman-MacLaren, Vicki Saunders, Cathy O'Mullan, and Jenni Judd. All rights reserved)

of Aboriginal people in mental health care are usually told in ways that others now describe as deficit discourses.

Re-covering methodologically

There are many ways to ask a question
    And many questions to ask
    The trick to seeking answers
    Is knowing which answer you want at the start
    But questions have a habit
    An irritating trend
    An inevitable growing spiral
    With no beginning and no end

The what of questions asked
    Comes from the questions why
    And to have the question answered
    depends on who it is asked by.
    How answers are found
    Is all about where and when
    And from the answers, you already know
    Ultimately is where "new knowledge" is located
    in the end.

But knowing and knowledge is a funny thing
    In the world of Indigenous science
    Especially in the field of research about those
    named Aboriginal or Indigenous mental health clients
    In the "mental health" arena—
    to be Indigenous is mainly deemed a curse
    In the discourses of "health,"
    it seems nothing is counted nor countered worse.
    Indigenous questions are all about Who
    And how our stories are related
    And answering unasked questions
    About how knowledge is used and how "truths" are created

Being human
    is to story that which we deem "real."
    About the truths that we know
    and can't separate from those which we feel.
    Where whose reality? is the central question
    In the field defining the "real" that gets heard
    To ask Indigenous questions
    makes an attempt to find "a 'real' answer" faintly absurd

To be able to ask
    My first questions come from the heart
    Do I have the courage?
    How will my words be used?
    And how do you express in words of science
    Questions better asked of spirit and through art?

At mental health's so-called cultural interface
   Where "knowledge" and "truth" are impossibly blurred
   Only questions bound in the "logic of care,"
   Cognitocentrism and pathology tend to emerge.
At heart the Indigenous quest is critical
   It's challenge—a way of seeing
   how knowing relates to doing
   and what this means for being
   a human researched being.

11.4   Discussion

While each of the four case studies used different ABR methods, collectively the case studies raise methodological and ethical issues for health promotion practitioners and researchers, including matters of differing aspirations, expectations, agendas, and power. However, there is a commonality that underpins all of these issues. At the heart of all four case studies was a commitment to relational epistemology within a participatory paradigm. Each case foregrounds or focuses on knowledge drawn from building relationships and dialogue between researchers, community organizations, and participants. In the case of *IT ALL BEGINS WITH LOVE*, there was a core group of co-researchers comprising artists, a counselor, and a university researcher who shared the decision making. In the IMPACT case, the university researchers partnered with support workers and case managers to work through the ethical issues that arose. The storyboarding case highlighted the need for the researchers to work in a culturally appropriate way in partnership with communities. The poetic inquiry case demonstrated how a researcher embedded within complex social and cultural relationships responded to the ethical and moral demands of working with Indigenous stories in cross-cultural and cross-disciplinary research. Not all ABR projects are located within a participatory paradigm. However, given health promotion's focus on social justice, social activism, and creating social change, it is not unusual that there is a propensity toward participatory ABR. As Foster (2012) suggests, arts activism can offer a platform for marginalized groups and help facilitate a different way of thinking to challenge oppression.

However, there are several implications for health promotion when relationality is privileged in ABR. First, considerable time is required to build relationships of trust that reflect genuine collaboration and shared decision-making (for further theoretical discussion of collaborative functioning in health promotion research, see Chap. 21, this volume). As highlighted in our case studies, when using ABR, health promotion researchers and practitioners may need to spend time understanding the variety of perspectives and language. Likewise, when working in a cross-cultural context, especially one in which roles and relationships are viewed from differing perspectives, considerable effort is needed to learn what is culturally appropriate.

Consequently, universities, partner organizations, or funding bodies may query the amount of time spent on participatory ABR projects, particularly regarding "returning benefits"—that is, the outcomes or outputs gained in comparison to the time and effort invested. There are challenges in evidencing relational outcomes or outcomes of the time spent building shared understandings with research partners and co-researchers. These outcomes are often intangible and only become visible over time; addressing these challenges means putting a priority on quality and social and relational dimensions of research results rather than quantity. The importance of a cultural guide/mentor advisor in projects with cultural diversity is a key element for research with other cultural groups. In research focused on contributing to grass-roots social change (see Capous-Desyllas and Morgaine 2018 for multiple examples), changes can be quite slow, with evidence of change often emerging outside the usual timeframes allowed for in research data collection. For example, each of the projects required a significant time investment at the beginning of the project; the *IT ALL BEGINS WITH LOVE* project involved three years of community consultation, with the evaluation component introduced at the end of that process.

The second implication is that of determining whose agenda or voice is being heard. Participatory ABR projects enable a range of people to be involved, many of whom have been excluded from participating in the research process in the past (although they have often been the objects of research). We (Cathy and Jenni) in the IMPACT project needed to adopt a flexible approach to be able to capture the voices of people with cognitive and physical disabilities. As Tina Cook and Pamela Inglis (2012) note, gaining the perspectives of those with disabilities can enable new understandings if we take a participatory, collaborative, and recursive approach. Adapting the photovoice methodology to suit the participants, and omitting customary interviews to explore the ideas further, allowed *their* stories to be told. The storyboarding and poetic inquiry cases both demonstrated how ABR enabled the inclusion of voices not always heard. Indeed, those who continue to live under the oppression of colonization are conscious that their stories may be filtered through the lenses of the colonizers (Smith 2012). In the poetic inquiry case study, ABR allowed Indigenous stories to be told directly by Indigenous voices.

Thus, the third implication is that of power and participation. Traditional research practices privilege those with numeracy, literacy skills, and knowledge, in both researchers and those who form the focus of research. People who come from oral knowledge traditions or whose cognitive processes act as barriers to participation in research projects are at a disadvantage in what is researched, how it is investigated, and what happens with data when they are collected. Participatory ABR helps to reduce power differences using genuine decision-sharing processes, inclusive data generation processes, collaborative analysis, and dissemination (Capous-Desyllas and Morgaine 2018; Ledwith and Springett 2010). Building and maintaining relationships of trust as well as a commitment to redressing power imbalances are critical for more effective health promotion research (Madsen and O'Mullan 2018).

11.5 Conclusion

While ABR practices are inherently aesthetic in that they emphasize arts processes and art products, the specific outcomes illustrated in these case studies demonstrate that ABR can also address issues of power and trust and amplify local knowledge and voices. Thus, there is a strong resonance between ABR practices and the values and actions within the Ottawa Charter (World Health Organization 1986) that provide a strong foundation for this work. ABR practices can enable different understandings of health promotion, well-being, and research, and can help reshape the traditional role of researcher from objective observer to co-participant/co-facilitator/co-researcher. While the outcomes from each of the case studies were unique, central to the success of all of them were the iterative, organic research processes and practices that responded to priorities of communities. Dedicating the necessary time to building trust and partnerships is what enabled these projects to succeed, and ABR was a critical part of this process. The ABR practices used in these case studies reinforced group potential and local knowledge, often within challenging social environments in which participants had little control over external or internal factors.

For the authors of this chapter, the value of using ABR practices in health promotion research lies in how it aligns with and reframes our positions as health promotion practitioner-researchers. ABR processes are juxtaposed with traditional research processes, including assumptions underpinning reasoning, validity, data construction, and interpretation. Importantly, ABR uses aesthetics to bridge the gap between researchers and the communities in which they work by generating new knowledge that is not only valid and useful, but also beautiful and aesthetically and emotionally rich.

References

Abadian, S. (2006). Cultural healing: When cultural renewal is reparative and when it is toxic. *Pimatisiwin: A Journal of Aboriginal and Indigenous Community Health, 4*(2), 5–28.

Archibald, J. A. (2008a). *Indigenous storywork: Educating the heart, mind, body, and spirit.* Vancouver: UBC Press.

Archibald, J. A. (2008b). An Indigenous storywork methodology. In *Handbook of the arts in qualitative research: Perspectives, methodologies, examples, and issues.* Thousand Oaks: Sage Publications.

Ashley, A. J. (2015). Beyond the aesthetic: The historical pursuit of local arts economic development. *Journal of Planning History, 14*(1), 38–61.

Banks, M. (2007). *The Sage qualitative research kit, 8 vols: Using visual data in qualitative research.* London: Sage.

Bessarab, D., & Ng'andu, B. (2010). Yarning about yarning as a legitimate method in indigenous research. *International Journal of Critical Indigenous Studies, 3*(1), 37–50.

Blomkamp, E. (2015). A critical history of cultural indicators. In *Making culture count* (pp. 11–26). London: Palgrave Macmillan.

Butler-Kisber, L. (2017). *Lynn Butler-Kisber defines poetic inquiry [streaming video]. SAGE research methods*. Retrieved from http://methods.sagepub.com/video/lynn-butler-kisber-defines-poetic-inquiry. Accessed 16 Nov 2018.

Butler-Kisber, L., & Stewart, M. (2009). The use of poetry clusters in poetic inquiry. In M. Prendergast, C. Leggo, & P. Sameshima (Eds.), *Poetic inquiry: Vibrant voices in the social sciences* (pp. 3–12). Rotterdam: Sense Publishers.

Capous-Desyllas, M., & Morgaine, K. (2018). Preface. In M. Capous-Desyllas & K. Morgaine (Eds.), *Creating social change through creativity: anti-oppressive arts-based research methodologies* (pp. vii–xix). Cham. Palgrave Macmillan.

Cluley, V. (2017). Using photovoice to include people with profound and multiple learning disabilities in inclusive research. *British Journal of Learning Disabilities, 45*(1), 39–46.

Cook, T., & Inglis, P. (2012). Participatory research with men with learning disability: Informed consent. *Tizard Learning Disability Review, 17*(2), 92–101.

Dassah, E., Aldersey, H. M., & Norman, K. E. (2017). Photovoice and persons with physical disabilities: A scoping review of the literature. *Qualitative Health Research, 27*(9), 1412–1422.

Daykin, N., & Stickley, T. (2016). The role of qualitative research in arts and health. In S. Clift & P. M. Camic (Eds.), *Oxford textbook of creative arts, health, and wellbeing: International perspectives on practice, policy and research* (pp. 73–81). Oxford: Oxford University Press.

Foster, V. (2012). What if? The use of poetry to promote social justice. *The International Journal of Social Work Education, 31*(6), 742–755.

Fraser, K. D., & al Sayah, F. (2011). Arts-based methods in health research: A systematic review of the literature. *Arts & Health, 3*(2), 110–145.

Graham, G. (2005). *Philosophy of the arts: An introduction to aesthetics* (3rd ed.). London: Routledge.

Hassan, N. (2017). Re-voicing: Community choir participation as a medium for identity formation amongst people with learning disabilities. *International Journal of Community Music, 10*(2), 207–225.

Kovach, M. (2010). *Indigenous methodologies: Characteristics, conversations, and contexts*. Toronto: University of Toronto Press.

Ledwith, M., & Springett, J. (2010). *Participatory practice: Community-based action for transformative change*. Bristol: Policy Press.

Lyall, M. (2014). Method emerging: A statement of poetics for a project-based PhD. *Qualitative Research Journal, 14*(2), 134–149.

Madsen, W. (2018). Raising social consciousness through verbatim theatre: A realist evaluation. *Arts & Health, 10*(2), 181–194.

Madsen, W., & O'Mullan, C. (2018). Power, participation and partnerships: Reflections on the co-creation of knowledge. *Reflective Practice, 19*(1), 26–34.

Pittaway, E., & Bartolomei, L. (2012). *Community consultations using reciprocal research methodologies*. Sydney: Centre for Refugee Research, University of New South Wales.

Pollock, V. L., & Paddison, R. (2014). On place-making, participation and public art: The Gorbals, Glasgow. *Journal of Urbanism: International Research on Placemaking and Urban Sustainability, 7*(1), 85–105.

Prendergast, M. (2009). "Poem is what?" Poetic inquiry in qualitative social science research. *International Review of Qualitative Research, 1*(4), 541–568.

Redman-MacLaren, M., Mills, J., Tommbe, R., MacLaren, D., Speare, R., & McBride, W. J. H. (2017). Implications of male circumcision for women in Papua New Guinea: A transformational grounded theory study. *BMC Women's Health, 17*(53), 1–10.

Salazar, L. F., Crosby, R. A., & DiClemente, R. J. (2015). *Research methods in health promotion*. San Francisco: John Wiley & Sons.

Saunders, V. -L. (2016). "...": Using a non-bracketed narrative to story recovery in aboriginal mental health care. PhD thesis: James Cook University.

Scott, K., Rowe, F., & Pollock, V. (2018). Creating the good life? A wellbeing perspective on cultural value in rural development. *Journal of Rural Studies, 59*, 173–182.

Seed, N. (2016). Photovoice: A participatory approach to disability service evaluation. *Evaluation Journal of Australasia, 16*(2), 29–35.

Smith, L. T. (2012). *Decolonizing methodologies: Research and indigenous peoples*. London: Zed Books.

Stroud, S. R. (2014). The art of experience: Dewey on the aesthetic. In *Practicing pragmatist aesthetics: Critical perspectives on literature and the arts*. Amsterdam: Rodopi.

Van Luyn, A., Gair, S., & Saunders, V. (2016). 'Transcending the limits of logic': Poetic inquiry as a qualitative research method for working with vulnerable communities. In *Sharing qualitative research* (pp. 95–111). London: Routledge.

Wang, C., & Burris, M. A. (1997). Photovoice: Concept, methodology, and use for participatory needs assessment. *Health Education & Behavior, 24*(3), 369–387.

Webb, D. (2014). Placemaking and social equity: Expanding the framework of creative placemaking. *Artivate: a Journal of Entrepreneurship in the Arts, 3*(1), 35–48.

World Health Organization. (1986, November 17–21). *The Ottawa charter for health promotion: An international conference on health promotion: The move towards a new public health*. Ottawa.

Chapter 12
A Kaleidoscope of Words and Senses to (Re)Think the Chagas Problem: Experiences in Argentina and Brazil

Carolina Amieva, Carolina Carrillo, Cecilia Mordeglia, María Cecilia Gortari, María Soledad Scazzola, and Mariana Sanmartino

12.1 Introduction

Chagas is a complex socio-environmental health problem with a direct and indirect impact on millions of people all over the world (Coura and Viñas 2010). The degree of advancement in scientific knowledge about the biological, medical, and

C. Amieva
Grupo de Didáctica de las Ciencias, IFLYSIB, CONICET - UNLP. Grupo ¿De qué hablamos cuando hablamos de Chagas?, La Plata, Buenos Aires, Argentina
e-mail: caro.amieva@gmail.com

C. Carrillo (✉)
Instituto de Ciencias y Tecnología Dr. César Milstein, CONICET, Grupo ¿De qué hablamos cuando hablamos de Chagas?, Buenos Aires, Argentina
e-mail: ccarrillo@centromilstein.org.ar; carolina.carrillo@conicet.gov.ar

C. Mordeglia
Grupo de Didáctica de las Ciencias, IFLYSIB, CONICET – UNLP, Facultad de Ciencias Naturales y Museo, UNLP Grupo ¿De qué hablamos cuando hablamos de Chagas?,
La Plata, Buenos Aires, Argentina
e-mail: cmordeg@fcnym.unlp.edu.ar

M. C. Gortari
Epidemiología y Salud Pública Básica, Facultad de Ciencias Veterinarias, UNLP, Grupo ¿De qué hablamos cuando hablamos de Chagas?, La Plata, Buenos Aires, Argentina
e-mail: mcgortari@fcv.unlp.edu.ar

M. S. Scazzola
Museo de La Plata, Facultad de Ciencias Naturales y Museo, UNLP. Grupo ¿De qué hablamos cuando hablamos de Chagas?, La Plata, Buenos Aires, Argentina
e-mail: scazzolasol@fcnym.unlp.edu.ar

M. Sanmartino
Grupo de Didáctica de las Ciencias, IFLYSIB, CONICET - UNLP. Grupo ¿De qué hablamos cuando hablamos de Chagas?, La Plata, Buenos Aires, Argentina
e-mail: mariana.sanmartino@conicet.gov.ar

epidemiological aspects of Chagas over the last 100 years has not translated into an equivalent increase in the welfare of people affected by Chagas (Sanmartino 2015). Thus, the complexity of the problem requires an innovative and interdisciplinary approach that recognizes the value of understanding the multiplicity of factors involved. In this sense, within the framework of the group *"What are we talking about when we talk about Chagas?"* (*¿De qué hablamos cuando hablamos de Chagas?*), we aim to make the topic visible in different educational and community contexts, critically reflecting with work team members and society to promote the exchange of knowledge and ways of thinking among the highest possible number and diversity of social actors. To accomplish this goal, we organized a variety of activities, including trainings and workshops, proposing a multidimensional approach to the topic where art, science, and other "sub-universes" (Good 1994) engage in dialogue to situate the Chagas problem beyond dichotomies and traditional approaches (Carrillo et al. 2018; Mordeglia et al. 2015; Sanmartino 2015). In this context, we share this chapter as a contribution to the collective fabric woven by speaking words about the Chagas problem in particular, health promotion in general, and art(s) as a tool and bridge to overcome barriers in the search for social transformation (Chap. 1, this volume).

12.2 What Are We Talking About When We Talk About Chagas?

As mentioned above, Chagas is much more than a disease; it represents a complex socio-environmental health issue in which elements of a different nature converge and interact with each other (Sanmartino 2015). However, the way in which the Chagas problem is generally addressed—in literature, prevention and control actions, awareness and education strategies, etc.—is focused on and limited to some specific aspects, particularly the biomedical perspectives. As a consequence of this partial and static understanding, as if it were a "monochromatic kaleidoscope" with few fixed pieces, the progress made in some disciplines has not had a proportional effect on the health and welfare of those affected by Chagas. For this reason, our group discusses and works on Chagas from an innovative and comprehensive perspective from at least four dimensions: *biomedical, epidemiological, socio-cultural,* and *political.* As we will highlight, each dimension offers and adds groups of unique pieces or "colored beads," with their special shapes and peculiar colors that interact and complete the others in a "kaleidoscopic puzzle" (see Fig. 12.1). In a kaleidoscope, every little bead with its own shape, color and size, is essential to forming a diverse and enriching image: a dynamic image that results from a unique conjunction of all the parts (Carrillo et al. 2018). In fact, the kaleidoscopic model implies movement of its pieces!

As with all puzzles, all the pieces—in this case called *dimensions*—contribute the same weight to the image we want to assemble/observe, and if one of them is missing, we cannot access the whole figure. Similarly, in all kaleidoscopes, the

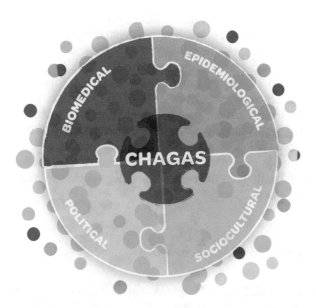

Fig. 12.1 Chagas problem represented as a "kaleidoscopic puzzle". (Design: Ruth Oño)

richness of the images we observe is made possible by the contribution of each and every one of the colored beads—in this case, every component of each dimension, every actor, and every bit of knowledge involved. For this reason, we believe that components of all four of the dimensions briefly described below are necessary when approaching the Chagas problem because they constitute the aforementioned "kaleidoscopic puzzle," and they make sense if we analyze them as a whole from the dynamic interrelationships existing among them.

12.2.1   Biomedical Dimension

This point of view—one of the most common means of addressing the topic—focuses on Chagas as the parasitosis caused by the unicellular parasite *Trypanosoma cruzi* (*T. cruzi*). One of the main routes of transmission of *T. cruzi* is the so-called "vector route," in which infected blood-sucking insects (triatomines, which in Argentina and other countries from the Southern Cone are known by their Quechuan name "vinchucas" and, in English, "kissing bugs") transmit the parasite through their stool. However, it can also be transmitted during pregnancy or delivery (vertical or congenital transmission), through the transfusion of blood or the transplant of some organs of infected donors, through the consumption of foods or beverages containing the parasite, or by laboratory accidents of people working in health or scientific fields. Chagas disease has an acute stage, when the parasite enters the organism, which can either be characterized by symptoms like malaise, prolonged fever, and vomiting or be asymptomatic. After approximately 1 month, the chronic stage starts. Although 70% of people with a chronic Chagas infection may not present any symptoms throughout their lives, 30% of them may develop heart, digestive, and—in very unusual cases—neurological problems 20 or 30 years after becoming infected. The available treatments are partially effective, and the sooner the diagnosis, the more effective the treatment. However, although there are good detection methods, it is estimated that only one out of ten people has been diagnosed (Coura and Viñas 2010), which directly affects both individual and public health. We usually approach both points of view, biological and medical, together as a unique kaleidoscopic puzzle piece: the *"biomedical dimension"* (Sanmartino et al. 2012), which has traditionally been the common and hegemonic approach to addressing this complex problem.

12.2.2 Epidemiological Dimension

This dimension considers that Chagas disease is endemic to Latin America and originally spread out from rural areas in the southern United States to Patagonia (Argentina and Chile). There are currently at least eight million people infected with *T. cruzi* in the world, mainly in Latin America (with at least 1.5 million people in Argentina, the authors' home country) (WHO 2012). Nevertheless, the epidemiological picture has become more complex due to the migratory movements of the last few decades as well as the urbanization and globalization phenomena and climate change. As a result, Chagas disease is no longer exclusively a rural problem or only a Latin American reality (Briceño-León and Méndez Galván 2007). We are currently facing a problem that is present in both rural and urban contexts around the world.

Biomedical and epidemiological dimensions are undoubtedly important; however, they are not enough to represent all the complexity involved in the "kaleidoscopic problem" of Chagas. That is why we have added components ("colored beads") from at least two more dimensions to this dynamic puzzle to better comprehend the Chagas complexity.

12.2.3 Socio-cultural Dimension

This aspect involves "cosmovisions" or worldviews and cultural practices of directly or indirectly implied actors; management of the environment; particularities of rural and urban contexts; social representations; stereotypes; prejudices; and social assessments (discrimination and stigmatization, among others).

12.2.4 Political Dimension

Lastly, we add this dimension that involves issues related to public management and health decision-making, education, and legislative topics at local, regional, and global levels. This dimension also includes public and private administrations, whose economic resources directly or indirectly affect this problem. Furthermore, this dimension encompasses personal, civil, and community points: the decisions that each one of us—as individuals or as a group, from our civil and professional roles (in research, teaching, communication, health care, etc.)—actively or passively assumes when we think (or not) about Chagas from a certain perspective.

12.3 Brief Thoughts on the Art-Chagas Problem Dialogue

We are convinced of the necessity of going beyond "preventing and curing the disease" to focus on the practice of health promotion to improve people's quality of life. With this purpose in mind over more than 7 years of work, our multidisciplinary group has approached the Chagas problem from an integrated, innovative, and "kaleidoscopic" way in different educational and social contexts: schools, museums, fairs, universities, and social organizations. Our aim is to integrate multiple aspects, perspectives, and languages from the four dimensions (biomedical, epidemiological, socio-cultural, and political) into a collaborative work in permanent dialogue with different social actors to create and encourage various ways of looking at, understanding, and approaching the complexity of Chagas to ultimately produce positive synergy in outcomes (see Chap. 21, this volume, for further background on synergy in health promotion initiatives).

In this sense, as proposed by Ros (2004), art is a language—among multiple languages—that expresses and communicates the ideology, subjectivity, and vision of people's reality. In addition, art is a specific way of knowing, analyzing, and interpreting our environment through different symbolic languages (body, sound, visual, dramatic, and literary). For this reason, we believe that different artistic expressions summon, communicate, and sensitize people differently, providing sensitivity and depth in the interpretation and analysis of complex topics such as Chagas (Sanmartino and Ale 2011). In agreement with Aranda Zamudio, we are convinced that science and technology offer us the possibility of understanding and transforming the world, showing us its limits, whereas art allows us to break these limits and go beyond them, challenging reality and ourselves (Aranda Zamudio 2011).

In this way, along our path, the artistic languages explicitly nourished the collective fabric around the Chagas problem in all the possible dimensions. In our experience, we have created and encouraged the deliberate promotion of spaces, instances, and productions where different expressions of visual arts, music, audiovisual arts, literature, and performing arts take on special importance (Mordeglia et al. 2015). Many of these productions emerged from learning spaces (such as the one presented in this chapter) and, at the same time, became resources to promote discussions, reflections, critical viewpoints, and even new artistic expressions.

In this chapter, we aim to advance the systematization process of the art-Chagas axis that crosses practically all the proposals we have developed (and continue to develop) in the group *"What are we talking about when we talk about Chagas?"* We focus on the analysis of the literary productions elaborated by different actors (teachers, degree and/or postgraduate students, and professionals, among others) after having participated in multiple training opportunities (courses, meetings, workshops) between the years 2012 and 2018 in Argentina and Brazil. In this analysis, we evaluated the different dimensions of the Chagas problem that were included in these texts and also characterized the actors, identifying the characters' roles and the strategies posed to approach the topic in each case.

12.4 "Brushstrokes" About the Theoretical Context That Guides and Inspires Our Work

Throughout these years of work, we progressively recognized the potential of systematizing our experiences, both to learn from our practices and to advance findings in a way that allows us to share our learnings with others (Sanmartino et al. 2014). The "systematization of experiences" is a process of reflection and critical interpretation about and from the practice, performed from the reconstruction and structuring of the objective and subjective factors that are part of an experience to extract learnings and be able to share them (Jara 2012). Thus, as Torres and Cendales (2006) propose, we assumed systematization as a research practice with its own identity, and not as a moment or stage in research; it is not an assessment, because its intention is not to evaluate the accomplishment or the impact of a planned objective, but instead to recover the knowledge and meanings of the experience to make it stronger. As a qualitative-critical investigation in which the processes of reconstruction, interpretation, and transformation of the experience are simultaneously developed, "systemization of experiences" implies an engaged participation of their constituents at the same time as it contributes to their formation (Torres Carrillo 1996).

We are also interested in incorporating into our readings and interpretations certain contributions from the so-called *Epistemologies of the South*, which propose approaches for the construction and validation of knowledge developed by social groups as part of their struggles and resistance against the injustices and oppressions generated by capitalism, colonialism, and patriarchy (De Sousa Santos 2014). Particularly for the purposes that underlie these pages, we worked using the *Ecology of Knowledge* as an organizing framework. This perspective assumes that all the practices of relationships among human beings, as well as between human beings and nature, imply more than one way of knowledge and, thus, of ignorance. It consists, on the one hand, of exploring alternative scientific practices that are made visible through the plural epistemologies of the scientific practices and, on the other hand, of promoting the interdependency between scientific and non-scientific knowledge (De Sousa Santos 2014). In other words, it is an ecology based on the recognition of the plurality of heterogeneous knowledges (where modern science is one of them) and on the continuous and dynamic interconnections among these kinds of knowledge without compromising their autonomy. Hence, as opposed to a rooted monocultural perspective, the *Ecology of Knowledge* understands knowledge as an intervention in reality more than as a hierarchy of occidental knowledge over other ways of knowing. That is, this perspective does not consider knowledge in abstraction but rather as practices of knowledge that allow or prevent certain interventions in the real world.

In this frame, we believe that promoting a kaleidoscopic approach of the Chagas problem implies putting into practice the *Ecology of Knowledge*, which would allow us to reach a *Cognitive Justice* (De Sousa Santos 2014). De Sousa Santos states that from the conquest and the beginning of modern colonialism, there has been a kind of injustice that founds and contaminates all the other kinds of injustices we have acknowledged in modernity; whether they are socio-economic, sexual, racial, historical, or generational injustices, it is all about cognitive injustice. In this sense, it is evidenced throughout the work that among the different kinds of injustices related to the Chagas problem (political, economic, social, cultural, sanitary), there is a transverse injustice directly related to knowledge because, as we mentioned earlier, the biomedical/epidemiological knowledge is recognized almost exclusively as the only valid one.

12.5 Presentation of the Case Example—Where Did These Texts Come from?

The literary texts analyzed here were produced, as we have already mentioned, in diverse courses, workshops, and/or meetings held between 2012 and 2018 in different locations in Argentina and Brazil. The first time we performed the literary writing exercise about Chagas was in August 2012 within the framework of the first "Month of Chagas" that we organized in the Museum of La Plata (Buenos Aires Province, Argentina). There, we delivered a teacher training course consisting of seven meetings (21 hours in total) for ten kindergarten teachers. At the closure of the course, the participants were asked to write a story about the Chagas problem in first person, inspired by an image provided by the course coordinators that showed a group of people of different ages, as a family group, but without giving details about relationships between them, about rural or urban context, or about their social or economic position. The ten texts resulted in such beautiful literary expressions that we decided to gather them in a publication. To give the texts some color, at the end of the same year we organized a "Meeting of Illustrators" in the Municipal Ecological Park of La Plata. Numerous artists (professional and amateur) from the area were invited to be inspired by and to illustrate the teachers' texts. The literary and visual beauty obtained through these activities about the Chagas problem was condensed in the book *"We talk about Chagas: stories and strokes to think of a complex problem"* (Sanmartino et al. 2013; free at https://hablamosdechagas.org.ar/recursos-libros/); the book, beyond its value as a cultural object, resulted in an inspiring tool to approach the topic in new contexts or with new actors. From that first and pleasant experience onward, we decided to replicate the literary text production exercise in other scenarios, given the potential of the activity and the excellent reception of the participants turned into "authors."

The other texts analyzed here corresponded to the following six contexts:

1. Workshop: *"Art and Chagas: expressions to think of a complex problem"* (4 hours work) within the framework of the I Brazilian Symposium of Cultural Entomology, May 2013, Feira de Santana, Brazil. Recipients: students of natural sciences and professionals devoted to the study of insects and their link with diverse aspects of culture (four texts).

2. Talk-Workshop: *"A kaleidoscopic proposal to think of Chagas today"* (5 hours work) within the framework of the seminar "Chagas disease: conscience and sensitization" (Iniciar for Global Action Foundation), June 2014, University of Buenos Aires, Argentina. Recipients: Research professionals and people interested in the Chagas topic in general (six texts).

3. Teacher Training Course: *"What are we talking about when we talk about Chagas?"* (15 hours work) within the framework of the Month of Chagas, September 2014, Museum of La Plata, Argentina. Recipients: teachers from all educational levels and university students (Degree Complementary Activity—National University of La Plata) (ten texts). The texts are published in the Appendix of the book *"We talk about Chagas: Contributions to (re)think the problem with a comprehensive view"* (Sanmartino 2015).

4. Workshop: *"(Re)Thinking the Chagas problem from a kaleidoscopic perspective"* (3 hours work) within the framework of the Annual Meeting of the Research Platform in Chagas Disease, Drugs for Neglected Diseases Initiative—Latin America (DNDi), August 2015, Buenos Aires, Argentina. Recipients: specialists from diverse disciplines, mainly biomedical ones, professionally related to the Chagas problem (seven texts).

5. Postgraduate Course: *"Educating in health from a comprehensive perspective: The multidimensionality of problems such as Chagas and illnesses transmitted by mosquitoes"* (Chagas block: 4 hours work), National University of Río Cuarto, June 2017, Río Cuarto, Córdoba, Argentina. Recipients: university teachers, postgraduate students, and students from other educational levels in courses related to education and health (four texts).

6. Postgraduate Course: *"Tools to understand and approach the multidimensionality of regional health problems"* (Chagas block: 4 hours work), National University of El Litoral, June 2018, Santa Fe, Argentina. Recipients: postgraduate students, teachers, researchers, and professionals related to health (four texts).

For all cases, the following instruction was provided to inspire the literary productions about Chagas:

With a family image as a trigger, in groups (of no more than six members), write a text (story, poem, letter, news story, etc.) in first person from the role assigned by the workshop coordinator (according to the features of the context where the activity is being developed, the roles might be: kissing bug, children, mother, father, neighbor, teacher, doctor, ruler, employer, journalist), considering the peculiarity that one of the family members in the image has Chagas disease (it does not matter who, but it is worth mentioning that the text must report that information in some way).

The 45 analyzed productions—with no directions about format or style (there were stories, letters, news stories, interviews, speeches, dialogues between different characters, play scripts, monologues, songs, and poems)—were written by 216 people of whom 80% were women, 17% were men, and 3% were an undeclared gender. With regard to their professional or academic activities, 49% were teachers from different educational levels, 32% were professionals and/or researchers, and the remaining 19% were degree and postgraduate students.

12.6 Some Methodological Considerations

Within our main goal of approaching the Chagas problem in a "kaleidoscopic" way by considering the arts as tools and bridges to go beyond the limits of typical approaches to addressing scientific questions, this work was centered on two particular objectives about the aforementioned literary texts: (1) to visualize and describe the conceptual representation of the different dimensions of Chagas, and (2) to characterize the actors, their roles, and their strategies to approach the problem depicted in the texts. We chose a qualitative methodology, since it allowed us to approach the social experience of the subjects and their links with "others" and with different ways of knowledge/power (Vasilachis de Gialdino 2007). Thus, on our first approach to the compiled texts, we made an individual reading prior to the formal analysis, acknowledging the appearance of the proposed characters and of other ones who were incorporated spontaneously as well as of the four-dimensional fabric that we proposed as the model to approach the Chagas problem. Then, we addressed our two objectives with specific methodologies.

12.6.1 Objective One: Conceptual Representations

For the objective related to analyzing the different dimensions of the Chagas problem, we used the *systemic network technique* proposed by Bliss et al. (1983) and the *word cloud/tag cloud generation technique* (McNaught and Lam 2010).

12.6.1.1 Systemic Network Technique

Systemic networks allow for structuring qualitative data according to a categorization previously determined or elaborated from the obtained words in the texts to be studied (Bliss et al. 1983). As a whole, the networks collect all the meanings to be analyzed and represent them in the form of an ordinary graphic language. For the network structuring, we pre-established, as primary categories, each of the four dimensions we proposed for the Chagas problem approach (biomedical, epidemiological, socio-cultural, and political). Then we started the readings and, according to their appearance, we defined the subcategories of conceptual organization included in each dimension. The level of subcategories emerged naturally, in accordance with the depth reached in the texts for each dimension. Hence, we considered that the appearance of different subcategories or deepness levels accounts for the dependence or independence among ideas, feelings, and values expressed in the texts. In this sense, every built structure or network is one among many possible others, related to the analyst's interpretation (Sanmartí 1993).

12.6.1.2 Word Cloud

The concepts systematized in each dimension of the systemic network were represented according to their frequency of appearance through a word cloud or tag cloud (excluding those that appeared only once or twice). The word cloud is a graphical representation of text data that assigns to each included word a size relative to its prominence in terms of frequency of appearance, obtaining a "quick and visually rich" shape (McNaught and Lam 2010). The platform used for the elaboration of the word cloud was WordArt (2009).

12.6.2 Objective Two: Actors Characterization

With the particular aim of characterizing the actors, their roles and their strategies, and the frequency of appearance of each them in the texts, we applied Content Analysis (CA) (Bardin 1977). The process started with a first "floating reading" (i.e., a reading that focuses on structures rather than deeply on the content) to identify the main analysis variables (Cea D'Ancona 1996)—for example, "type of character" or "role in the text" and their correspondent self-built categories system (see Table 12.1). Next, during the step of "material utilization," we assigned codes to each variable and each defined category to load them into the IBM SPSS Statistics 23 program. This process permitted us to generate simple characteristics of the text samples—i.e., to count frequency of appearance for each variable and each category (for example, times in which "mother" was presented as the main character in "type of character").

Table 12.1 Coding variables and their categories system

Variable	Description of variables with their categories system
Type of character	In all cases, the main character was provided by the exercise instructions; then, the authors decided freely whether to introduce (or not) more characters. The characters mentioned in the texts were: doctor, member of a family (aunt or uncle, daughter or son, niece or nephew, cousin, grandparent, children, mother, father), kissing bug, teacher, employer, mayor, journalist, neighbor, scientist (biologist), and people in general (men and women)
Role in the text	We classified characters into active or passive. Active characters were those in charge of decision-making and situation-solving; passive characters performed the activities the others had decided on (without questioning)
Attitude toward the problem presented by active characters	According to the situations posed in the texts, we identified the following attitudes: to provide biomedical information as well as diagnosis and treatment of the disease, to look for biomedical information, to advocate for more involvement of the state (via resources and/or campaigns), to deliver informative talks at school, to generate discrimination situations (especially in work environments), and to report discrimination situations in the media
Focus of the problem for active characters	We identified the following categories as the focus of the problem for active characters: lack of biomedical information, desire for better access to certain resources, little involvement of the government in providing budget and resources, and lack of information about legal rights
Recipients of the problem-solving strategies for active characters	We found the recipients of problem-solving strategies for active characters to be the following: people without information, patients, the community in general, doctors, interdisciplinary teams (doctors, social workers, field technicians, psychologists, and lawyers, among others), people infected in general, people infected who are not apt for work, media, and people who are not aware of their legal rights
Focus of the problem for passive characters	We identified the following categories as the focus of the problem for passive characters: lack of biomedical information, little presence of the state, lack of medical knowledge, little presence of the school, discrimination at work, people in general and their prejudices, knowledge within the family, and specialized Chagas-trained field technicians
Recipients of the problem-solving strategies for passive characters	We found the recipients of problem-solving strategies for passive characters to be the following: doctors, teachers, politicians, the community in general, and employers
Position in the strategy posed by passive characters	We identified the positions in the strategy posed by passive characters to be the following: waiting for answers and action plans posed by others (if there is a solution, the character accepts it); waiting for answers and action plans posed by others but, in certain cases, showing a certain degree of initiative at the time of asking for information and the necessary help; and the victim's position

12.7   What These Written Words Do (and Do Not) Say

12.7.1   About the Dimensions Crossing the Texts

The word cloud obtained from the analyzed literary productions provided us with an initial overview (see Fig. 12.2). Out of the 43 concepts present at least three times, 31 belonged to the nucleus of biomedical/epidemiological dimensions: *disease* was the predominant term, followed by *diagnosis, transmission routes*, and *treatment*. In the word cloud—as well as in the systemic network—we found that the biomedical and epidemiological dimensions formed a conceptual entity difficult to separate because there are concepts that, depending on the scale and context, could be included in one or the other dimension. Even when considering them separately, they had a predominant presence over the socio-cultural and political dimensions.

In the systemic network and considering both majority dimensions separately, we found that the biomedical dimension (red words in Fig. 12.2) was predominant, represented mainly by the concepts of *disease, vector*, and *transmission routes*, and secondarily by *disease stages* and *parasite*. Among them, *disease* was the most represented concept, related to diagnosis, symptoms, and treatment. *Vector (vinchuca)* was a subcategory also represented with great depth and detail, in particular regarding its feeding habits, refuge, and life cycle. In turn, the concept of *transmission routes* was often represented by the vectorial transmission.

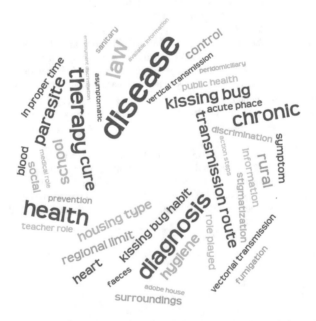

Fig. 12.2 Word cloud obtained from the analyzed literary productions. Color reference: Red/Biomedical dimension, Orange/Epidemiological, Green/Socio-cultural, Light blue/Political

Focusing on the epidemiological dimension (orange words in Fig. 12.2), although it was not present in all of the texts, it was the second most important dimension according to the frequency of appearance and level of detail. Its components were condensed into four subcategories: *geographical distribution* of the disease in certain provinces in the north of Argentina, *epidemiological indicators*, *population* (or *migratory*) *movements*, and *prevention* and *vector control*, in agreement with the relevance assigned to the vectorial transmission in the biomedical dimension.

The socio-cultural dimension (green words in Fig. 12.2) appeared to be next in importance, represented by five concepts: *housing* (type and condition), *social representations* (for example, the roles of doctor and teacher), *discrimination* (both at work and among social classes and strongly linked to the concept of stigmatization), *person* or *migrant group*, and *quality of life*. In all cases, it was evident that the strong symbolic value assigned to certain social actors reflected the existence of hegemonic and stereotypical roles.

Lastly, the political dimension (light blue words in Fig. 12.2) included the common concepts of *public health*, *information/disinformation*, *citizen role*, and *education content*, and, to a lesser extent, the *legal framework* in Argentina (Ley 26.281, 2007). These concepts are centered in the role of the public policy—present or absent—and the state as the only ones responsible for it, whereas the appropriation of the personal political responsibility as citizens was barely represented by a tangential acknowledgment of the degree of disinformation of certain actors, even when it was a specific topic discussed in the courses.

As a general observation, we found that the conceptual structure of biomedical and epidemiological dimensions is hierarchically organized and is condensed in technical terms of high repetition (for example, the term *disease* represented, in turn, by the subordinate categories *acute disease, chronic disease, neglected disease*). In contrast, socio-cultural and political dimensions do not present a defined conceptual structure, being represented by a great diversity of concepts mentioned few times without hierarchical organization among them. We think that word diversity without hierarchy reveals the absence of a previous conceptual structure about the socio-cultural and political dimensions in the participants, because these points of analysis are not familiar to people who do not work in topics related to Chagas and social or political sciences.

12.7.2   About the Characters Present in These Texts

Considering the types of actors represented in the texts, in 60% of the cases main or secondary characters were embodied by members of the *family*, and in 40% of the texts the *doctor* figure was also included (in only one case, it was a female doctor). The *teacher* (female in all of the cases) appeared in 20% of the texts, the same as the *vinchuca*—considered as a main character with the ability to express itself. Finally, the characters of *employer* (male), *mayor* (male), *journalist* (male), *neighbor* (male), *member of the family*, and *scientist/biologist* (male) appeared in at least 10% of texts.

In most of the cases, active roles were embodied either by characters with professions recognized as "holders of knowledge"—*doctor* (35%), *teacher* (14%), *journalist* (6%), and *biologist* (2%)—or by characters with a favorable position within an asymmetric power relationship, namely *employer* (8%) and *mayor* (8%). Characters without an explicit stamp of power (either of authority or of knowledge), such as *neighbor* (8%), had an active role in only a few cases; on the contrary, all the passive roles were held by these actors' profiles, frequently described as family members (*mother*, *father*, *child*). These findings suggest that perhaps these passive but familiar characters might be viewed as lacking the pertinent knowledge/power necessary for action.

12.7.2.1   Active Characters

Regarding the analysis of active characters, we focused on four axes: (1) attitude toward the problem, (2) problem focus, (3) role in their strategy, and (4) recipients of the strategies.

In the first axis, most (90%) of the attitudes toward the problem were constructive or "positive"; that is, they posed a concrete and specific solution for it. In this sense, doctors were identified as those in charge of providing biomedical information and diagnosing and treating those who needed it. Teachers were also acknowledged as providers of biomedical information at schools. We understand that these evaluations respond to a stereotypical view regarding the competencies of these professions. On the contrary, "negative" attitudes, such as discrimination toward an affected person by an employer and/or neighbor, appeared in a small proportion of texts (10%). Characters aimed at individual and personalized solutions did not consider, for example, the option of organizing themselves and/or contacting the existing organizations related to the problem. As an exception, there was one text—out of 45—where Chagas was recognized as a social problem (referred as "Chagas involves all of us" and "it is a problem for everyone"), although in this case there was not a manifested reference to a collective search for responses.

In the second axis, the focus of the problem for these characters was primarily centered (89%) in people's lack of biomedical information. In only a small percentage (4%) was it mentioned that the role of the state was as a central actor, the one that must administer budgets and/or organize prevention campaigns.

Similarly, in the third axis of analysis, the strategies adopted by the active characters to face the problem were, on the one hand, those of sources of biomedical knowledge (44%) and, on the other hand, those of sources of power (41%) in charge of performing, managing, and/or organizing the posed strategies.

In the last axis of analysis, the recipients of the strategies were mostly individuals (89%) who, as we have already mentioned, lacked knowledge and power. In only a small proportion (11%) were the recipients doctors, media, and/or interdisciplinary work teams. Can we infer then that biomedical knowledge (of active characters present in the texts) constitutes a unidirectional, categorical, and non-dialogic knowledge that must be transmitted only by certain specialized actors? Are "ordinary" people "mere receptors" of that knowledge in this uneven knowledge relationship, with no valid knowledge of their own to contribute to the understanding of the problem? (Sanmartino 2015).

12.7.2.2 Passive Characters

Regarding the analysis of passive characters, we focused on three axes: (1) focus of the problem, (2) position in the proposed solving strategy, and (3) recipients of the strategies.

In the first axis, we found that the focus of the problem for these characters was related to individual actions, centered frequently (67%) in the lack of biomedical information. On the other hand, 30% of these characters mentioned the state, doctors, school, and workspaces as places where there should be a search for solutions to the problem.

With respect to passive characters, we found that they were frequently (65%) in the position of waiting for responses or action plans elaborated by "others," generally recognized as active characters. Only one-third of passive characters, although waiting for responses from active characters, showed initiative to ask for solutions and be in charge of accomplishing them. For example, we frequently found that some characters consulted a doctor about their possible positive Chagas disease diagnosis because they had been looking for information and knew about the existence of treatment. In these cases, although they had the initiative of looking for information and undergoing the existing treatments, they needed a doctor to confirm and decide the treatment. Among these passive characters, people carrying the infection were characterized by fear, uncertainty, and/or worry, persisting in their characterizations a certain degree of stereotyped and/or prejudiced assumptions toward them. It should be noted that a minority (3%) of these characters positioned themselves as "motionless victims" who neither accepted a solution nor performed actions to change "their fate."

Finally, the responses of both active and passive characters complemented each other regarding who was identified as a recipient of problem-solving strategies. As we have already mentioned, active characters identified "ordinary" people as the main recipients; conversely, passive characters pointed out mostly *doctors* (75%), *teachers* (11%), *politicians* (8%), and *employers* (7%) as the recipients of such strategies. This result complements the analysis previously performed that represented active characters as not only the sources of knowledge and power, but also as the main (and only) responsible parties for permanent training, researching, informing, and assigning resources to and about the topic. The analysis positioned passive characters as "non-actors" in the Chagas puzzle, because they were not recognized by others or by themselves as holders of valuable knowledge or facilitators of concrete actions (of their own and others) to face the Chagas problem.

12.8   Final Words: What This Kaleidoscope of Words and Senses Left Us With

During the process of kaleidoscopic analysis of these diverse literary productions, we faced some difficulties that are worthwhile to consider for future experiences.

The first challenge pertains to dimensions. The conceptualization and categorization into one or another dimension was a difficult task in terms of simplifying into four categories a complex multidimensional matrix, whose dynamic and diffuse boundaries—depending on the subject and the situation—in many cases are blurred in the analysis. Furthermore, because of the literary nature of the texts, we found that there were not only explicit but also implicit or metaphorical aspects to be included. On the other hand, in the task of classifying complex concepts, we found in many cases an additional difficulty based on the abstract descriptions of the scenarios and/or the characters' situations. For example, several times there were references to provinces in the north of Argentina—made by authors who do not live in that region—as vaguely defined scenarios, without distinction between urban and rural realities and that put forward assumptions based on lack of knowledge and/or prejudice. In these cases, we assumed that when referring to a "place in the north" or a "north province" the authors were considering a rural setting typically related to Chagas distribution.

Another difficulty we faced was related to the characters and their strategies. We discussed both the level of detail that analysis categories should have as well as the possibility of losing the text richness when "reducing" its interpretation to predetermined categories. Because of this challenge, we left the categories open so that they could be revised, enriched, and/or redefined if necessary. We also debated quantifying certain aspects in this qualitative analysis process, eventually deciding to have a quantitative review first (by examining descriptive statistics) that later would allow us to develop more complex results. Certainly, we did not want to forget that this categorization was the product of a constant process of qualitative construction aimed at responding to work objectives and that we should be careful not to make broader generalizations. In this sense, as we have focused on some specific words, we are aware that part of the richness of the analyzed texts – in terms of their literary and/or artistic character – were left out to focus on the categorizations and descriptions that we present in this chapter.

According to Alderoqui and Pedersoli (2011), "the mirrors inside kaleidoscopes let us see the colored and multi-shaped beads contained within them multiplied, thus forming different images every time we rotate them. In this sense, building kaleidoscope views are to favor the observation of the same, integrating different viewpoints so that the overlapping of different partial images allows us to build a more complex and richer image than the one we isolatedly had about the topic." In particular, a kaleidoscope view about the Chagas problem invites us to acknowledge the relevance of adopting different approaches for its complex analysis. At the same time, it is essential to recognize the dynamism of the built images because they emerge from the interaction among the considered components that, in turn, depend both on the viewpoint of the different actors involved and in the great number and variety of conditioning related to the characteristics of the context (Sanmartino 2015).

Throughout these years working on this complex problem, different arts, sciences, and popular knowledge have been combined to create a kaleidoscope with beads of multiple shapes and colors whose objective is to overcome the dichotomies such as "sick/healthy," "rich/poor," and "rural/urban." We are sure that both arts and education, in a broad and inclusive sense, are key elements to shorten the distance between formal and non-formal knowledge and build alternatives that impact and transform reality. For this reason, we promote joint work among researchers, teachers, students, and the community in general at all educational levels (school as well as technical and professional training levels) and in all possible contexts (rural/urban, formal/informal, where there are/are not vector insects, etc.) with the purpose of engaging a greater number and diversity of voices talking about Chagas (Carrillo et al. 2018). We also aim to make our work a source of inspiration to approach other complex issues that affect different communities by encouraging critical and inclusive reflections of diverse voices and looks.

Beyond the results shared here (and its limitations), we recovered the value of the words woven by the authors of the 45 analyzed texts as multicolored beads that contribute to this collective kaleidoscope. We agree with Saavedra Rey, who claims that the construction of a narrative transcends a mere writing exercise. This process is linked to the human experience, which gives the words new meaning by adding to the human condition novel interpretations that can be expressed and shared by diverse people as an aesthetic experience and, as such, a vital experience (Saavedra Rey 2011). Although the literary text produces a world alternative to the "real" one, it also reproduces logics of knowledge and power and makes visible (even between the lines) the history and its fights for consolidating a sense of the hegemonic world. It is undoubtable, then, that in every text analyzed there was intentionality, because the one who writes assumes a particular position and builds knowledge about reality from his/her own perspective. Because of these factors, we value the potentiality of the literary production, not only on what those words say and do not say about Chagas.

Finally, we are convinced that for the complex topic we are considering here, the *Epistemologies of the South* (De Sousa Santos 2014) are one of the most fertile frameworks to incorporate new realities and analytical spaces to collect from the transforming and liberating scenarios that, within the context of health care and the biomedical hegemonic approach of Chagas, have been forgotten or simply disregarded. In this sense, although various aspects of the conventional social imagination (centered in rural issues, poverty, vectorial transmission, and ignorance, among others) that emerge from the aforementioned *cognitive injustice* had a strong presence in the analyzed texts, we believe that the work of symbolic deconstruction and resignification of the value of political and socio-cultural dimensions proposed in the courses and workshops allowed the emergence of concepts usually infrequently noticed. Enabling and/or making visible other voices—in particular ordinary, local, and non-specialized knowledge—brings us closer to the conceptual richness offered by the *Ecology of Knowledge*, necessary for an effective and kaleidoscopic approach toward the Chagas problem.

References

Alderoqui, S., & Pedersoli, C. (2011). *La educación en los museos. De los objetos a los visitantes.* Buenos Aires: Paidós.

Aranda Zamudio, M. R. (2011). Ciencia, arte y creatividad: creando vínculos a través de experiencias educativas. Boletín de la Comunidad de Educadores para la Cultura Científica, OEI. http://www.oei.es/divulgacioncientifica/spip.php?article217. Accessed 4 Nov 2018.

Bardin, L. (1977). *Análisis de contenido.* Madrid: Akal.

Bliss, J., Monk, M., & Ogborn, J. (1983). *Qualitative data analysis for educational research.* Londres: Coom Helm.

Briceño-León, R., & Méndez Galván, J. M. (2007). The social determinants of Chagas disease and the transformations of Latin America. *Memórias do Instituto Oswaldo Cruz, 102*(Suppl 1), 109–112.

Carrillo, C., Sanmartino, M., & Mordeglia, C. (2018). Education, communication, and lots of creativity: A good combination to face complex problems like Chagas. *Social Innovation Journal, 45.* www.socialinnovationsjournal.org/75-disruptive-innovations/2775-education-communication-and-lots-of-creativity-a-good-combination-to-face-complex-problems-like-chagas. Accessed 4 Nov 2018.

Cea D'Ancona, M. A. (1996). *Metodología cuantitativa: estrategias y técnicas de investigación social.* Madrid: Ed. Síntesis S.A.

Coura, J. R., & Viñas, P. A. (2010). Chagas disease: A new worldwide challenge. *Nature, 465*(Suppl 7301), S6–S7.

De Sousa Santos, B. (2014). *Epistemologies of the south: Justice against epistemicide.* New York: Paradigm Publishers.

Good, B. J. (1994). The body, illness experience, and the lifeworld: A phenomenological account of chronic pain. In Cambridge University Press (Ed.), *Medicine, rationality, and experience: An anthropological perspective* (pp. 116–134). Cambridge: Cambridge University Press.

IBM SPSS Statistics for Windows, Version 23.0. Armonk: IBM Corp.

Jara, O. (2012). *La sistematización de experiencias, práctica y teoría para otros mundos posibles.* Costa Rica: Centro de Estudios y Publicaciones Alforja. Consejo de Educación de Adultos de América Latina e Intermon Oxfam.

Ley 26.281. (2007, August 8). Ley de prevención y control de todas las formas de transmisión de la enfermedad de Chagas. Boletín Oficial de la República Argentina. Buenos Aires, Argentina. http://servicios.infoleg.gob.ar/infolegInternet/anexos/130000-134999/131904/norma.htm. Accessed 8 Nov 2018.

McNaught, C., & Lam, P. (2010). Using Wordle as a supplementary research tool. *The Qualitative Report, 15*(3), 630–643.

Mordeglia, C., Sanmartino, M., Amieva, C., Del Re, C., Gortari, M. C., Scazzola, M. S., et al. (2015). Arte y Chagas: recorrido por una galería de intercambio y producción colectiva. In *Libro de Memorias del XIV Congreso RedPop, Arte, tecnología, ciencia Nuevas maneras de conocer* (pp. 761–770). Colombia: Medellín.

Ros, N. (2004). El lenguaje artístico, la educación y la creación. *Revista Iberoamericana de Educación.* (ISSN: 1681-5653)*, 35,* 1–8.

Saavedra Rey, S. (2011). La creación literaria en el ámbito educativo: de la estructura superficial a la construcción narrativa de la realidad. *Lenguaje, 39*(2), 395–417. http://www.scielo.org.co/scielo.php?script=sci_arttext&pid=S0120-34792011000200005&lng=en&tlng=. Accessed 8 Nov 2018.

Sanmartí, N. (1993). *Las redes sistémicas: construcción y aplicaciones. Documento de trabajo.* Departament de Didàctica de la Matemàtica i de les Ciencies Experimentals. España: Universitat Autònoma de Barcelona.

Sanmartino, M. (coordinación). (2015). Hablamos de Chagas. Aportes para (re)pensar la problemática con una mirada integral. Contenidos: Amieva, C., Balsalobre, A., Carrillo, C., Marti,

G., Medone, P., Mordeglia, C., et al. Buenos Aires: CONICET. https://hablamosdechagas.org. ar/wp-content/uploads/2019/12/hablamosdechagas_aportes_para_re_pensar.pdf. Accessed 15 Sept 2020.

Sanmartino, M., & Ale, M. E. (2011). "Arte, Ciencia y Chagas: miradas posibles, diálogos necesarios. Memorias de un comienzo..." Edición Especial Coleccionable N°1. El latir de los equipos. Plan Nacer Entre Ríos.

Sanmartino, M., Mengasini, A., Menegaz, A., Mordeglia, C., & Ceccarelli, S. (2012). Miradas Caleidoscópicas sobre el Chagas. Una experiencia educativa en el Museo de La Plata. *Revista Eureka sobre Enseñanza y Divulgación de las Ciencias, 9*(2), 265–273.

Sanmartino, M., Mordeglia, C., Menegaz, A., & Zucchi, M. (Coord). (2013). *Hablamos de Chagas. Relatos y trazos para pensar un problema complejo.* ¿De qué hablamos cuando hablamos de Chagas? La Plata. ISBN 978-987-29223-0-6. https://hablamosdechagas.org.ar/wp-content/uploads/2020/04/Libro_Hablamos_de_Chagas.pdf. Accessed 4 Nov 2018.

Sanmartino, M., Mordeglia, C., Menegaz, A., Carrillo, C., Marti, G., Echazarreta, D., et al. (2014). Educación y Chagas: sistematización de experiencias innovadoras en la Región de La Plata (Buenos Aires, Argentina). Actas del Congreso Iberoamericano de Ciencia, Tecnología, Innovación y Educación (Buenos Aires, Argentina), Organización de Estados Iberoamericanos (OEI) y el Ministerio de Educación de la Nación.

Torres Carrillo, A. (1996). La sistematización como investigación interpretativa crítica: entre la teoría y la práctica. Seminario Internacional sobre sistematización y producción de conocimiento para la acción. Conferencia. Santiago, Chile.

Torres, A., & Cendales, L. (2006). *La sistematización como experiencia investigativa y formativa* (Vol. 23, pp. 29–38). La Piragua.

Vasilachis de Gialdino, I. (2007). La investigación cualitativa. In I. Vasilachis de Gialdino (coord.), *Estrategias de investigación cualitativa* (pp. 23–64). Barcelona, España: Gedisa.

WordArt.com. (2009). https://wordart.com/. Accessed 2 Nov 2018.

World Health Organization. (2012). Research priorities for Chagas disease, human African trypanosomiasis and leishmaniasis. *WHO Technical Report Series, 975,* 11–14.

Chapter 13
Mapping the Discourse on the Health-Promoting Impacts of Community Arts

Charlotte Lombardo

13.1 Introduction

Art-making and creative expression are powerful tools for personal and social learning, growth, and transformation. This rationale is at the essence of the practice of community arts (CA). CA have been defined as artistic activity based in a community setting and characterized by dialogue and co-creation with the community (Novak 2012). CA programs cite goals ranging from improving the social and emotional well-being of participants (Carson et al. 2007; Hampshire and Matthijsse 2010) to promoting civic dialogue and community building (Kelaher et al. 2014; Rhodes and Schechter 2012). CA initiatives are increasingly being understood as "whole person" approaches for improving health at individual and community levels, drawing on holistic conceptualizations of health that are not just physical or disease-specific, but rather emphasize broader concepts of mental and social well-being (Macnaughton et al. 2005) and thus aim to promote synergy within health promotion initiatives (for further theoretical background of synergy in health promotion, see Chap. 21, this volume).

The use of the arts within diverse health-related endeavors has been identified as an emerging field of "arts and health." This comprises arts-infused practice within a range of settings and approaches, including in therapeutic initiatives and health care practices, as a method for conducting and/or disseminating health research, or as an intervention strategy for community development and health promotion (Cox et al. 2010). This chapter seeks to investigate the latter—to unpack the current state of knowledge on the health-promoting impacts of CA. Health promotion refers to the conceptualization and specialized field of public health practice grounded in a social model of health that recognizes the wider social, economic, and environmental determinants of health (Rootman and O'Neill 2017; Chap. 1, this volume). The

C. Lombardo (✉)
Faculty of Environmental and Urban Change, York University, Toronto, ON, Canada
e-mail: charl@yorku.ca

© The Author(s) 2021
J. H. Corbin et al. (eds.), *Arts and Health Promotion*,
https://doi.org/10.1007/978-3-030-56417-9_13

structural determinants and conditions of daily life, marked by the unequal distribution of power, income, goods, and services, constitute the social determinants of health and are responsible for a major part of health inequities (CSDH 2008; Marmot 2015; Raphael 2016).

A growing body of literature seeks to substantiate the impacts of arts and health initiatives. There is no shortage of individual initiative evaluations. As the evidence base grows, there are now academic and lay synthesis publications detailing various forms of reviews (APPGAHW 2017; Bungay and Vella-Burrows 2013; Daykin et al. 2008; Zarobe and Bungay 2017). This work, however, has been hampered by complexities of practice and by contention regarding what constitutes the best or most valid forms of evidence (Clift 2012; Putland 2008; Raw et al. 2012). This chapter explores the discourse on the health-promoting impacts of CA, seeking to map current knowledge and debate in relation to CA and impacts on social determinants of health, in the English language literature.

13.2 Methods

A search was undertaken between April and August of 2018 to identify and synthesize peer-reviewed and grey literature on community arts and health promotion. Literature was identified through English language database searches (using the keywords "community arts" AND "health" OR "social impact"), reference lists of key articles, key informants, conferences, and workshops. For the purposes of mapping, emphasis was placed on articles identifying and summarizing outcomes of CA interventions, and on articles directly discussing or theorizing CA impacts. The goal here was not an exhaustive review, but rather a mapping of the central arguments and key tensions across the discourse on CA and health promotion in the English language literature.

One hundred and fifteen articles were initially identified, and 39 were found to meet the inclusion criteria (i.e., a focus on CA and impacts related to the social determinants/social model of health). CA was conceptualized as the participatory practice of art-making in groups within community settings. Articles were excluded if their primary focus was individually oriented and/or not community-based, such as therapeutic initiatives (e.g., arts-therapy, hospital/clinic-based interventions or supports), school-based arts education (arts engagement in formal curricula), and more general engagement in arts and culture (e.g., museum attendance, audience participation in music or performing arts, personal art-making or instruction). Articles were also excluded if their main focus was arts-based research (ABR), such as arts-based methods employed primarily in the context of a research project. ABR and CA are similar and related; the key differentiation lies in the overarching approach. While much ABR is participatory and socially motivated, arts-based activities/methods in ABR are undertaken primarily in the service of a pre-defined research question/program (Boydell et al. 2012). (For a detailed discussion of ABR, please see Chap. 11 (Madsen et al. 2021) in this volume). CA are community-based arts programs/interventions that seek to engage participants broadly in creative expression for the purpose of plural knowledge and cultural production (Novak 2012). Though generally not the expressed focus, CA approaches can be understood and leveraged as a form of research. Leading CA practitioner and theorist Deborah Barndt (2004) identifies processes of CA broadly as collaborative and participatory research, explaining: "When people are given the opportunity to tell their own stories, they bring their bodies, minds, and spirits into a process of communicating and sharing their experiences; they affirm their lives as sources of knowledge, and they stimulate each other in a synergistic process of collective knowledge production" (p. 354). While ABR methods are becoming increasingly recognized and integrated into research paradigms, less attention has been paid to more emergent CA approaches, hence the emphasis of this chapter.

Sixteen primary studies, eight review articles, and 15 practice commentaries were included and analyzed. Primary studies and review articles were so classified as they describe clear data collection and analysis methods. Practice commentaries, as opposed to reporting or synthesizing research, focus instead on discussing practice-based issues related to impact and evaluation, exploring practitioner perspectives on particular challenges, or reviewing and discussing epistemological tensions. The majority of the literature stems from Western contexts—notably the United Kingdom, Australia, and Canada—where policy agendas explicitly seeking to leverage CA approaches for health and/or community development have recently proliferated (Badham 2010; Clift et al. 2009; Cox et al. 2010). Table 13.1 provides a short description of each article.

The identified literature was further organized using an ecological mapping of micro-, meso-, and macro-level findings. Ecological analysis and mapping is a way of approaching issues that accounts for interrelationships between persons and settings, with the goal of exploring and unpacking dynamic interactions between individuals and their environment (Kingry-Westergaard and Kelly 1990). Increasingly utilized in public health and health promotion, such models explore health issues through multiple, interdependent levels of influence, from individual (micro), to interpersonal/communal (meso), to broader social (macro) levels (Richard et al. 2011).

13.3   Ecological Analysis of CA Health-Promoting Impacts

The following ecological analysis seeks to map and discuss health-promoting impacts of CA within a dynamic social context that should be read as complex and interrelated (Sallis et al. 2015). While locating issues or outcomes with a key ecological level, the whole system is understood as fluid and reciprocal. See Fig. 13.1 for a graphic depiction of this ecological mapping.

Table 13.1 Summary of articles included

Citation	Article type	Location	Key findings
Angus (2004)	Review (63 studies)	UK	Diverse CA projects, impacts on awareness raising, personal and social development, aesthetic improvement
APPGAHW (2017)	Review (16 roundtables)	UK	Diverse CA projects, place-based impacts on community, life course effects from childhood to end of life
Badham (2010)	Practice commentary	Australia	Critiques emphasis on instrumental benefits of CA and lack of critical attention to intrinsic artistic values
Belfiore (2006)	Practice commentary	UK	Discusses CA evaluation dilemmas, issues of causality, opportunity cost, outcome vs. outputs, anecdotal evidence
Belfiore (2002)	Practice commentary	UK	Discusses CA as means of alleviating social exclusion, in particular critiquing "instrumentalist" cultural policy
Belfiore and Bennett (2010)	Practice commentary	UK	Calls for humanities approach to assessing CA impacts, challenging perceived reductionist evaluation approaches
Böhm and Land (2009)	Practice commentary	Various	Critiques focus on capital benefits of culture, such as creativity and innovation, employability, social inclusion
Bungay and Vella-Burrows (2013)	Review (20 studies)	Various	Youth CA projects, impacts on sexual health, obesity, mental health, and emotional well-being
Cameron et al. (2013)	Primary study (100 projects)	London, England	CA in disadvantaged areas, impacts on well-being, mental health, wider participation in the arts
Carson et al. (2007)	Primary study (31 participants)	Victoria, Canada	CA center, demonstrates impacts on community capacity, enhanced health-promotion initiatives
Clift et al. (2009)	Practice commentary	England	Discusses practice, research, and policy developments, in particular research methods, theoretical considerations
Clift (2012)	Practice commentary	Various	Identifies hierarchy of evidence, values diverse methods, calls for need for more robust controlled studies
Cohen (2009)	Primary study (300 participants)	USA	CA music projects with older adults promote healthy aging through sense of control and social support
Cox et al. (2010)	Practice commentary	Canada	Overview of arts and health-related policy and practice, for individual and community health promotion
Cuypers et al. (2011)	Review (67 studies)	Norway, Sweden	Diverse CA projects, impacts on social capacity, psychological development, and mental health

(continued)

Table 13.1 (continued)

Citation	Article type	Location	Key findings
Daykin et al. (2008)	Review (104 studies)	Various	CA performing arts for youth, impacts on social skills, empowerment, sexual health, drug use
Daykin et al. (2017)	Primary study (26 participants)	UK	Study on evaluation challenges of CA, identifies need for shared frameworks
Galloway (2009)	Practice commentary	Various	Discusses challenges evaluating CA, theory-based evaluation as alternative understanding of causation
Gaztambide-Fernández (2013)	Practice commentary	Various	Critiques positivistic arts impact discourse, suggesting this masks complexity of arts practices and processes
Goulding (2014)	Primary study (8 participants)	England, UK	Explores CA evaluation challenges, tensions evaluating health and arts pieces, and demonstrates cost-savings
Hacking et al. (2008)	Primary study (62 participants)	England, UK	Youth CA projects demonstrate improvements in youth empowerment, mental health, social inclusion
Hamilton et al. (2003)	Practice commentary	Various	Discusses need for more formal evaluation to move beyond anecdote and opinion
Hampshire and Matthijsse (2010)	Primary study (64 participants)	UK	CA community singing impacts on children's social and emotional well-being, and social capital
Johnson and Stanley (2007)	Primary study (3 projects)	Australia	CA impacts on individual and community engagement, self-determination, social inclusion, and cohesion
Kelaher et al. (2012)	Primary study (1473 participants)	Australia	CA promote civic dialogue, challenging perceptions and providing space for communal reflections
Khan (2013)	Primary study (1 project)	Australia	CA impacts examined using theories of cultural capital, emphasis on new kinds of capital produced through CA
Macnaughton et al. (2005)	Primary study (1 project)	UK	CA visual arts project demonstrated enhanced social relationships and social capital
Matarasso (1997)	Primary study (90 projects)	UK	CA impacts on personal development, social cohesion, empowerment, local identity, imagination, health
Newman et al. (2003)	Review (8 studies)	Various	CA impacts on personal change, social change, economic change, educational change
Purcell (2007)	Review (12 studies)	Various	CA photography projects' impacts on community development, cultural practice, and regeneration
Putland (2008)	Practice commentary	Various	Discusses tensions between "health/scientific perspectives" and "arts perspectives"

(continued)

Table 13.1 (continued)

Citation	Article type	Location	Key findings
Raw et al. (2012)	Practice commentary	Various	Discusses tensions in developing evidence base, calls for increased description, analysis, and theorizing of practice
Rhodes and Schechter (2012)	Primary study (1 project)	Hartford, USA	CA center placed-based impacts on resilience, prosocial relationships, social capital, protective factors
Secker et al. (2011)	Primary study (37 participants)	UK	Diverse CA projects demonstrate impacts on mental health, well-being, and social inclusion
Sonn and Baker (2016)	Practice commentary	Various	Discusses and theorizes CA impacts as community pedagogies that challenge oppression and exclusion
Spiegel and Parent (2017)	Primary study (4 projects)	Quebec, Canada	CA circus arts' impacts on personal transformation, community, and personal development
Staricoff (2006)	Practice commentary	Various	Discusses approaches to CA evaluation, calls for need to know what, when, and how to use various art forms
White (2006)	Primary study (3 projects)	England, S. Africa	CA impacts on environment, social relationships, and psychological and physical health
Zarobe and Bungay (2017)	Review (8 articles)	Various	Youth CA projects demonstrate enhanced resilience through self-confidence, relationship building, belonging

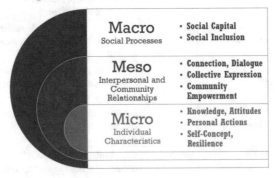

Fig. 13.1 Health-promoting impacts of community arts: an ecological model. (Reproduced with permission from author. Copyright © 2021 Charlotte Lombardo. All rights reserved)

13.3.1 Micro-level Impacts

At the micro level, CA impacts map to individually oriented constructs of health-related knowledge, attitudes, and personal actions (Angus 2004; Bungay and Vella-Burrows 2013) and to aspects of self-concept, i.e., beliefs about oneself (Baumeister 1999). Several initiatives report improved mental/psychological health (Cuypers et al. 2011; Hacking et al. 2008; Secker et al. 2011; White 2006). CA programs have reported life course effects from childhood through to end of life (APPGAHW 2017). In youth, CA programs have been found to promote intrinsic resilience in the form of a sense of belonging, identify formation, confidence, and self-esteem (Zarobe and Bungay 2017), and to have positive effects on social skills, awareness raising, and behavior change in relation to health issues such as HIV/AIDS and drug use (Daykin et al. 2008). In older adults, participation in CA has produced evidence of improvements in physical well-being and morale, as well as reductions in loneliness, doctor visits, falls, and medication use (Cohen 2009).

13.3.2 Meso-level Impacts

At the meso level, interpersonal and community-related impacts are explored through "upstream" health determinants, e.g., psychosocial mechanisms such as social support and social engagement (Berkman and Glass 2000). CA initiatives have reported increased community connection, creativity, social support, and civic dialogue and have been highlighted as asset-based spaces for communal reflection, value exploration, and community development (Cameron et al. 2013; Carson et al. 2007; Kelaher et al. 2014; Purcell 2007; Rhodes and Schechter 2012). Supporting ecological concepts of reciprocity, CA evaluations have found interrelated individual and community empowerment outcomes related to imagination and vision, positive risk taking, and strengthened sense of place (Hacking et al. 2008; Matarasso 1997). Micro-level impacts of personal transformation have been found to be reinforced by meso-level impacts of collective creative expression and cathartic experience (Spiegel and Parent 2017).

13.3.3 Macro-level Impacts

At the macro level, CA impact analyses explore societal structures and systems, understood to be dynamic and operating within and across levels, with individual and interpersonal constructs dependent upon—and interacting with—broader social and economic processes (Johnson and Stanley 2007; Newman et al. 2003; Spiegel and Parent 2017). Here conceptualizations of social capital in particular are employed, building on foundational theorists Bourdieu (1997) and Putnam (2000) and exploring bonding (within community) and bridging (between community) forms of capital such as social networks and norms/processes of cohesion or exclusion (Hampshire and Matthijsse 2010; Khan 2013; Macnaughton et al. 2005).

13.4   Goals and Epistemologies of CA Impact Analyses

Across the evolving discussion of CA outcomes are epistemological, methodological, and theoretical considerations and debates with regards to what constitutes valid evidence of impact. With growing interest in arts-based approaches, as well as the need to justify return on investment, CA initiatives are increasingly feeling pressure to evaluate and substantiate their work using empirical methods (Clift 2012; Hamilton et al. 2003). However, alongside broad calls for "better evidence" are questions and tensions related to the feasibility and fit of positivist approaches (Daykin et al. 2017). With an inherent emphasis on artistic and community-driven process, many CA investigators and practitioners locate themselves within more constructivist and qualitative-oriented perspectives (Goulding 2014; Putland 2008). A lack of theory-driven and theory-based evaluations and frameworks has also been frequently noted (Galloway 2009; Sonn and Baker 2016). This section discusses three distinct themes uncovered in the literature related to the goals and epistemologies of CA impact analyses: (1) making the case/scaling up, (2) articulating and uncovering process, and (3) mapping mechanisms and building testable theories.

13.4.1   Making the Case/Scaling Up

The increasing interest in and uptake of arts-based interventions has generated efforts and calls for more attention to the evidence base for this work. This perspective is often rooted within hierarchies of evidence-based practice, ascribing some value to case studies, qualitative research, and participant testimonies while calling for controlled studies quantitatively substantiating health outcomes, in order to scale up CA interventions to population-level impacts (Clift 2012). To this end, methodologies often center on the use of surveys or standardized scales to test individuals before and after exposure to a CA experience, ideally in comparison to some control group.

Arts therapy and clinical initiatives have been successfully measured using "gold standards" of evidence-based medicine, such as randomized controlled trials and meta-analyses, but this approach has been more challenging for CA initiatives, which often consist of small sample sizes with no obvious control group (APPGAHW 2017). Though there is some agreement regarding "encouraging" findings, systematized reviews of the CA evidence base consistently report issues with methodological rigor, citing concerns such as lack of validated outcome measures, issues with response rates and attrition, and lack of statistical power (Bungay and Vella-Burrows

2013; Clift 2012; Merli 2002; Zarobe and Bungay 2017). Consequently, there is an overall appraisal of the evidence as lacking robustness and multiple calls for higher-quality studies, which Hamilton et al. (2003) characterize as "still searching for the holy grail." In contrast, some question whether positivist approaches are appropriate for CA initiatives, with their focus on participatory and creative process (Daykin et al. 2017). Raw et al. (2012) caution that attempts to gain visibility alongside dominant healthcare research can lead to a problematic "conflation of professionalized, clinically based arts and health practice and non-professionalized, participatory, community-based practice" (p. 100). These discussions emphasize the complex nature of CA interventions, rooted in the "open systems of the real world," as well as related challenges in areas such as data collection, selection of appropriate outcome measures, and ability to synthesize findings (Daykin et al. 2008).

13.4.2 Articulating and Uncovering Process

Reflecting the tensions described above, many CA analyses emphasize qualitative investigations that focus on intervention and change processes, as opposed to empirical substantiation of outcomes (Clift 2012, p. 123). There is a significant body of peer-reviewed qualitative research on CA impacts, which highlights the role of such methods—including focus groups, interviews, and participant observation—in uncovering deeply contextual and relational effects and processes (Staricoff 2006). Macnaughton et al. (2005) suggest this is of particular importance in the evaluation of social capital goals of CA, framing evaluation in such cases as a "process of discovery, not proof" (p. 336). Of note is the recent proliferation of "mixed methods" designs, utilizing quantitative methods to explore specific impacts alongside qualitative methods to deepen the analysis and critically interpret findings (Spiegel and Parent 2017). Many CA initiatives rely on testimonials and case reports, often published in the form of grey literature reports by programs, funders, or policy makers (Galloway 2009; Putland 2008). Such publications can be influential, while also critiqued for lack of formal or rigorous evaluation measures (Hamilton et al. 2003). One of the first large-scale CA evaluations, *Use or Ornament*, utilized case studies to investigate CA initiatives across Britain (Matarasso 1997). The report details a host of individual and social outcomes and was a key element in an ongoing health policy agenda employing CA approaches in the UK. However, it has come under criticism for lack of internal and external validity, as well as its overall inability to prove causation in relation to the reported effects (Belfiore 2006; Merli 2002).

13.4.3   Mapping Mechanisms and Building Testable Theories

In an effort to recognize, but not necessarily reconcile, epistemological challenges related to evaluation and impact, some practitioners are calling for more efforts toward theorizing CA practice. Such perspectives argue that attention is needed toward theorizing the mechanisms by which CA interventions achieve impact, both as a basis for understanding and actualizing the findings of impact studies, and for moving beyond repeated debates on the quality of the evidence base (Raw et al. 2012, p. 105). Some believe that as long as the mechanisms of impact remain a mystery, evidence will fail to contribute to the field gaining the status desired (Cohen 2009; Sonn and Baker 2016). A small body of work is rooted in critical social science perspectives. Exploring the use of circus arts with equity-seeking communities, Spiegel and Parent (2017) take up the work of social theorist Guattari (1995) on "aesthetic paradigm"—art as a means of altering ways of seeing and engaging with the world, and experimenting with different kinds of social configurations. Spiegel and Parent (2017) draw on Guattari's ideas to explore concepts of "social subjectivities and collectivities" (p. 2) in circus arts' participants. Theory-based evaluation on the social effects of the arts seeks to counter the critique of the evidence base rooted in a "dominant rationalist-modernist paradigm" that emphasizes methodology rather than theory as the basis of "good evaluation" (Galloway 2009). Growing in popularity, "Theory of Change" approaches (Mayne 2015) seek to provide rigorous models of causality rooted in an embrace of complexity rather than experimental design (Galloway 2009). Though relying heavily on qualitative and first-person accounts, theory-based evaluation approaches seek to counter the view of self-report data as anecdotal by utilizing participant testimony as way of confirming, refining, or falsifying theory, and by providing an explicit methodological framework for data analysis.

13.5   Key Themes and Tensions

Given the dominant discourse on the need for more "robust and credible" evidence, there are growing attempts to support research and evaluation on CA practice through a proliferation of toolkits and frameworks. Such resources seek to provide enough detail on a range of methodological options to allow practitioners to employ them effectively. Some, however, critique what they refer to as over-reliance on a toolkit mentality, problematizing the oversimplification inherent in seeking to identify a method of impact evaluation that is easily replicable across contexts and equally applicable to diverse art forms and audiences (Belfiore and Bennett 2010, p. 122). Also questioned are the perceived benefits of generating more and "better" evidence; despite the goals of evidence-informed policy making, evidence is infrequently the main driver of policy action (Goulding 2014). Rather, well-focused theory and advocacy may be more effective than resource-intensive attempts to generate more evidence.

A key tension is emerging between the more instrumentalist approach, which positions the arts activity as a tool to fulfill policy objectives (Belfiore 2002), and a creative or transformational approach "that trusts in the arts process itself to deliver outcomes" (Macnaughton et al. 2005, p. 336). Artists often report feeling marginalized by research and evaluation discourse, which can be perceived to have a reductive focus on outputs and products, as opposed to artistic process (Daykin et al. 2017). As Badham (2010) contends, "Socially engaged arts are inherently transformational because they are collaborative and engaging, especially when lead artists are determined to uphold the artistic integrity of the work. It is the art more than the social policy outcome that results in transformation, yet there has been limited discussion in the literature on these kinds of artistic processes" (p. 91).

Reductionism can impact not only how community arts projects are valued and evaluated, but also project design and implementation. Consider the shift in emphasis from a discovery-oriented artistic process to "social policy" outcomes such as improved self-esteem or decreased social isolation; how might such changes impact the way an intervention is conceptualized or delivered? Might the more intentional, instrumental approach even diminish the potential for self-esteem to emerge as a more natural product of the collective process? Some fear this emphasis may be "throwing arts projects off track," in particular through a shift in emphasis toward outcome evaluation "with a consequent devaluing of other forms, such as process evaluation and reflective practice" (Daykin et al. 2017, p. 133).

Returning to the ecological perspective, a change in discourse has been noted from an emphasis on the direct economic contributions of cultural industries, such as increased tourism and job creation, to more indirect economic benefits, such as creativity and innovation, employability, social inclusion, and community cohesion (Böhm and Land 2009). This may be due to a view of the product of artistic and cultural activity as capital—human, social, and cultural—within "the simultaneous recognition of the value of culture and the difficulty of measuring that value" (Böhm and Land 2009, p. 77). Some question whether "it may seem like positivism gone mad to expect the arts to justify their existence on scientific grounds" (Hamilton et al. 2003, p. 402). Further problematizing notions of impact, Gaztambide-Fernández (2013) challenges the construction of the arts as a definable naturalistic phenomenon that is available to be observed and measured, arguing that diverse art forms and practices are "processes of cultural production…evolving within both symbolic and material conditions that constrain but do not predefine how individuals engage each other. In other words, rather than thinking about the arts as *doing something to people,* we should think about artistic forms as *something people do*" (p. 225–226). Further research on, with, and through CA—which embraces explorations of artistic and social processes, as opposed to more individually oriented notions of output and impact—would be well positioned to engage and deepen this dialogue.

13.6   Potential Ways Forward

How to reconcile these diverse perspectives and approaches? Perhaps the key—for funders, researchers, and practitioners alike—is in not seeking to do so, in resisting the urge to espouse one particular standard for all CA practice and to live instead in the tensions and complexities. Such thinking can be found in the rising popularity of "whole system" approaches to impact and evaluation that embrace complexity theory and explore impacts at more macro levels and/or across multiple initiatives (APPGAHW 2017). Collective Impact (CI), for example, has gained traction as an approach to social impact analysis based on an embrace of complexity principles. CI seeks to move beyond standard evaluations of individual initiatives (termed "isolated impact") toward a focus on relationships between organizations and progress toward shared objectives (Kania and Kramer 2011). CI takes a complexity, systems-oriented perspective rooted in the belief that the process and results of social innovation are emergent rather than predetermined, and that adoption often happens simultaneously across many different organizations (Kania and Kramer 2013). CI-oriented research on CA would provide an interesting opportunity to further illuminate both approaches, as well as systems and complexity thinking in general.

A way forward that also embraces plurality of thought and approach lies in the call for more attention to theory development, building on the recent attention paid to theory-based evaluation and Theory of Change approaches (Galloway 2009; Mayne 2015). Deeper attention to theorizing practice can build on foundational artists and cultural theorists such as Augusto Boal, Paulo Freire, and Jan Cohen-Cruz and can draw on interdisciplinary perspectives, incorporating disciplines such as geography, anthropology, and psychology (Raw et al. 2012). Within such directions are discussions on the need for more explicit attention to issues of equity and cultural production. A shift in discourse has been noted from "a 'top-down' welfare-like approach of helping disadvantaged communities, to the embracing of cultural democracy: the recognition of unique, valuable and plural communities' right to control the creation and trajectory of their own culture" (Badham 2010, p. 86). Such narratives suggest an important role for harnessing and actualizing theoretical frames that can help operationalize values and principles like participatory practice, anti-oppression, and Indigenous ways of knowing.

More research in general is needed that seeks to view and build upon CA as an intrinsic form of knowledge production, for example through the use of artistic outputs of CA initiatives to theorize and/or evaluate programs and to explore impacts on both direct participants and broader communities. CA approaches may also provide a unique space to explore the growing interest in implementation research, an emerging discipline that seeks to link research and practice to adopt and integrate evidence-based health interventions within specific settings (Theobald et al. 2018). Implementation research investigates what, why, and how interventions work in "real world settings," working within these conditions rather than trying to control or remove their influence as causal effects (Peters et al. 2013). Principals of implementation research include a critical reflection on contextual and power dynamics, equitable knowledge production, and engagement of marginalized communities (Wallerstein and Duran 2010)—all of which are key elements of the CA discourse. Finally, potential synergies may be found in strengthening linkages between CA and ABR. Similar needs and tensions exist in ABR in relation to problematization of impact as fluid, emergent, non-linear, and highly complex (Parsons et al. 2017), which could be co-explored for shared meaning making.

13.7   Conclusions and Limitations

This chapter describes increasing attention in both academic and community settings to the role of CA in promoting health and well-being at multiple levels, from the personal to the social. Within the widening discourse on CA approaches, disagreements exist in relation to state of the evidence base and on what is most needed to move this work forward. The current analysis suggests that promising directions involve resisting instrumentalist approaches and embracing plurality of thought in relation to knowledge and theory building. This chapter does not provide a comprehensive review of all relevant literature (for example, of note is the lack of attention to the rich body of thought and literature on aesthetics). It is also very important to note that the literature identified is primarily from Western sources and lacks detailed input from the very rich and diverse traditions of community-based art from majority world and Indigenous contexts. This chapter seeks to provide an initial roadmap for ongoing work and discussion, which—despite inherent tensions—suggests fertile ground for further study and praxis.

References

All-Party Parliamentary Group on Arts, Health and Wellbeing (APPGAHW). (2017). *Creative health: The arts for health and wellbeing*. London: Health Development Agency.
Angus, J., & University of Durham, Centre for Arts and Humanities in Health and Medicine, NHS Health Development Agency. (2004). *A review of evaluation in community-based art for health activity in the UK*. London: Health Development Agency.
Badham, M. (2010). The case for "socially engaged arts": Navigating art history, cultural development and arts funding narratives. *Identity, Security, Community, 7*, 84–99.
Barndt, D. (2004). By whom for whom: Intersections of participatory research and community art. In A. Cole, L. Nielson, J. G. Knowles, & T. Luciani (Eds.), *Provoked by art: Theorizing art-based inquiry*. Toronto: Backalong Books and Centre for Arts Informed Research, OISE.
Baumeister, R. F. (Ed.). (1999). *The self in social psychology*. Philadelphia: Psychology Press (Taylor & Francis).
Belfiore, E. (2002). Art as a means of alleviating social exclusion: does it really work? A critique of instrumentalist cultural policies and social impact studies in the UK. International *Journal of Cultural Policy, 8*(1), 91–106.
Belfiore, E. (2006). The social impact of the arts—myth or reality. In *Culture vultures: Is UK arts policy damaging the arts?* London: Policy Exchange Limited.

Belfiore, E., & Bennett, O. (2010). Beyond the "toolkit approach": Arts impact evaluation research and the realities of cultural policy-making. *Journal for Cultural Research, 14*(2), 121–142.

Berkman, L. F., & Glass, T. (2000). Social integration, social networks, social support, and health. In L. F. Berkman & I. Karachi (Eds.), *Social epidemiology* (pp. 137–173). New York: Oxford University Press.

Böhm, S., & Land, C. (2009). No measure for culture? Value in the new economy. *Capital & Class, 33*(1), 75–98.

Bourdieu, P. (1997). The forms of capital. In A. H. Halsey, H. Lauder, P. Brown, & A. Stuart Wells (Eds.), *Education: Culture, economy, society* (pp. 46–58). Oxford: Oxford University Press.

Boydell, K. M., Gladstone, B. M., Volpe, T., Allemang, B., & Stasiulis, E. (2012). The production and dissemination of knowledge: A scoping review of arts-based health research. *Forum: Qualitative Social Research, 13*, 1.

Bungay, H., & Vella-Burrows, T. (2013). The effects of participating in creative activities on the health and well-being of children and young people: A rapid review of the literature. *Perspectives in Public Health, 133*(1), 44–52.

Cameron, M., Crane, N., Ings, R., & Taylor, K. (2013). Promoting well-being through creativity: How arts and public health can learn from each other. *Perspectives in Public Health, 133*(1), 52–59.

Carson, A. J., Chappell, N. L., & Knight, C. J. (2007). Promoting health and innovative health promotion practice through a community arts centre. *Health Promotion Practice, 8*(4), 366–374.

Clift, S. (2012). Creative arts as a public health resource: Moving from practice-based research to evidence-based practice. *Perspectives in Public Health, 132*(3), 120–127.

Clift, S., Camic, P., Chapman, B., Clayton, G., Daykin, N., Eades, G., et al. (2009). The state of arts and health in England. *Arts & Health, 1*(1), 6–35.

Cohen, G. (2009). New theories and research findings on the positive influence of music and art on health with ageing. *Arts & Health, 1*(1), 48–62.

Commission on the Social Determinants of Health (CSDH). (2008). *Closing the gap in a generation: Health equity through action on the social determinants of health.* Geneva: World Health Organization.

Cox, S. M., Lafrenière, D., Brett-MacLean, P., Collie, K., Cooley, N., Dunbrack, J., et al. (2010). Tipping the iceberg? The state of arts and health in Canada. *Arts & Health, 2*(2), 109–124.

Cuypers, K. F., Knudtsen, M. S., Sandgren, M., Krokstad, S., Wikström, B. M., & Theorell, T. (2011). Cultural activities and public health: Research in Norway and Sweden: An overview. *Arts & Health, 3*(1), 6–26.

Daykin, N., Orme, J., Evans, D., Salmon, D., McEachran, M., & Brain, S. (2008). The impact of participation in performing arts on adolescent health and behaviour: A systematic review of the literature. *Journal of Health Psychology, 13*(2), 251–264.

Daykin, N., Gray, K., McCree, M., & Willis, J. (2017). Creative and credible evaluation for arts, health and well-being: Opportunities and challenges of co-production. *Arts & Health, 9*(2), 123–138.

Galloway, S. (2009). Theory-based evaluation and the social impact of the arts. *Cultural Trends, 18*(2), 125–148.

Gaztambide-Fernández, R. (2013). Why the arts don't do anything: Toward a new vision for cultural production in education. *Harvard Educational Review, 83*(1), 211–237.

Goulding, A. (2014). Arts on prescription for older people: Different stakeholder perspectives on the challenges of providing evidence of impact on health outcomes. *Journal of Applied Arts & Health, 5*(1), 83–107.

Guattari, F. (1995). *Chaosmosis: An ethico-aesthetic paradigm.* Sydney: Power Publications.

Hacking, S., Secker, J., Spandler, H., Kent, L., & Shenton, J. (2008). Evaluating the impact of participatory art projects for people with mental health needs. *Health & Social Care in the Community, 16*(6), 638–648.

Hamilton, C., Hinks, S., & Petticrew, M. (2003). Arts for health: Still searching for the Holy Grail. *Journal of Epidemiology & Community Health, 57*(6), 401–402.

Hampshire, K. R., & Matthijsse, M. (2010). Can arts projects improve young people's wellbeing? A social capital approach. *Social Science & Medicine, 71*(4), 708–716.

Johnson, V., & Stanley, J. (2007). Capturing the contribution of community arts to health and well-being. *International Journal of Mental Health Promotion, 9*(2), 28–35.

Kania, J., & Kramer, M. (2011). Collective impact. *Stanford Social Innovation Review,* 36–41.

Kania, J., & Kramer, M. (2013). Embracing emergence: How collective impact addresses complexity. *Stanford Social Innovation Review,* 1–7. https://ssir.org/articles/entry/social_progress_through_collective_impact.

Kelaher, M., Berman, N., Dunt, D., Johnson, V., Curry, S., & Joubert, L. (2014). Evaluating community outcomes of participation in community arts: A case for civic dialogue. *Journal of Sociology, 50*(2), 132–149.

Khan, R. (2013). Rethinking cultural capital and community-based arts. *Journal of Sociology, 49*(2–3), 357–372.

Kingry-Westergaard, C., & Kelly, J. G. (1990). A contextualist epistemology for ecological research. In P. Tolan, C. Keys, F. Chertok, & L. Jason (Eds.), *Researching community psychology* (pp. 23–41). Washington, D.C.: American Psychological Association.

Macnaughton, J., White, M., & Stacy, R. (2005). Researching the benefits of arts in health. *Health Education, 105*(5), 332–339.

Madsen, W., Redman-MacLaren, M., Saunders, V., O'Mullan, C., & Judd, J. (2021). Reframing health promotion research and practice in Australia and the Pacific: The value of arts-based practices. In J. H. Corbin, M. Sanmartino, E. A. Hennessy, & H. B. Urke (Eds.), *Arts and health promotion: Tools and bridges for practice, research, and social transformation.* Springer, in press.

Marmot, M. (2015). The health gap: The challenge of an unequal world. *The Lancet, 386*(10011), 2442–2444.

Matarasso, F. (1997). *Use or ornament?: The social impact of participation in the arts.* Stroud, Glos: Comedia.

Mayne, J. (2015). Useful theory of change models. *Canadian Journal of Program Evaluation, 30*(2), 119–142.

Merli, P. (2002). Evaluating the social impact of participation in arts activities. *International Journal of Cultural Policy, 8*(1), 107–118.

Newman, T., Curtis, K., & Stephens, J. (2003). Do community-based arts projects result in social gains? A review of the literature. *Community Development Journal, 38*(4), 310–322.

Novak, P. (2012). *Community arts in community health: (re)Making ME.* Toronto: SKETCH.

Parsons, J. A., Gladstone, B. M., Gray, J., & Kontos, P. (2017). Re-conceptualizing "impact" in art-based health research. *Journal of Applied Arts & Health, 8*(2), 155–173.

Peters, D. H., Taghreed, A., Olakunle, O., Agyepong, I. A., & Nhan, T. (2013). Implementation research: What is it and how to do it. *BMJ, 347,* f6753.

Purcell, R. (2007). Images for change: Community development, community arts and photography. *Community Development Journal, 44*(1), 111–122.

Putland, C. (2008). Lost in translation: The question of evidence linking community-based arts and health promotion. *Journal of Health Psychology, 13*(2), 265–276.

Putnam, R. (2000). *Bowling alone: The collapse and revival of American community.* New York: Simon.

Raphael, D. (2016). *Social determinants of health: Canadian perspectives* (3rd ed.). Toronto: Canadian Scholars' Press.

Raw, A., Lewis, S., Russell, A., & Macnaughton, J. (2012). A hole in the heart: Confronting the drive for evidence-based impact research in arts and health. *Arts & Health, 4*(2), 97–108.

Rhodes, A. M., & Schechter, R. (2012). Fostering resilience among youth in inner city community arts centers. *Education and Urban Society, 12,* 1.

Richard, L., Gauvin, L., & Raine, K. (2011). Ecological models revisited: Their uses and evolution in health promotion over two decades. *Annual Review of Public Health, 32*(1), 307–326.

Rootman, I., & O'Neill, M. (2017). Key concepts in health promotion. In I. Rootman, A. Pederson, S. Dupéré, & M. O'Neill (Eds.), *Health promotion in Canada: Critical perspectives on practice* (pp. 20–43). Toronto: Canadian Scholars' Press.

Sallis, J. F., Owen, N., & Fisher, E. (2015). Ecological models of health behavior. In K. Glaz, B. K. Rimer, & K. Viswanath (Eds.), *Health behavior: Theory, research, and practice* (pp. 43–64). San Francisco: Jossey-Bass.

Secker, J., Loughran, M., Heydinrych, K., & Kent, L. (2011). Promoting mental well-being and social inclusion through art: Evaluation of an arts and mental health project. *Arts & Health, 3*(1), 51–60.

Sonn, C., & Baker, A. (2016). Creating inclusive knowledges: Exploring the transformative potential of arts and cultural practice. *International Journal of Inclusive Education, 20*(3), 215–228.

Spiegel, J. B., & Parent, S. N. (2017). Re-approaching community development through the arts: A 'critical mixed methods' study of social circus in Quebec. *Community Development Journal, 53*(4), 1–18. https://academic.oup.com/cdj/issue/53/4

Staricoff, R. L. (2006). Arts in health: The value of evaluation. *The Journal of the Royal Society for the Promotion of Health, 126*(3), 116–120.

Theobald, S., Brandes, N., Gyapong, M., El-Saharty, S., Proctor, E., Diaz, T., et al. (2018). Implementation research: New imperatives and opportunities in global health. *Lancet, 392*, 2214–2228.

Wallerstein, N., & Duran, B. (2010). Community-based participatory research contributions to intervention research: The intersection of science and practice to improve health equity. *American Journal of Public Health, 100*(S1), S40–S46.

White, M. (2006). Establishing common ground in community-based arts in health. *The Journal of the Royal Society for the Promotion of Health, 126*(3), 128–133.

Zarobe, L., & Bungay, H. (2017). The role of arts activities in developing resilience and mental wellbeing in children and young people: A rapid review of the literature. *Perspectives in Public Health, 137*(6), 337–347.

Part IV
Arts and Health Promotion: Tools and Bridges for Social Transformation

Chapter 14
Art and Co-creation for the Community Promotion of Affective Sexual Health in Catalonia

Jordi Gómez i Prat, Isabel Claveria Guiu, Mario Torrecillas, Arturo Solari, and Hakima Ouaarab Esadek

14.1 Approaching Affective Sexual Health and Cultural Diversity

Applying a health promotion approach in the sphere of international health care and immigrant populations—in which the subjects covered are often associated with significant cultural baggage and emotional burdens—requires leveraging social construction processes from an intercultural and gender perspective. In doing so, the participating population abandons its role as a potentially ill or at-risk population and instead becomes an agent for the transformation of its health condition. These processes, especially with regard to affective sexual health (ASH), are influenced by a number of different biological, psychological, social, cultural, economic, historic, religious, and spiritual determining factors (Health Department, 2013). Working across all of these dimensions is a challenge that requires participative, innovative, and creative methodologies within the community through co-creation processes,

J. Gómez i Prat (✉) · I. C. Guiu · H. O. Esadek
Hospital Universitari Vall d'Hebron. Unitat de Salut Internacional Drassanes. Equip de Salut Pública i Comunitària. PROSICS, Barcelona, Catalunya
e-mail: j.gomez@vhebron.net; iclaveria@vhebron.net; houaarab@vhebron.net

M. Torrecillas
Pequeños Dibujos Animados (PDA-films), Barcelona, Catalunya
e-mail: info@pda-films.com

A. Solari
Private Practice in Expressive Arts Therapist, Girona

Collaborator at the Unitat de Salut Internacional Drassanes-Vall d'Hebron, Barcelona, Catalunya
e-mail: thehealingproject@hotmail.com

© The Author(s) 2021
J. H. Corbin et al. (eds.), *Arts and Health Promotion*,
https://doi.org/10.1007/978-3-030-56417-9_14

with the goal of producing citizens who are capable of expressing themselves, identifying their problems and needs, drafting proposals, and contributing to decision-making with regard to health jointly with health care services and other sectors of civil society.

Artistic expressions are inherent to and essential for humans, and they offer a broad range of highly valuable and powerful tools to express feelings and communications between individuals and groups and to achieve change in people's lives. Art is a part of community life (see Chap. 1, Sect. 1.1). Deliberate, methodological use of these expressive outlets promotes health and self-knowledge among people for mental, emotional, physical, spiritual, and social well-being (Ganim 1999; Gysin and Sorín 2011; Knill et al. 2005; Solari 2015).

The Diverxualitat program emerged from the melding of art and co-creation in the fields of international health care, affective sexual health, and interculturality. Diverxualitat is a part of the innovative Espictools-Actua health promotion program—from the ESPiC team (equip salut pública i comunitària/community and public health team) of the International Health Unit Drassanes – Hospital Universitari Vall d'Hebron (Barcelona)—which generates evidence-based educational tools (Espictools) through a scientific-based process of *artistic co-creation* with the communities and in which different art forms are used throughout its different phases (Avaria Saavedra and Gómez i Prat 2008; Gómez i Prat et al. 2001; Gómez i Prat et al. 2015; Ouaarab Essadek et al. 2017; Sanmartino et al. 2015). These educational tools are a part of the community intervention strategies that can be combined with different informative, educational, or communicative actions (Claveria Guiu et al. 2017; Essadek et al. 2018).

Before delving into the details of the Diverxualitat Espictools program, we provide some background on the Espictools-Actua model to elaborate on the framework that guides the co-creation process in this program.

14.2 Espictools-Actua

Espictools-Actua (educational tools – community interventions) is a model developed by the authors in 2017 that uses art and culture as instruments to facilitate the creation of new tools and strategies to promote health through a process of artistic co-creation among migrant populations, local artists, and members of the health team. It is especially focused on immigrant populations facing a situation of vulnerability by supporting their own development, based, in turn, on the theories of co-creation (Beran et al. 2018; Holmboe et al. 2016), peer education, and communications models as strategies for social change (Boyle et al. 2011; Kirby et al. 2006; Sriranganathan et al. 2010). Espictools-Actua is structured in two phases, described below.

14.2.1   Phase 1—Espictools: Creating the Educational Tool

To begin, it is worth discussing needs analyses and asset analyses. One of the most common errors when it comes to starting community interventions is to believe that we (the health team members) are the community's only resource or its most important resource, and that health is the community's main center of interest; in reality, the community has many other concerns, and educational, social, cultural, or leisure resources may play an even more relevant and prominent role than health care. Self-knowledge and knowledge of others, the environment, extant policies and programs, active organizations, social spaces, available means of communication, and a "mapping" of the relationships maintained by different figures of society throughout the area allows us to carry out an analysis of the landscape from another point of view, helping to define potential areas for change and providing individuals and groups with assistance when it comes to discovering their potential and that of others. Therefore, based on any needs that have been detected, educational tool development is carried out in two stages as follows.

Participative research study This study is conducted through workshops/focus groups carried out in the educational, health care, and community fields. Each workshop or focus group is facilitated by different professionals (e.g., art therapists, community workers, nurses, community health agents, physicians, and anthropologists). Recruitment for these groups is carried out by all the people involved in the program, taking into account the profile of the people they are working with and their needs. These workshops are intended to provide a forum for creativity and mutual exchange in which resources that may contribute to improving or maintaining their well-being can be brought to light. Through different exercises, projects, and forms of artistic expression, participants approach the core subject of the work by exposing their personal and group realities and discovering new possibilities to approach them, along with offering tools that help promote health with regard to the topic being discussed. At the end of this stage, the attitudes and responses from the participants are collected, in a structured way.

Designing and creating an educational tool These tools may be created by professionals who participated in the first stage (using the results that have been obtained). Alternatively, workshops can be organized with participants from the first phase, conducted by a team of professionals with expertise in community work and health care educational materials. Throughout these workshops, new tools (e.g., educational videos, animation videos created by participants using mobile applications, and board games) are produced from an intercultural point of view in collaboration with participants. These new tools stem from the entirety of the information and results that were collected throughout the first phase and take into account the proposals concerning the format, content, and structure of the type of tool that could help improve access to the subject in question and its quality in the participants' environment. At the end of this stage, a number of workshops are carried out with different community groups, as well as a pilot test to assess the effectiveness of the tools and to rate their impact through several surveys. Once the effectiveness of the newly created tools has been assessed, they will be used in the next phase of action by participants and by professionals from the subject areas in their environments.

14.2.2 Phase 2—Espictools-Actua: Actions and Implementation of the Tools in the Community

Based on the results of the first phase, the following stages are carried out in Phase 2 of Espictools-Actua.

Training in the use of the new tools This training involves a basic training action intended for *health care professionals* in order to qualify them to use this tool in their professional practice, as well as another broader training program intended for active members of the community in order to qualify them as *peer educators* so that they may act in their environments using the newly created tools.

Interventions and actions with and for the community Trained participants carry out a number of workshops and activities at the individual, group, and community levels through the action plan, using the new tools for the promotion of health—especially in the covered subject area—from an intercultural and gender perspective, in their environments.

Throughout these phases, questionnaires are used to assess participants' satisfaction. At the end of the process, a joint assessment report with all the parties involved in the project is drafted concerning the most relevant aspects to be maintained, improved, or modified in the future with regard to the design and development of the program.

14.2.3 The Espictools-Actua Programs: Different Educational Tools for Different Needs

Espictools-Actua is currently developed through different health promotion programs in the international and immigration health spheres, mainly in the city of Barcelona and in Catalonia. Each program contains a variety of educational tools on subjects of interest that can be established and adapted as appropriate to different community groups, and which are provided to professionals and active members of the community working in this field. The following is a list of the available programs and educational tools (www.espictools.cat):

1. The XarChagas (ChagasNet) program, which is intended to guarantee access to comprehensive care for Chagas disease. It contains the following Espictools:

   - Music: "El viatge de l'heroi" (The Hero's Trip) (Catalan); "A vida da gente poder ser melhor" (Our Lives Can Be Better) (Portuguese); and "Las palabras no dan miedo" (Words Are Not Scary) (Spanish). These songs have been composed specifically to raise awareness about Chagas disease and its reality.
   - Documentary film: "Saber o no saber: me siento bien, dicen que tengo la enfermedad de Chagas" (To Know or Not to Know: I Feel Good, They Say that I Have Chagas Disease). Through the experiences of the characters in the film (people affected by Chagas disease), viewers can learn about the reality of the disease far from their countries of origin.
   - Spots: "Accessibilitat al diagnòstic i tractament de la malaltia de Chagas" (Accessibility to the Diagnosis and Treatment of Chagas Disease) and "Transmissió congènita malaltia de Chagas" (Congenital Chagas Disease Transmission). These two spots—with the participation of a public figure (football/soccer player Leo Messi)—are used to reflect on the reality of Chagas disease in the world and raise awareness of the subject.

2. The "Tbactiva't" (TB activation) program, which is intended to strengthen networking for active surveillance against tuberculosis. This program contains the following Espictools:

   - Video: "TB" (available in Spanish, Arabic, Urdu, Chinese, and Romanian), an educational film with a fictional story that provides knowledge about tuberculosis and its determining factors, assisting in detection and follow-up for affected people. It is structured around two parts: a 30-minute fictional story and a 7-minute guide video in which a number of subjects to be discussed are proposed based on specific questions.
   - Teaching guide: "Manual TB" (available in Spanish, Arabic, Urdu, Chinese, and Romanian), a teaching guide intended to promote understanding of tuberculosis. It has been drafted as a companion document to the video "TB."

3. The "Around Me" program seeks to put all aspects related to the determining factors of health on the table through collective reflection. It contains the Espictool "Around Me," a game that covers the determining factors of health in a dynamic way. It is available in Catalan, Spanish, English, French, and Italian.

4. The Diverxualitat (diversity and sexuality) program, intended to improve access to affective sexual health. This program will be explained in detail in the next section and contains the following Espictools:

   - Animated features: "Broken Condom" and "The Photograph"
   - Board game: "SIDAJoc"
   - Teaching support tool: "Heparjoc"

14.3 The Diverxualitat Program: Improving Access to ASH

The Diverxualitat program is intended to improve access to ASH within the various communities of immigrants residing in Barcelona and Catalonia. Diverxualitat is focused on the process of co-creation with the community based on the methodological framework of the Espictools-Actua model aforementioned. It is grounded in two principal concepts: The first is the fact that the definitions and perceptions of the community exert significant influence on the context of the affective sexual health of the population. Aspects such as fostering women's ability to make decisions affecting their health or improving the perception of preventive measures such as condoms are clear examples of actions to be carried out at both the individual and community levels. The second concept is the use of expressive arts from an intercultural perspective in the scope of ASH that is available to most of the population, thus generating creative processes led by the community and giving rise to a number of highly valuable and effective tools based on both scientific knowledge and the humanities—namely, Diverxualitat Espictools.

14.3.1 Diverxualitat Espictools: The Tools of the Diverxualitat Program

The following Espictools have been created for the Diverxualitat program:

1. *SIDAJoc* (available in Catalan, Spanish, English, French, and Portuguese) is a game based on pictures and questions to gain in-depth knowledge about different situations associated with HIV/AIDS in order to promote reflection and knowledge of this disease. It is intended for immigrants, especially those from sub-Saharan Africa. It emerged from a need that was detected during daily practice for educational support material to provide engaging information and education in order to improve testing and promote healthy attitudes toward prevention. The research process that was the basis for this educational tool emerged as a consequence of an initiative to train African women as community health agents—through the Drassanes-Vall d'Hebron International Health Unit (ICS) and ACSAR (Catalan Association of Solidarity and Assistance to Refugees) in Barcelona; AIDS & Mobility in Amsterdam; the Service Social des Étrangers in Brussels; and AIDES (www.aides.org) in Paris—between the years 1999 and 2000, with the support of the EEC (European Commission) and the AIDS Prevention and Assistance Programme of the Ministry of Health of the Catalan Regional Government.

   SIDAJoc is among the first HIV/AIDS prevention materials that are provided to African women residing in Barcelona after their immigration. We know that, in a relaxed and dynamic working environment, participants are much more open when it comes to verbalizing their beliefs and doubts. This is especially relevant when it comes to covering subjects such as HIV/AIDS, which often evoke significant emotional and cultural baggage. That is why *SIDAJoc* is intended to draw people closer together through its visual format (drawings representing different situations such as sexual relations, pregnancy, and drugs, all of which are related to the situations to be covered when delving into the reality of HIV/AIDS) (Fig. 14.1), thus allowing people to identify with the different situations being put forth.

This game is intended to facilitate dynamic, playful health information sessions while assessing the knowledge of participants. In addition, it provides a tool that is able to consider and adapt to the peculiarities of the cultural differences of various ethnic groups. This tool is most commonly used in the context of workshops.

2. *HEPARJoc* (available in Spanish and English and including an animation video available in Spanish, English, Catalan, Urdu, Arabic, French and Romanian) is a game based on pictures and questions whose purpose is to share knowledge about viral hepatitis, especially hepatitis B (HB), and to raise awareness of the importance of diagnosing these infections early on. It is a teaching support tool in digital format to raise awareness among immigrant populations and to promote the detection of hepatitis among vulnerable groups. It emerged from a need that was detected due to the high prevalence of HB in the sub-Saharan immigrant population in Barcelona (Manzardo et al. 2008). *HEPARJoc* was created based on qualitative research carried out through a number of groups drawn from the

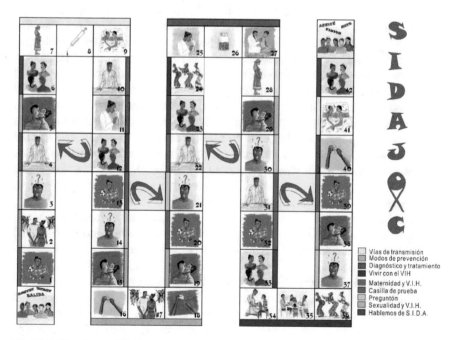

Fig. 14.1 Board game *SIDAJoc*

sub-Saharan African immigrant population. A qualitative, descriptive, and interpretive study with a phenomenological focus was conducted in May 2015
through focus groups (Ouaarab Essadek et al. 2017). Immigrants of different
ages and genders from sub-Saharan Africa who reside in Catalonia were recruited
through community health agents. Their knowledge and opinions on HB were
analyzed, along with strategies to motivate people from their community to
undergo screenings. Conclusions included messages to be worked on and a lack
of knowledge of basic facts, modes of contagion, diagnosis, treatment, and
means for prevention.

   HEPARJoc features a "kit" of five dynamic activities that are carried out in a
workshop lasting approximately one hour. The first four activities are games
based on pictures that participants must associate with or identify. The fifth
activity is an animation feature that was produced to promote hepatitis screenings (Fig. 14.2). The workshop is based on guided participation by a group coordinator who involves participants in the processes of the game in a fun and
dynamic way. *HEPARJoc* requires a monitor (health care personnel, normally a
community health agent), as well as access to diagnosis for vulnerable
populations.

3. *DIVERXUAL* is geared toward full integration by improving access to ASH
   among the immigrant population in Catalonia and providing practical knowledge
   and tools to health care professionals. It emerged from the need to draw health
   care services closer to the immigrant population with regard to ASH. It contains
   the animation videos "The Photograph" (Fig. 14.3) and "Broken Condom"
   (available in Catalan, Spanish, and English). The videos are the result of a
   research process based on a qualitative, descriptive pilot study whose objective
   was to evaluate health care approaches for access to sexual and reproductive
   health rights for women of reproductive age and of immigrant origin in Catalonia
   (Gómez i Prat et al. 2015). In order to create these videos, a diagnosis was carried
   out through interviews and discussion groups with a number of professionals and
   the immigrant population from September to November 2014. This diagnosis
   gave rise to the following: 1) the creation of a guide whose goal is to provide
   access to the proper tools for health care professionals to improve access to ASH
   for immigrant men and women, and 2) the creation of the two animation videos
   mentioned above. Both videos are geared toward health care professionals and
   those who cover cases of violence (from a health care perspective) who seek to
   allow access to sexual and reproductive health rights for these women.

These animation videos were created with the writer and screenwriter Mario
Torrecillas, his PDA (*Pequeños Dibujos Animados* – Small Cartoons) team, and
its artists and animators. The animations were voiced and the script was completed through an eight-hour workshop with young immigrants of different ori-
gins. Through this workshop, the PDA-FILMS production company, with the
technical cooperation of the Community Health Unit of Salut Internacional
Drassanes – Vall d'Hebron, considered the barriers that young immigrants face
when it comes to accessing affective sexual and reproductive health. A group of
ten young people from different countries (Morocco, Pakistan, Romania, Bolivia,

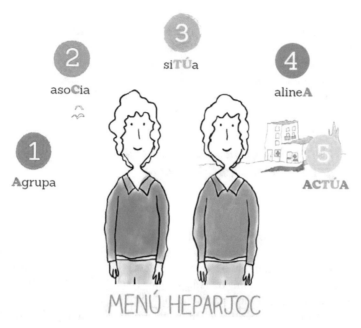

Fig. 14.2 The *HEPARJoc* menu

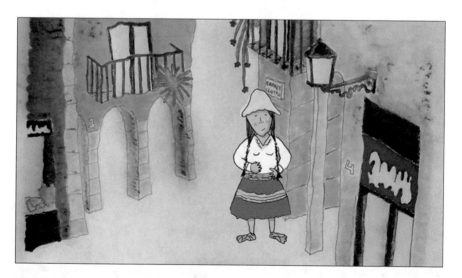

Fig. 14.3 A frame from the animation video. ("The Photograph" (2015))

Ecuador, Senegal, and Equatorial Guinea) were selected for the purpose of creating the materials (Fig. 14.4). The definition of access to affective sexual and reproductive health provided by the WHO (2007) was used as the common thread for the workshop, as well as the scripts that were suggested.

The videos reflect the barriers and difficulties confronted by both immigrants attempting to access affective sexual and reproductive health care, and by health care professionals when they perform sexual health tasks with immigrants. This unique material reflects two different experiences of the same encounter. The purpose of the two pilot videos is to draw the attention of both immigrants and professionals so that they have a chance to reflect on the stories told in the animation videos.

14.3.2   Diverxualitat Actua: The Interventions of the Diverxualitat Programs

14.3.2.1   Train to Act

In order to transform perceptions and attitudes—both in people and in communities (territories in which a determined population lives, has certain requests and needs, and which may or may not rely on given resources)—it is necessary to have an educative process that supports this transformation. The intention is to achieve the generation of another reality and paradigm by parting from a previous reality and paradigm (Diaz Bordenave 1998). This work in the community should gradually

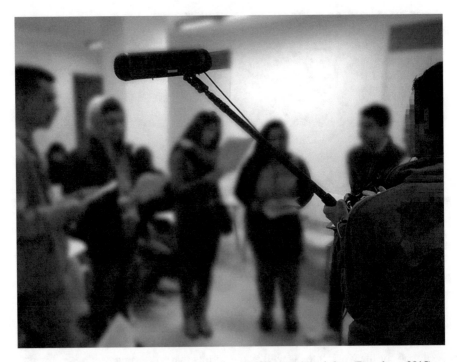

Fig. 14.4 Voice recording with young people from the Diverxual workshop (Barcelona, 2015)

improve the acceptability of the health care system to its people, which consequently will cause access to the health care system to improve (Tanahashi 1978).

The different Espictools from the Diverxualitat program (*SIDAJoc*, *HEPARJoc*, and the animation videos) or from other programs (e.g., the song "Las palabras no dan miedo") are designed, within the framework of a community intervention, to educate. From the standpoint of community health teams, it is important to train health care professionals—including active community members and peer educators— in processes of artistic co-creation and intercultural competences so that they are able to carry out the different community interventions in health based on co-creation processes to promote affective sexual health along with entities of civil society. For this purpose, our team created "Train to Act" in 2008 with the goal of training peer educators in the use of the different educational tools (Espictools) so that they may serve in the community with their peers.

Health professionals   Training health professionals is a key factor when it comes to integrating health in the community. One training strategy used is a workshop on sexual health and cultural diversity. The workshop begins by viewing the two animated videos aforementioned to later generate a discussion space. By providing health care professionals with knowledge and practical tools related to ASH, they have the opportunity to change their attitudes toward cultural diversity. This, in turn, allows health system users to be treated with more understanding. In 2018, three cycles of training were performed for primary health care professionals in the city of Barcelona. Over 300 professionals attended the course; one of the topics covered was sexuality and cultural diversity. There was a significant level of interaction from participants, and there are numerous examples of interactions from the debate forum of the two videos that have reinforced the role of artistic expression in knowledge acquisition. One participant said:

> It is true that, in our daily life, we occasionally contact people from different countries and ethnicities. Communication is sometimes difficult, as they cannot understand what we are attempting to explain to them and we cannot understand what they are telling us, as words, expressions and needs are different for both of us. This often makes providing quality care difficult if nobody is around to help us 'interpret' each other. We should never underestimate the knowledge, doubts or fears of our patients; this will make us better professionals and allow us to provide better care, earn their trust and encourage them to return whenever they have problems, especially with regard to sexual health, which is still a taboo among many people nowadays. It is important to attend [to] people as a whole.

Another participant said:

> We often put ourselves in other people's shoes but we fail to take cultural values into account. Some things that are very simple for us may be baffling to someone else. This has made me think.

Finally, another participant stated:

> These videos invite us to reflect on the person in front of us and in whose shoes we sometimes fail to put ourselves. We should be able to understand their bio-psycho-social situation and be open to interculturality.

Peer educators Training peer educators is the key to reaching the most vulnerable groups and empowering the community. This training is aimed at different groups of vulnerable immigrants. The objective is to intervene in the community using educational tools formed through a co-creation process inside of the community. In 2018, the project "Pilot Hepatitis C Micro-Elimination Strategy in Pakistani Immigrants in Catalonia through the Implementation of a Community Intervention" began, with the goal of implementing and assessing the acceptability, effectiveness, and costs of a community intervention based on HCV prevention and screening and linking to care (LTC) focused on Pakistani immigrants in Catalonia. In order to do this, two people from the Pakistani community (one community health agent and one peer educator) were trained through the program "Train to Act." Their goal was to carry out community interventions with their respective peers through a one-hour workshop using the educational tool *HEPARJoc*, and administer quick tests afterward for hepatitis C (Fig. 14.5a).

The way the program is conducted currently, using the development of *HEPARJoc* in 2015 as a starting point, people in the community are detected through community health agents and peer educators, who were previously trained to conduct a workshop using the *HEPARJoc* tool (Fig. 14.5b, c). They involve different entities of civil society in the Pakistani community throughout the entire process of this project.

14.3.2.2 Community Actions

Once they have been trained in the use of the educational tools in the Diverxualitat program (*SIDAJoc* and *HEPARJoc*), peer educators and community health agents conduct a number of workshops and activities at the individual, group, and community levels, using the educational tools for which they have been trained in order to promote affective sexual health from an intercultural and gender perspective with their peers in their own environments. Normally, through social networks (associations, parties, family homes, and public places), community health agents call people to attend the different workshops. Figure 14.6 shows one example of one workshop with *SIDAJoc* (Fig. 14.6). These strategies allow us to reach hard-to-access populations, thus promoting affective sexual health among vulnerable populations that operate on the margins of the health care system with regard to these subjects.

14.4   Conclusion

The Espictools-Actua program is a model for an innovative and dynamic co-creation artistic process that promotes an intercultural, global, and interdisciplinary/intersectoral educational approach—involving peer educators, community health agents, community workers, anthropologists, sociologists, art therapists, artists, the community, designers, community nursing, epidemiologists, and medical doctors. It is a

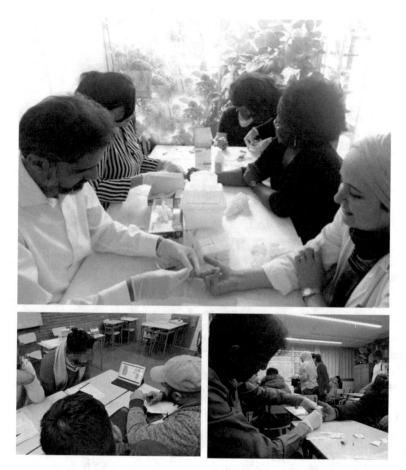

Fig. 14.5 (**a**) Preparation of the community health agent to administer the quick test (top); community intervention: (**b**) *HEPARJoc* workshop (bottom, left, 2018) and (**c**) execution of quick test (bottom, right, 2019)

program that is adapted to the needs and particularities of each specific community for more integral, fair, and sustainable care. Incorporating art in both research and in the tool itself implies added value that opens new approaches for the promotion of health.

Each phase of Espictools-Actua takes into account a point of return to the community, either by organizing dissemination exhibitions of project participants' artistic creations, or by carrying out community interventions using the tools created based on community proposals. These actions may allow for the creation of a network of community assets for fair affective sexual health promotion using these educational tools. In addition, the fact that this approach allows for a boost in the capacity of the target population to start from its own needs and realities to understand and manage what is happening (including the effects of inequality), to face these needs and realities by becoming aware of their own capabilities and of what

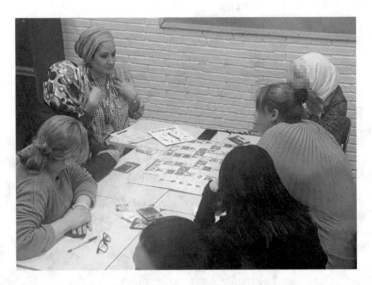

Fig. 14.6 *SIDAJoc* workshop with a Pakistani peer educator trained in the workshops

must be changed, and to work jointly with professionals and other assets from different sectors will ensure that the approach will endure over time.

The specific features of this experience may be applied to other groups by tailoring the length, methodology, and tools to suit the specific needs of the population being acted upon (according to age, gender, type of group, place of residence, etc.).

These interventions have been framed within broader work on information, education, and communication, which has been conducted since the beginning of the current study in ESPiC. This education process becomes necessary to overcome the psycho-social and cultural barriers that are present. Programs like this, with community health agents, have also been used successfully for other diseases such as HIV in adolescents and in other types of health care, such as primary care and mother/child health care (Austin-Evelyn et al. 2017; Koon et al. 2013; Mwai et al. 2013). This suggests that the presence of community health agents improves the effectiveness of community interventions.

In any case, we have been able to verify how difficult it is to incorporate this approach systematically. Despite the variety of experiences that point toward art as a key element in the success of health programs through community empowerment, there is still a need for more studies that describe their results in detail. This situation reflects one of the problems that appears in different studies that discuss the lack of clear evaluative criteria, and whether or not these can be interpreted as an effect of art. Because of this, it is necessary to evaluate the success of these community interventions further than their impact on health by examining their social effects on the community and analyzing their consequences for promoting autonomy. It is also necessary to strive to standardize, as much as possible, a methodology that guarantees maximum correlation between the objectives and the results.

As we highlighted at the beginning of this chapter, we know that artistic expressions are inherent and essential to humans, and that art of all forms are a part of community life. For this reason, the bio-psycho-social and multidisciplinary approach of these community interventions requires a multidisciplinary team. Community-based interventions, involving community health teams with a holistic approach, are highly useful in improving access to screening, increasing knowledge of ASH, and combating the psycho-social and cultural barriers to diagnosis. The intervention explained in this chapter is a viable way to work dialogically between health teams and communities.

References

Austin-Evelyn, K., Rabkin, M., Macheka, T., Mutiti, A., Mwansa-Kambafwile, J., Dlamini, T., et al. (2017). Community health worker perspectives on a new primary health care initiative in the Eastern Cape of South Africa. *PLoS One, 12*, e0173863.

Avaria Saavedra, A., & Gómez i Prat, J. (2008). "Si tengo Chagas es mejor que me muera". El desafío de incorporar una aproximación sociocultural a la atención de personas afectadas por Enfermedad de Chagas. *Enfermedades Emergentes, 10*(S1), 40–45.

Beran, D., Lazo-Porras, M., Cardenas, M. K., Chappuis, F., Damasceno, A., Jha, N., et al. (2018). Moving from formative research to co-creation of interventions: Insights from a community health system project in Mozambique, Nepal and Peru. *BMJ Global Health, 3*(6).

Boyle, J., Mattern, C. O., Lassiter, J. W., & Ritzler, M. S. (2011). Peer 2 peer: Efficacy of a course-based peer education intervention to increase physical activity among college students. *Journal of American College Health, 59*(6), 519–529.

Claveria Guiu, I., Caro Mendivelso, J., Ouaarab Essadek, H., González Mestre, M. A., Albajar-Viñas, P., Gómez, i., & Prat, J. J. (2017). The Catalonian expert patient programme for Chagas disease: An approach to comprehensive care involving affected individuals. *Journal of Immigrant and Minority Health, 19*(1).

Diaz Bordenave, J. E. (1998). *Estratégias de Ensino Aprendizagem*. Petrópolis: Vozes.

Essadek, H. O., Mendioroz, J., Guiu, I. C., Barrabeig, I., Clotet, L., Álvarez, P., et al. (2018). Community strategies to tackle tuberculosis according to the WHO region of origin of immigrant communities. *Public Health Action, 8*(3), 135–140.

Ganim, B. (1999). *Art and healing: Using expressive art to heal your body, mind, and spirit.* New York: Three Rivers Press.

Gómez i Prat, J., Ros Collado, M., Ndiaye, A. M., Ouaarab, H., Djibaou, K., Raja, S., et al. (2001). Investigación y promoción de los utensilios y métodos innovadores en la lucha contra la tuberculosis destinado a las comunidades de inmigrantes: entrevistas en grupo para la realización de un vídeo-guía sobre el conocimiento de la tuberculosis en comunidades inmigrantes. *Gaceta Sanitaria, 15*(Suppl 3), 39.

Gómez i Prat, J., Garreta, G., Ouaarab, H., Ghali, K., Claveria, I., Torrecillas, M., et al. (2015). Diverxualitat: A model of comprehensive intervention to improve access to affective sexual and reproductive health in a multicultural context. *Tropical Medicine and International Health, 20*(Suppl 1), 286.

Gysin, M., & Sorín, M.. compilers(2011). In ISPA Edicions (Ed.), *El arte y la persona: esa hierbita verde*. Barcelona.

Health Department, Catalonian Government. (2013, February). *Pla de salut afectiva i sexual (PSAS) Promoció i prevenció en la infància i l'adolescència, amb especial èmfasi en la població vulnerable*. Edita Agència de Salut Pública de Catalunya. Departament de Salut 1a edició Barcelona. http://hdl.handle.net/11351/1277

Holmboe, E. S., Foster, T. C., & Ogrinc, G. (2016). Co-creating quality in health care through learning and dissemination. *Journal of Continuing Education in the Health Professions, 36*(Suppl 1), S16–S18.

Kirby, D., Obasi, A., & Laris, B. A. (2006). The effectiveness of sex education and HIV education interventions in schools in developing countries. *World Health Organization technical report, 938*, 103–150; discussion 317–341.

Knill, P. J., Levine, E. G., & Levine, S. K. (2005). *Principles and practice of expressive arts therapy: Toward a therapeutic aesthetics.* London/Philadelphia: Jessica Kingsley Publishers.

Koon, A. D., Goudge, J., & Norris, S. A. (2013). A review of generalist and specialist community health workers for delivering adolescent health services in sub-SaharanAfrica. *Human Resources for Health, 11*, 54.

Manzardo, C., Treviño, B., Gómez, i., Prat, J., Cabezos, J., Monguí, E., Clavería, I., et al. (2008). Communicable diseases in the immigrant population attended to in a tropical medicine unit: Epidemiological aspects and public health issues. *Travel Medicine and Infectious Disease, 6*(1–2), 4–11.

Mwai, G. W., Mburu, G., Torpey, K., Frost, P., Ford, N., & Seeley, J. (2013). Role and outcomes of community health workers in HIV care in sub-Saharan Africa: A systematic review. *Journal of the International AIDS Society, 16*(1), 18586.

Ouaarab Essadek, H., Caro Mendivelso, J., Claveria Guiu, I., Salomón Bisobe, A., Gómez i Prat, J. (2017, October 23–25). Equip de Salut Pública i Comunitària. Unitat de Salut Internacional Vall D'Hebron - Drassanes-Institut de recerca (VHIR). HEPARJOC "ACTUA": Investigación; promoción de herramientas y métodos innovadores a través un proceso de co-creación para promover el cribado de la Hepatitis B en inmigrantes vulnerables. X Congreso SEMTSI. Bilbao.

Sanmartino, M., Avaria Saavedra, A., Gómez, i., Prat, J., Parada Barba, M. C., & Albajar-Viñas, P. (2015). Que no tengan miedo de nosotros: el Chagas según los propios protagonistas. *Interface: Comunicação Saúde Educação, 19*(55), 1063–1075.

Solari, A. (2015). La llave del espacio-tiempo. Revista "El Duende" n° 16 (Revista del Máster de Arteterapia Transdisciplinaria y Desarrollo Humano), Barcelona.

Sriranganathan, G., Jaworsky, D., Larkin, J., Flicker, S., Campbell, L., Flynn, S., et al. (2010). Sexual health education: Interventions for effective program evaluation. *Health Education Journal, 71*(1), 62–71.

Tanahashi, T. (1978). Health service coverage and its evaluation. *Bulletin of the World Health Organization, 56*(2), 295–303.

World Health Organization & United Nations Population Fund. (2007, March 13–15). National-level monitoring of the achievement of universal access to reproductive health: Conceptual and practical considerations and related indicators. Report of a WHO/UNFPA technical consultation, Geneva.

Chapter 15
ArtScience for Health Awareness in Brazil

Tania C. de Araújo-Jorge, Roberto Todor, Rita C. Machado da Rocha,
Sheila S. de Assis, Cristina X. A. Borges, Telma T. Santos, Valeria S. Trajano,
Lucia R. de La Rocque, Anunciata C. M. Braz Sawada,
and Luciana Ribeiro Garzoni

15.1 Introduction

Promoting health awareness is important but challenging for ensuring public health. Recent examples include the need to control the *Aedes aegypti* to reduce urban transmission of dengue, Zika, chikungunya, and yellow fever (Fonseca 2016). The summers of 2015, 2016, and 2017 were especially alarming in Brazil, since a triple epidemic arose with these arbovirus fevers (Nunes et al. 2018). To add to the complexity faced, a sylvatic yellow fever reemerged in the country at the same time (Moreira-Soto et al. 2018), people were actively called to receive yellow fever vaccinations, the only available immunization.

The Brazilian education system promotes a fairly narrow view of health as an absence of disease (Assis and Araújo-Jorge 2018). This is a view of health that has been contested by the World Health Organization (WHO) since 1946 (Nielsen 2001) because of fails to acknowledge the social context in which health is created. Educational initiatives based on even this traditional narrow view of health have not been plentiful nor effective enough to address this situation. Vertical models of communication in use since the 1980s have failed successively to combat dengue epidemies in Brazil. These models use strategies involving mass communication campaigns and authoritative/prescriptive education actions that displace governmental responsibilities to the accountability of the most vulnerable populations (Assis and Araújo-Jorge 2018; Valla 2000). Thus, the academic community has

T. C. de Araújo-Jorge (✉) · R. Todor · R. C. Machado da Rocha · S. S. de Assis
C. X. A. Borges · T. T. Santos · V. S. Trajano · L. R. de La Rocque · A. C. M. Braz Sawada ·
L. R. Garzoni
Laboratory of Innovations in Therapies, Education and Bioproducts, Oswaldo Cruz Institute
(LITEB-IOC/Fiocruz), Oswaldo Cruz Foundation (Fiocruz), Rio de Janeiro, Brazil
e-mail: taniaaj@ioc.fiocruz.br; roberto.todor@ioc.fiocruz.br; rita.rocha@ioc.fiocruz.br;
sheila.assis@ioc.fiocruz.br; valeria.trajano@ioc.fiocruz.br; luroque@ioc.fiocruz.br;
sawada@ioc.fiocruz.br; luciana.garzoni@fiocruz.br

© The Author(s) 2021
J. H. Corbin et al. (eds.), *Arts and Health Promotion*,
https://doi.org/10.1007/978-3-030-56417-9_15

been challenged to generate new strategies and actions that can engage education actors (teachers, public health vigilance agents, health management services, and academic centers) as well as the general population in expanding health awareness.

Despite the general distribution of *Aedes aegypti* in broad urban areas (Ferreira and Chiaravalloti Neto 2007; Mulligan et al. 2015), the consensus is that social determinants have a great impact on arbovirus epidemics (Ali et al. 2017; WHO 2012). Poor housing, inadequate garbage collection, and the absence of a continuous water supply (leading to the need to accumulate water in domestic reservoirs) create favorable conditions for the *Aedes* life cycle development and characterize dengue, Zika, and chikungunya infections as neglected diseases associated with poor living conditions in general.

At the Laboratory of Innovations in Therapies, Education, and Bioproducts in the Oswaldo Cruz Foundation (Fiocruz), our group adopted the concept and definitions of the ArtScience Manifesto (Root-Bernstein et al. 2011) and introduced ArtScience activities into education strategies to foster health and creativity. ArtScience is an interdisciplinary concept that hybridizes science and art practices and methods designed to favor creativity and innovation (Araújo-Jorge et al. 2018). It focuses on processes rather than on products, having the latter as a consequence of multiple engagements of awareness-raising, reasoning, and emotion of activity participants. Our goal was to address the difficulties that people of less-favored neighborhoods in Rio de Janeiro have when facing those epidemics, both with the general public and particularly with local schoolteachers (Araújo-Jorge et al. 2018). The activities converge to connect ArtScience workshops and courses with concepts of health promotion, dialoguing with the Brazilian National Policy of Health Promotion (Brazilian Ministry of Health 2010; Malta et al. 2018) and other policies that impact health. Our approach is based on the Ottawa Charter and Adelaide Statement, addressing health in all policies and the social determinants of health (WHO, Adelaide Statement on Health in All Policies 2010; WHO, Ottawa Charter for Health Promotion 1986).

Health promotion is simultaneously a field of knowledge and a field of practice, converging to reach and to improve quality of life. In the current context, health promotion has been reinforced with the goals of the United Nations' 2030 agenda (UN 2015), in which its sustainable development objectives strengthen the need for a global pact to improve the quality of life on the planet.

In this context, to achieve the aforementioned goals, the center of our strategy is the use of the ArtScience approach in socially vulnerable communities, mixing multiple artistic languages and socially accessible digital technologies. We always start the first workshop by playing Rita Lee's "Saúde" ("Health"), a popular Brazilian rock-and-roll song (www.youtube.com/watch?v=zEPXOQvN6vM) that immediately introduces discussions of health promotion. Following this, we begin developing and facilitating activities such as board and computer games, sustainability and art workshops (using reusable and recyclable materials), music for health awareness (with people of various ages and diverse pathologies), dialogic circles on science fiction, production of materials for health care communication in the training of health care agents, and contributing to the "ecology of knowledge" of teenagers and adults in socio-environmentally vulnerable areas with a high disease prevalence. We integrate the activities in the context of (1) basic and translational research on health and education, (2) "university extension" (the social link between academy and society), and (3) education (not only training) to empower the target population of the activities in a real praxis of social activism as defended by Paulo Freire's pedagogy of autonomy for popular education (Borg and Mayo 2000). Dialogue, emancipation, reflexive capacity, hope, passion, critical analysis, and awareness about their own living conditions and the conditions of the whole planet are essential elements of this pedagogy. Other essential elements are respect toward people's diversity of knowledge and cultures; confidence in the mutual construction of new knowledge that emerges from these dialogues, known as "ecology of knowledge" (Bowen 1985; Santos 2007); and the search for collaborative and creative solutions for the present problems (Araújo-Jorge et al. 2018; Root-Bernstein et al. 2011).

15.2 Project and Methods

15.2.1 Approach

The ArtScience project (CienciArte©) has been under development in our laboratory for 20 years (Araújo-Jorge et al. 2018), dating from the first PhD thesis that was presented in 1998. In Fig. 15.1, we present the project logo (a) as well as its mobile/itinerant version (b)—used when courses and workshops are literally "on the road," outside the walls of Fiocruz campus and immersed directly in communities. The project applies a qualitative research, exploratory, and descriptive approach that focused initially on science education (Araújo-Jorge et al. 2004) and more recently on health promotion and health surveillance with popular participation (Garzoni et al. 2018). We developed a variety of workshops using science and art (Araújo-Jorge et al. 2004) and recognized in our practices intensive exercising of the 13

Fig. 15.1 (**a**) Logomark of the project; (**b**) logomark of the mobile version "on the road" ("na Estrada," in Portuguese). (Logos created by the designer and PhD ArtScience student R. Todor)

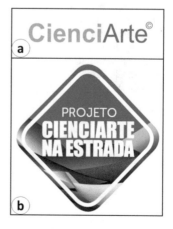

cognitive categories summarized by Robert and Michelle Root-Bernstein (2001) as their 13 creative thinking tools to foster creativity (see Box 15.1).

We adopted the term CienciArte© as a free translation for the neologism ArtScience, created and defended in the ArtScience Manifesto (Root-Bernstein et al. 2011). We recognize ArtScience as a transdisciplinary new field that transforms discoveries and inventions into innovations (Fig. 15.2) through the intensive work of making connections and driven by the necessity of applying relevant knowledge and creating social technology. History is being written with the merging of science and art in different countries (Sanders 2009; Welch 2011), and in the United States, acronyms are prevalent. The 1950s saw the birth of the now already-old STS (Science-Technology-Society) approach (Auler and Bazzo 2001; Iglesia 1997), and nowadays the new versions—STEM (science, technology, engineering, and mathematics) and STEAM (science, technology, engineering, arts, and mathematics)— are under intense debate (Malina et al. 2018; Sawada et al. 2017). The "taxonomy" of this area is still confusing; a Google search on December 30, 2018 recovered thousands of results using the following words: ArtScience (644,000), SciArt (386,000), STEAM education (586,000), and STEM education (4,860,000). In our experience, it is easier to work with the neologism "CienciArte," which in Portuguese blends the single "a" in both words—"ciência" and "arte"—and thus intuitively sparks the interdisciplinary concept of interfaces and interceptions among those fields. We refer to ArtScience as an "approach" rather than a "method" (Siler 1999), since replication is possible but results always depend on the type and depth of participant engagement.

Fig. 15.2 A general scheme for the ArtScience approach; the curved arrows form a continuous circle starting on imagination, following through making connections (through the intense use of the 13 cognitive categories to inspire discoveries) that support inventions, which can be applied and generate innovation. (Source: CienciArte© collection)

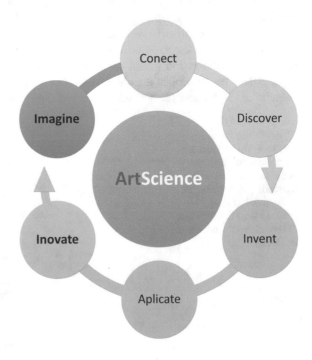

In the general ArtScience scheme in Fig. 15.2, the first three steps—imagine, connect, discover—are the foundation for basic research in all science and humanity fields; discoveries continuously feed the scientific literature. However, only when discoveries are converted into inventions that serve different applications—translating knowledge into products, processes, and tools—will they be characterized as innovations, meaning something representing a novelty, either totally or partially new; something causing an impact of any nature in the social context; and something adding value, either tangible or intangible.

15.2.2   ArtScience Workshops

Focused on the goal of creating awareness for health promotion, we developed courses that innovate both with the target public (vulnerable populations affected by neglected diseases such as Chagas disease and dengue fever) and with the ArtScience pedagogical approach. In this chapter, we will describe the activities promoting health with ArtScience to prevent arbovirus spreading through *Aedes aegypti* infestation. Three courses were performed at Manguinhos neighborhood in Rio de Janeiro (the geographic region where Fiocruz is located), directly in the community areas (February 2016 and 2017) and in a public secondary school (2018). Two adaptations of this course were also prepared, one for the arid rural zone of Quixeramobim, Ceará state in northeastern Brazil in October 2016, and the other for an industrial area at the Atlantic forest of Rio de Janeiro state in the city of Itaguaí in March 2017.

15.2.2.1   Target Public and Characteristics of the Courses

These workshops were run with adolescents (15–18 years old, in the secondary schools) and with adults (19–62 years old, in the community courses). Participants were invited by social media releases detailing the course period and conditions. The project was supported by two FAPERJ grants (E-26/010.001855/2014 and E-26/201.838/2017), and the courses were completely free of charge, thus relying only on each participant's motivation to become a popular agent of health promotion and vigilance. The main course was named *Formation for Health and Vigilance popular agents: ArtScience in Aedes control* (in Portuguese, "*Curso de Formação de Agentes Populares de Saúde e Vigilância: CienciArte no controle do Aedes*"). The practical workshops were composed of face-to-face activities in house (classrooms) and field areas. All involved artistic expressions were conceived for practicing the 13 thinking tools described in Box 15.1.

> **Box 15.1 The 13 Creative Thinking Tools**
> 1. **Observing and registering**, not simply watching, and going beyond the visual aspect of seeing.
> 2. **Imaging**, evoking images, creating visual representations in the mind.
> 3. **Abstracting**, to take something and simplify it to its most important single element, to imagine what something could be that it is not yet.
> 4. **Recognizing patterns**, identifying what is common and what is unique.
> 5. **Forming patterns**, creating something different by combining two or more elements together.
> 6. **Making analogies**, finding a relationship in size, function, form, or other.
> 7. **Thinking with the whole body**, moving the body through space to let imagination flow.
> 8. **Empathizing**, putting oneself in someone else's position, changing the perspective and the point of view.
> 9. **Thinking in a dimensional way**, moving from 2D to 3D, 4D, or 5D, scaling, or altering the proportions and symbols.
> 10. **Modeling**, creating representation of something in a physical (and even functional) form.
> 11. **Playing**, simply for the fun and for the enjoyment of doing something.
> 12. **Transforming**, altering some thing or some tool into another thing or another tool.
> 13. **Synthesizing**, describing in few words or in a picture a complex and whole idea.

15.2.2.2 Workshops

The workshops (WS) were prepared and combined according to the specific plans of each course, depending on the available time schedule and motivation of the participants.

WS1:   What is ArtScience? Is the *Aedes* control a problem? Why ArtScience for *Aedes* control?

WS2:   Observing mosquitoes and discovering novelties: in practice.

WS3:   Observing the *Aedes* life cycle with the film: "O mundo macro e micro do mosquito *Aedes aegypti*: para combatê-lo é preciso conhecê-lo" (produced in Fiocruz 2015), available at: https://youtu.be/PqUB85cE4Ls; Exploring games about *Aedes* life cycle, available at: http://www.fiocruz.br/ioc/media/comciencia_05.pdf.

WS4:   Field work: active search for mosquitoes' larvae, eggs, and adults; photo documenting mosquitoes' breeders (any open water reservoir, especially large and clean water tanks; see Powell and Tabachnick 2013).

WS5:   Mapping the neighborhood region, recognizing and localizing *Aedes* breeders, and tracing strategies for control: why a week table control? How do the environmental determinants and the urban organization favor the presence of *Aedes* mosquitoes and the incidence of arbovirus fevers?

WS6:   Making stop-motion films and a TV news report sketch for a potential community channel where the community itself and its real context were presented.

WS7:   5D modeling of the major problems: collective construction of simple structured sculptured models presenting solutions to a challenging question and implicating more than only three dimensions, thus including time, movement, sound, tactile, or olfactory perceptions (fourth dimension), as well as symbolic elements expressing a fifth dimension (see Siler 1999).

WS8:   Garbage and life: a sensitive look at garbage in public and private spaces.

WS9:   Theater sketch: performing the problem and its solutions.

WS10:   Synthesis: what have you learned? How will you use what you have learned?

As mentioned, all the workshops exercised one or more of the 13 cognitive categories (Box 15.1), with "Observing" the first and most continuous one. Figure 15.3a–e show different moments during the workshops. A recent paper showed in more detail some of the images used in WS1 (Garzoni et al. 2018). The different courses combined one or more workshops depending on the time available. Due to a lack of space, we will describe in detail WS5–WS10 in other publications.

WS1 (What is ArtScience? Is the *Aedes* control a problem? Why ArtScience for *Aedes* control?) introduced the subject, the problem, and the methodology. In a sequence of 30 slides, the participants were invited to think and to present their own view of the arbovirus problem. We explored the free association of words and of images and the ability to draw and model with clay, as if they were back in kindergarten classrooms. Their impressions emerged as we talked about "What is ArtScience for you?"

> Talking in a fun way; learning in a scientific way about what matters, and with art, in a manner that we all can understand; getting awareness of what we are learning; putting on practice through the arts, an easier means for all to understand; in a practical and not theoretical way; art is dynamic and fun; art impacts people, their voices, the theater, the films; it is good that we do not keep the knowledge for ourselves, since this knowledge is affecting all of us (transcript of participants' answers in a workshop).

The participants also shared opinions and impressions about the ideas they discussed concerning dengue, Zika, and chikungunya fevers: "What are we talking about when we talk about *Aedes*?"

> Is to talk about how you feel when you get dengue, six days at home, without feeling like eating or drinking anything; about any knowledge related to the mosquito; about knowing

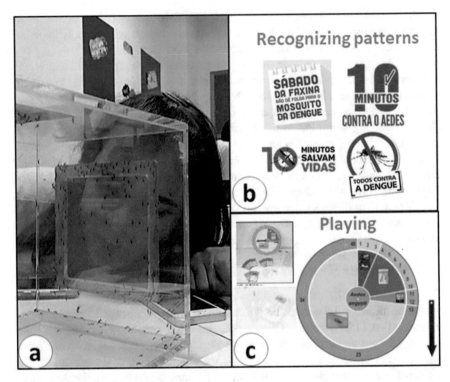

Fig. 15.3 (a) Moments and materials of workshops, showing activities of observing mosquitoes; (b) recognizing patterns by observing images of Aedes control campaigns. (Images from governmental sites (http://www.blog.saude.gov.br/index.php/combate-ao-aedes/50453-proteja-da-sua-casa-do-mosquito-da-dengue-antes-de-sair-de-ferias; http://www.ioc.fiocruz.br/dengue/textos/10minutos.html; https://www.vargemgrandedoriopardo.mg.gov.br/noticias/campanha-contra-dengue; http://www.10minutossalvamvidas.rj.gov.br/Site/Conteudo/Material.aspx); (c) playing with a game that shows the *Aedes* life cycle in a circle with 45 days (available in the material "Com Ciência na Escola #5" (www.fiocruz.br/ioc/media/comciencia_05.pdf))

how to fight it; about a problem that spread beyond Brazil; is to talk and trigger in people awareness about the risk of having a "deformed" generation of children attained by Zika; is to talk about sterilizing water, the environment must be clean; is to know more than just we have heard (transcript of participants' answers in a workshop).

The two major practical activities were conducted in WS2 (observing mosquitoes and discovering novelties) and WS4 (field work), mixing direct observation with video observations (WS3). Figure 15.3a shows a moment in WS2 when a young girl observes adult *Aedes* during an activity where all the mosquitoes' life cycle stages were presented to the participants. All the activities reinforce the first thinking tool ("observing") and are derived from it, thus attaining the main goal of the workshops: to exercise and sensitize the act of looking—to watch more than see.

In WS1, different slides provoke the participants. It is common to find errors in websites, such as mosquito images that are not *Aedes* in dengue control campaigns.

"Abstracting" (Box 15.1, tool #3) is another important tool that is exercised in the different workshops: what could this image represent besides that which it really is? The exercise of abstracting is not generally proposed in scholarly practices, yet it is an important tool to foster creativity in both art and science, as well as in the day-to-day lives of citizens. In many moments, we inserted "modeling" (Box 15.1, tool #10) and "synthesizing" (Box 15.1, tool #13) activities. An example of this is shown in Fig. 15.4, where we display the result of a 10-minute creative work by a group mixing 2D-image selection and collage with 3D modeling of *Aedes aegypti* exposure risk situations.

Following the 13 thinking tools (Box 15.1), we encouraged the participants to transform the available *Aedes* breeder control tables (Fig. 15.4b, c) into sources and inspiration materials to prepare their own individual tables (Fig. 15.4d). Two main criticisms were made regarding the table shown in Fig. 15.4b, in which 13 breeders are shown horizontally in images in the first line to be checked weekly: (1) not all the breeders are relevant for all the situations, and (2) the concept that all the relevant breeders should be actively surveilled for the presence of larvae for 8 weeks is not obvious from a simple reading of this material. A change was consequently introduced in the new version, constructed collectively with the WS participants (Fig. 15.4d): the eight-week period of vigilance was inserted in the horizontal lines and then highlighted.

Images, sounds, films, and texts on both the mosquito and the socio-environmental settings associated with the health care conditions for each group were used for awareness raising, encouraging questions and reflections on each theme. The participants produced drawings and photographs for stimulating the act of viewing under both a scientific and an artistic perspective, discussed texts, wrote folders on health care, engaged in handicraft production, and composed songs. The joint approach of science and art with the participants—using images, music, literature, and handicraft work as tools of observation, awareness raising, and mobilization—is innovative and resulted in active and critical participation. An intense and enriching dialogue took place between scientific and popular forms of knowledge, favoring the promotion of citizenship. The results produced allow for a reflection on social inequality and on the socio-environmental problems directly related to the disease carrier agents. A consequence is the proposal of collaborative and creative solutions, in a formative process of young people as multipliers for the control and prevention of diseases and health awareness promotion.

An important idea to highlight here is that such ArtScience events implicate active partnership of the community leaders involved. In the case of the Manguinhos area, the course was co-organized by the Community Intersectoral Management

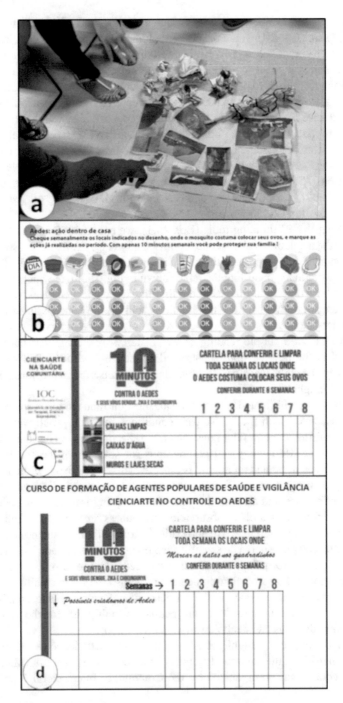

Fig. 15.4 Activities focusing on social determinants of health and of *Aedes* life cycle sustainability in the neighborhood where the courses were held, aiming to collectively build the concept of *mosquitoes' breeders* and the need for *active vigilance* of any small or large putative breeder.

Council, elected once a year and engaging all the civil society associations of the neighborhood as well as all the public sector involved in education and health services. In the case of the schools, the course involved the directors, the teachers, and the student representatives. After finishing the courses, the participants themselves became partners, since they received a Fiocruz certificate of "Popular Agent of Health Promotion and Vigilance." Participants also presented their own plan of action, a final work to complete the course, planning their interventions as "popular agents." Evaluation was based on this presentation. The study of these "interventions" is in our future objectives.

Our main concern relating to "what went wrong?" pertains to the infrastructural challenges in delivering the workshops outside the optimal conditions of the academic campus of Fiocruz. Deciding to go "on the road" (Fig. 15.1b) did not simply entail a different logo or catchphrase. To successfully engage all the partnerships necessary for the project in a specific locality, we had to grapple with the real problems of that neighborhood and maintain a focus on sensitive hearing, being open to change and adapting the content to that reality. Sometimes, to perform the course, we had to overcome simple infrastructure deficiencies such as lack of climatization (discomforting situations for the participants) or absence of Internet access for image and video searches. We learned the lesson that for any "on the road" course, all the partners should aggregate their talents and do their best. Organization was critical; everything needed should be previewed for the activities, without depending on screens, projections, or sounds from the hosting site. Furthermore, all of this is strongly dependent on the political, community, and organizational context. Thus, any dissemination of the project would always be limited by these conditions.

15.3 Discussion

ArtScience activities are not a new discovery or issue for education. In fact, STEAM, SciArt, ArtScience, Art & Science, Science-Art, and many other forms appear in the literature of creativity studies, and the evolution of STEM to STEAM-based curricula is in progress in many countries, as we stated in our introduction. The

---

Fig. 15.4 (continued) (**a**) Shows a 10-minute creative work mixing 2D-image selection and collage with 3D modeling of risk situations. (**b**) Shows part of the whole image available in the public material prepared for the "10 minutes campaign" (http://www.ioc.fiocruz.br/dengue/folder.pdf) that was used as a source for "observation." Two transformations were prepared during the courses: in Fig. 15.4c, the eight-week period of vigilance was inserted into and then highlighted in the horizontal lines, and the breeder figures were changed for clearer ones, placed vertically. In Fig. 15.4d, we developed a "do-it-yourself" control table, in which the participant chooses, draws, and describes the most relevant breeders toward which he/she has to sustain active vigilance during the eight-week period

innovation here is in ArtScience being applied to foster health awareness. The arts have been present in health education activities since the beginning of the Brazilian social movement known as Popular Education in Health (Stotz et al. 2005; Trezza et al. 2007), but they did not yet incorporate scientific concepts, images, or method-ologies. Efforts toward ArtScience mixing scientific images, principles, and prac-tices to build an actual new field (Araújo-Jorge et al. 2018; Sawada et al. 2017), are in practice at the Institute Oswaldo Cruz-Fiocruz, where educational materials are being continuously developed (http://www.fiocruz.br/ioc/cgi/cgilua.exe/sys/start. htm?sid=45). Moreover, ArtScience-based activities can contribute to achievement of the goals proposed in the 2030 Agenda for Sustainable Development (https:// www.un.org/sustainabledevelopment/sustainable-development-goals/).

Adopting for health promotion the foundations and principles exposed in the ArtScience manifesto (Root-Bernstein et al. 2011), we concluded that it can be a structuring idea in the global health education scene, as was also proposed by Dominiczak (2015). This approach is innovative and results in active and critical participation. A rich dialogue occurs between scientific and popular forms of knowl-edge, promoting citizenship. Social inequalities and environmental problems directly related to health conditions are debated. This allows for the reflection and proposal of collaborative and creative solutions, in a formative process of young people as multipliers for the control and prevention of diseases and for the promo-tion of health awareness. Its combination with the "ecology of knowledge" (Bowen 1985; Santos 2007) is a powerful tool in the exchange of knowledge with communi-ties. As one member of our team commented, "We went deep in Manguinhos...until the soul." We do not know which side of the partners learned more from the other—whether it was the "students" completing their course as "Popular Agents of Health Promotion and Vigilance," or whether it was the "teachers" that were transformed into more sensitive persons after interacting with Manguinhos inhabitants in the ArtScience practices. Converging with Paulo Freire's pedagogy, educators trans-form themselves as education transforms the society (Freire 1973, 1998). In this way, our ArtScience approach fits exactly with the general goal of this book, as stated in Chap. 1 of this volume.

15.4 Conclusion

The fundamentals of ArtScience can be applied to any health, scientific or artistic domain, which can evolve into a very powerful approach to empower and encourage participation in vulnerable communities. ArtScience can translate social, political, epidemiological and biomedical concepts into popular educational activities. It can contribute to the development of critical awareness, for example, around human rights including health, on an individual and collective level. From this work, we gained a profound understanding that ArtScience involves tools and bridges, by its transdisciplinary character, which can result in social transformation. ArtScience strategies have contributed to solving complex multidimensional problems such as emergent and re-emergent epidemics, making people face the social determinants of health in a creative and collaborative way.

Acknowledgements The authors thank Todd Siler, Harvey Seifter, and João Silveira and the team from the Laboratory of Innovations for Therapies, Education and Bioproducts – Oswaldo Cruz Institute, for interesting discussions that helped to improve this work. We also thank the Brazilian agencies CNPq, CAPES, and FAPERJ, as well as Fiocruz for funding the ArtScience activities.

References

Ali, S., Gugliemini, O., Harber, S., Harrison, A., Houle, L., Ivory, J., et al. (2017). Environmental and social change drive the explosive emergence of Zika virus in the Americas. *PLoS Neglected Tropical Diseases, 11*(2), e0005135. https://doi.org/10.1371/journal.pntd.0005135.

Araújo-Jorge, T. C., Cardona, T. S., Mendes, C. L., Henriques-Pons, A., Meirelles, R. M., Coutinho, C. M., et al. (2004). Microscopy images as interactive tools in cell modeling and cell biology education. *Cell Biology Education, 3*(2), 99–110. https://doi.org/10.1187/cbe.03-08-0010.

Araújo-Jorge, T. C., Sawada, A., Rocha, R. C. M., Azevedo, S. M. G., Ribeiro, J. M., Matraca, M. V. C., et al. (2018). CienciArte© no Instituto Oswaldo Cruz: 30 anos de experiências na construção de um conceito interdisciplinar. *Ciência e cultura, 70*(2), 25–34. https://doi.org/10.21800/2317-66602018000200010.

Assis, S. S., & Araújo-Jorge, T. C. (2018). O que dizem as propostas curriculares do Brasil sobre o tema saúde e as doenças negligenciadas? aportes para a educação em saúde no ensino de ciências. *Ciência & Educação (Bauru), 24*(1), 125–140. https://doi.org/10.1590/1516-731320180010009.

Auler, D., & Bazzo, W. A. (2001). Reflexões para a implementação do movimento CTS no contexto educacional brasileiro. *Ciência & Educação, 7*(1), 1–13. https://doi.org/10.1590/S1516-73132001000100001.

Borg, C., & Mayo, P. (2000). Reflections from a "third age" marriage: Paulo Freire's pedagogy of reason, hope and passion: An interview with Ana Maria (Nita) Freire. *McGill Journal of Education, 35*(2), 105–120. Available at http://mje.mcgill.ca/article/view/8521.

Bowen, M. (1985). The ecology of knowledge: Linking the natural and social sciences. *Geoforum, 16*(2), 213–225. https://doi.org/10.1016/0016-7185(85)90030-2.

Brazilian Ministry of Health. (2010). Política Nacional de Promoção da Saúde. Available at http://bvsms.saude.gov.br/bvs/publicacoes/politica_nacional_promocao_saude_3ed.pdf.

Dominiczak, M. H. (2015). Artscience: A new avant-garde? *Clinical Chemistry, 61*(10), 1314–1315. https://doi.org/10.1373/clinchem.2014.236992.

Ferreira, A. C., & Chiaravalloti Neto, F. (2007). Infestation of an urban area by *Aedes aegypti* and relation with socioeconomic levels. *Revista de Saúde Pública, 41*(6), 915–922. https://doi.org/10.1590/S0034-89102007000600005.

Fonseca, A. (2016). On the work and training of health agents in times of Zika. *Trabalho, Educação e Saúde, 14*(2), 327–335. https://doi.org/10.1590/1981-7746-sip00120.

Freire, P. (1973). *Pedagogy of the oppressed*. Harmondswoth: Penguin.

Freire, P. (1998). *Pedagogy of freedom*. Maryland: Roman and Littlefield.

Garzoni, L. R., Rocha, R. C. M., Todor, R., & Araújo-Jorge, T. (2018). Uso e produção de imagens em oficinas de CienciArte com Ecologia de Saberes para a promoção da saúde. *Em Aberto, 31*(103), 107–124. https://doi.org/10.24109/2176-6673.emaberto.31i103.

Iglesia, P. M. (1997). Una revisión del movimiento educativo Ciencia-Tecnología-Sociedad. Enseñanza de las Ciencias. *Barcelona, 15*(1), 51–57. Available at https://www.raco.cat/index.php/Ensenanza/article/view/21476.

Malina, R. F., Garcia, A. T., & Silveira, J. (2018). What is the evidence that art-science-technology collaboration is a good thing? *Leonardo, 51*(1), 2. https://doi.org/10.1162/LEON_e_01555.

Malta, D. C., Reis, A. A. C., Jaime, P. C., Morais Neto, O. L., Silva, M. M. A., & Akerman, M. (2018). Brazil's Unified Health System and the National Health Promotion Policy: Prospects, results, progress and challenges in times of crisis. *Ciência & Saúde Coletiva, 23*(6), 1799–1809. https://doi.org/10.1590/1413-81232018236.04782018.

Moreira-Soto, A., Torres, M. C., Lima de Mendonça, M. C., Mares-Guia, M. A., Rodrigues, C. D. S., Fabri, A. A., et al. (2018). Evidence for multiple sylvatic transmission cycles during the 2016–2017 yellow fever virus outbreak, Brazil. *Clinical Microbiology and Infection, 24*(9), 1019. https://doi.org/10.1016/j.cmi.2018.01.026.

Mulligan, K., Dixon, J., Sinn, C. L., & Elliott, S. J. (2015). Is dengue a disease of poverty? A systematic review. *Pathogens and Global Health, 109*(1), 10–18. https://doi.org/10.1179/2047773214Y.0000000168.

Nielsen, N. O. (2001). Ecosystem approaches to human health. *Cadernos de Saúde Pública, 17*(Suppl), 69–75. https://doi.org/10.1590/S0102-311X2001000700015.

Nunes, P. C. G., de Filippis, A. M. B., Lima, M. Q. R., Faria, N. R. C., Bruycker-Nogueira, F., Santos, J. B., et al. (2018). 30 years of dengue fatal cases in Brazil: A laboratorial-based investigation of 1047 cases. *BMC Infectious Diseases, 18*(1), 346. https://doi.org/10.1186/s12879-018-3255-x.

Powell, J. R., & Tabachnick, W. J. (2013). History of domestication and spread of Aedes aegypti: A review. *Memórias do Instituto Oswaldo Cruz, 108*(Suppl. I), 11–17.

Root-Bernstein, R., & Root-Bernstein, M. (2001). *Sparks of genius* (p. 401). New York: Houghton Mifflin.

Root-Bernstein, R., Siler, T., Brown, A., & Snelson, K. (2011). ArtScience: Integrative collaboration to create a sustainable future. *Leonardo, 44*(3), 192.

Sanders, M. (2009). STEM, STEM education, STEMmania. *The Technology Teacher, 68*(4), 20–26.

Santos, B. S. (2007). Para além do Pensamento Abissal: das linhas globais a uma ecologia de saberes. *Revista Crítica de Ciências Sociais, 78*, 3–46. (also published in *CEBRAP, 79*, 71–94, 2007).

Sawada, A. C. M. B., Ferreira, F. R., & Araújo-Jorge, T. C. (2017). Cienciarte ou ciência e arte? Refletindo sobre uma conexão essencial. *Revista Educação, Artes e Inclusão, 13*(3), 158–177. https://doi.org/10.5965/1984317813032017158.

Siler, T. (1999). *Think like a genius: The ultimate user's manual for your brain.* New York: Bantam.

Stotz, E. N., David, H. M. S. L., & Wong Un, J. A. (2005). Critical pedagogy and health: History, expressions and challenges of a Brazilian social movement. *Revista de APS, 8*(1), 49–60. Available at http://www.ufjf.br/nates/files/2009/12/EducacaoPopular.pdf.

Trezza, M. C. S. F., Santos, R. M., & Santos, J. M. (2007). Using art in popular health education, constructed in the daily nursing: An experience report. *Texto & Contexto Enfermagem, 16*(2), 326–334. Available at http://www.redalyc.org/articulo.oa?id=71416217.

United Nations. (2015). Transforming our world: The 2030 agenda for sustainable development. https://www.un.org/pga/wp-content/uploads/sites/3/2015/08/120815_outcome-document-of-Summit-for-adoption-of-the-post-2015-development-agenda.pdf.

Valla, V. V. (2000). Redes sociais, poder e saúde à luz das classes populares numa conjuntura de crise. *Interface—Comunicação, Saúde, Educação, 4*(7), 37–56. https://doi.org/10.1590/S1414-32832000000200004.

Welch, G. F. (2011). The arts and humanities and the 'English baccalaureate': STEAM not STEM. *Research in Teacher Education, 1*(2), 29–31. http://hdl.handle.net/10552/1415.

World Health Organization. (1986). The Ottawa charter for health promotion. Available at https://www.who.int/healthpromotion/conferences/previous/ottawa/en/.

World Health Organization. (2010). Adelaide statement on health in all policies moving towards a shared governance for health and well-being. Available at https://www.who.int/social_determinants/publications/isa/hiap_statement_who_sa_final.pdf?ua=1.

World Health Organization. (2012). Global strategy for dengue prevention and control 2012–2020. Geneva. Available at https://www.who.int/denguecontrol/9789241504034/en/.

Chapter 16
The Western Australian Indigenous Storybook Spins Special Yarns

Melissa Stoneham, Christina R. Davies, and Ray Christophers

16.1 Introduction

16.1.1 Storytelling, Yarning, and Storybooks

A storybook is a form of literature (Davies et al. 2012) that contains a narrative or collection of narratives. The West Australian Indigenous Storybooks (the Storybooks) contain a collection of autobiographical stories and artwork that showcase the achievements of Aboriginal and Torres Strait Islanders (herein referred to as Aboriginal Australians) and communities across Western Australia (HealthInfoNet 2011). Since colonization in 1788, Aboriginal Australians have experienced dispossession of traditional lands, genocidal policies, devastation of families via the forced removal of children (creating a "stolen generation"), and the

M. Stoneham (✉)
Public Health Advocacy Institute of Western Australia, School of Public Health, Curtin University, Perth, Australia

School of Public Health, Edith Cowan University, Joondalup, Australia

Menzies School of Health Research, Casuarina, Australia
e-mail: m.stoneham@curtin.edu.au

C. R. Davies
Health Humanities – Division of Health Professions Education, School of Allied Health, The University of Western Australia, Perth, Australia

Public Health Advocacy Institute of WA, Curtin University, Perth, Australia

The West Australian Arts and Health Consortium, Perth, Australia
e-mail: christina.davies@uwa.edu.au

R. Christophers
Nirrumbuk Environmental Health & Services, Nirrumbuk Aboriginal Corporation, Broome, Australia
e-mail: rchristophers@nirrumbuk.org.au

© The Author(s) 2021
J. H. Corbin et al. (eds.), *Arts and Health Promotion*,
https://doi.org/10.1007/978-3-030-56417-9_16

everyday stresses of racism (Bretherton and Mellor 2006; Dudgeon et al. 2010). In spite of such profound historical, cultural, emotional, and traumatic experiences, Aboriginal Australians and their communities have shown great resilience.

For Aboriginal Australians, the arts are an important way of building resilience, collaborating, passing on knowledge, and continuing traditions. This is especially the case for storytelling (Kovach 2009), or "yarning," a commonly accepted term for storytelling in Aboriginal culture. Yarning is a traditional communication tool that involves the sharing of stories and knowledge in a manner that is culturally prescribed, cooperative, and respectful (Walker et al. 2014). Building on this rich oral tradition and guided by an Aboriginal Steering Committee (of which author Ray Christophers is a member), the Storybooks are a strengths-based approach that extends storytelling into a written form. Storytelling is timely, accurate, appropriate, and culturally relevant for Indigenous people and their communities (Dei 2011; Iseke 2013). Traditional storytelling acts as a bridge for social transformation for Indigenous worldviews and shapes ethical, theoretical, methodological, and conceptual frameworks (Datta 2017). In the Australian context, Aboriginal knowledge of the land is embedded in the stories of the "Dreaming," which describe the creation of the world (Barrett 2013). Storytelling is ethically appropriate when engaging in projects with Aboriginal Australians and includes a range of practices that are community-based, collaborative, action-oriented, equitable, and grounded in sustained relationships of trust (Datta 2017; Simpson 2014).

16.1.2   A Background to Aboriginal Australian Health and Well-Being

To better understand the contemporary realities of Aboriginal life, a demographic, cultural, and health summary is provided below. As of June 2016, it was estimated that the Aboriginal Australian population was 798,400 people, or 3.3% of the total Australian population (100,512 people or 3.9% of the Western Australian population) (Australian Bureau of Statistics 2018). The Aboriginal population (median age 23 years) has a younger age structure than the non-Indigenous population (median age 38 years), with a larger proportion of young people and a smaller proportion of older people (Australian Bureau of Statistics 2018). It is estimated that one-third of Aboriginal Australians live in major cities, compared with three-quarters of the non-Indigenous population (Australian Bureau of Statistics 2018).

Aboriginal Australians are one of the most linguistically and culturally diverse populations in the world. At the time of colonization, there were approximately 260 distinct language groups and 500 dialects (Dudgeon et al. 2010). Aboriginal culture embraces family, the land (i.e., "country"), art, spirit, and "lore" (i.e., cultural beliefs). The relationship to family and country is an important part of Aboriginal life as are birthright, shared language, cultural obligations/responsibilities, and social and spiritual activities.

Aboriginal Australians have a holistic definition of health that acknowledges connection to culture, land, and spirit. There is little need for Aboriginal Australians to untangle the social determinants of health, as their holistic view of health is inclusive of all factors that impact well-being. The National Aboriginal Health Strategy defines Aboriginal health as not simply the physical well-being of an individual, but instead refers to the social, emotional, and cultural well-being of the whole community in which each individual is able to achieve their full potential, thereby bringing about the total well-being of their community. It is a whole-of-life view that includes the cyclical concept of life-death-life (National Aboriginal Health Strategy Working Party 1989). The Aboriginal Australian definition of health aligns with many of the core values of the Ottawa Charter (World Health Organization 1986), including a holistic view of health, participation, and equity. However, with higher rates of chronic disease and disability, the health status of Aboriginal Australians is much lower than that of non-Indigenous Australians (Sun and Buys 2015). While there are many statistics documenting the differences in health, the most telling is life expectancy. In 2010–2012, the estimated life expectancy at birth for Aboriginal males was 69.1 years and 73.7 years for females—this was approximately 10 years lower than the life expectancy for non-Aboriginal Australians (Australian Institute of Health and Welfare 2014). Overall, Western approaches to treating illness and promoting wellness have had limited success on Aboriginal health, primarily because they fail to take into account cultural issues of identity, kinship, family, community, and connection to country (Sun and Buys 2015). Other values that underpin the Ottawa Charter, such as social justice and empowerment, are captured within Aboriginal core values including Aboriginal self-determination principles, community ownership, and localized decision-making (Houston 2006).

16.2   The West Australian Indigenous Storybook Project

The West Australian Storybook was developed as one response to the amount of negative media relating to Aboriginal Australians in mainstream media. Negative media about Aboriginal Australians impacts their self-esteem and health and perpetuates racist stereotypes, prejudice, and discrimination (Balvin and Kashima 2012). Following on from a Public Health Advocacy Institute of Western Australia (PHAIWA) media analysis project that found that 74% of mainstream news coverage about Aboriginal Australians was negative (Stoneham et al. 2014), the need for a more balanced view of Aboriginal life was recognized. With the guidance of regional Elders and an Aboriginal Steering Committee (which has representation from most of the regions across Western Australia), the WA Indigenous Storybook project was initiated in 2011. Examples of the Storybook covers appear in Fig. 16.1. In the past, research and health projects facilitated by non-Indigenous agencies have often been a source of distress for Indigenous peoples because of the use of inappropriate methods and practices (Cochran et al. 2008). This was recognized in this project, and every effort was made to ensure that the processes occurred in a

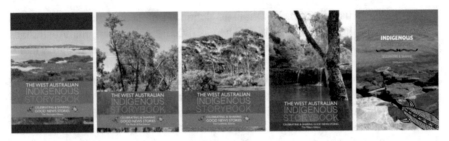

Fig. 16.1 Covers of past issues of the West Australian Indigenous Storybooks

culturally appropriate manner. Through consultation and collaboration, the project team, regional Elders, and the Aboriginal Steering Committee have worked together to:

1. Develop a storytelling process that empowers authors to write about their projects, events, and personal stories using their own words and language.
2. Enable a practice that encourages positive change via the use of positive rather than deficit language (e.g., using terms such as "excellence" and "success" instead of "disadvantage" or "closing the gap").
3. Empower authors to focus on elements that they hold dear to their spirits and hearts. Authors are offered all credit for the knowledge that is shared and have full editorial rights. This enables authors to use storytelling to promote social justice by amplifying their voice as discussed in Chap. 21.
4. Facilitate a practice whereby Aboriginal Elders, authors, and communities lead the storytelling process. For example, each edition of the Storybook focuses on a particular region of Western Australia where cultural similarities and language commonalities occur. At every stage, regional Elders are consulted (especially at the initial stages) to identify which community members should be approached by PHAIWA or which projects/events the community is particularly proud of or pleased with. Storytellers are also recruited via the Aboriginal Steering Committee and partner organizations (e.g., Aboriginal Medical Services, Aboriginal Corporations).
5. Encourage stories about projects and events that are community driven, developed, and implemented (Fletcher 2007), thereby recognizing the power Aboriginal methods can bring to a project/event and the benefits these stories can provide to other Aboriginal communities facing similar issues.
6. Enable stories that represent equity and discuss what is fair and just through an Aboriginal lens.

Through storytelling, authors reflect on and explain the rationale, implementation, outcomes, and potential future of their specific community project/event. The stories address a broad array of social and cultural determinants of health and embrace the holistic culture of Aboriginal Australians. Past story subject examples include art, mental health, preventive health, education, environmental sustainability, and sports programs/events. Stories also focus on individuals who are community leaders or emerging leaders who have achieved positive outcomes for their community.

To facilitate the storytelling process, a template was developed as a tool to provide guidance to potential authors. Figure 16.2 provides an example of how the stories look within each Storybook. The storytelling template was developed and pilot-tested with advice and guidance from the Aboriginal Steering Committee. The template is available electronically, in written form, or can be provided to the project team verbally. First, the template asks for information about the storyteller and their project/event/narrative (e.g., their name, project/event information, cultural background, organization, program partners, and the key people involved). Contact details for the authors are always provided to enable a reader to contact them directly. Second, the heading *"Once upon a time"* is presented to the storyteller and encourages the storytellers to reflect on the background or rationale for their story. This heading sets the context for the story and provides important details such as initiating factors, cultural considerations, or a brief history prior to the program/event. Third, the storyteller is presented with the heading *"And then one day."* This part of the template encourages the storyteller to focus on the issues the story is targeting. Fourth, the story heading *"And because of that"* provides the storyteller an opportunity to write about the outcomes of the project/event that has occurred. In this section, some stories also include a discussion of problems, limitations, barriers, or setbacks that arose during the project implementation under a sub-heading titled *"Unfortunately."* Lastly, the storyteller is presented with the heading *"And since that day,"* where the storyteller outlines the outputs, impacts, and outcomes they have achieved. Although this template could be considered a "Western" storytelling framework, the pilot testing, approval by the Aboriginal Steering Committee, evaluation, and subsequent publication of ten Storybooks over a period of 6 years demonstrates that this is an acceptable method and a holistic way to ensure that each story is written about in full and has an introduction, a middle, and an end.

Once complete, each Storybook has a regional launch where the storyteller is formally acknowledged and presented with a copy of the Storybook. Politicians, local leaders, and the media regularly attend these launches, which provide storytellers the opportunity to speak about their projects. The launch also allows PHAIWA to show its appreciation to the storytellers for their engagement and time in being involved in the storytelling process. The Storybook has its own website (https://www.phaiwa.org.au/indigenous-storybook/) and Facebook account (www.facebook.com/PHAIWA) and is tweeted from the PHAIWA account (@PHAIWA). The project has been funded since its inception by The Western Australian Health Promotion Foundation (Healthway).

ROEBOURNE ART GROUP

ORGANISATION NAME:
Roebourne Art Group

CONTACT PERSON:
Rex Widerstrom

EMAIL:
rex@roebourneart.com.au

PROGRAM / PROJECT PARTNERS:
Rio Tinto, Australian Government, Ministry for the Arts, Woodside Energy, Ngarluma Aboriginal Corporation, Museum of Contemporary Art, Aboriginal Arts Centre Hub of WA and Artsource

KEY STAFF / PEOPLE INVOLVED:
Rex Widerstrom, Violet Samson, Pansy Hicks

KEY WORDS:
Painting, art, culture, Country, hope, healing, collaboration

About the Storyteller...

Rex Widerstrom is the CEO at Roebourne Art Group.

About the Roebourne Art Group...

Roebourne Art Group is based in the Pilbara Region of WA. With a membership of around 70 artists of Aboriginal and Torres Strait Islander backgrounds, RAG is the region's only inclusive art group. In common with Aboriginal artists from other parts of Australia, our artists paint their stories from "when the world was soft" before creation, to contemporary pieces reflecting the reality of life today in one of the country's toughest, most remote locations. Roebourne Art Group represents Aboriginal and Torres Strait Islander artists working in an area that is home to many different language groups.

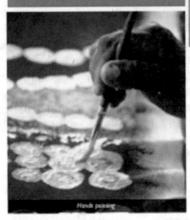

Hands painting

Once upon a time...

Roebourne Art Group (RAG) formed in 2007. At the time, local artists were painting independently in small clusters but all joined together under one roof which eventually became the Roebourne Art Group. In June 2017 we had the opportunity to move into the Roebourne Visitors Centre which is our current premises. This is the old Roebourne gaol and the building, which was built in 1886, has a sad history

which our people had to come to terms with. Some of our artists were a little bit wary when we were first offered this space, so I asked our Elders how they felt about it. One of our Elders, Aunty Violet said, "Well, if there are ghosts up there then they'll keep people away from stealing our art!" So we accepted that and it became our new home.

When we first moved in, there were a few issues to iron out before we could start functioning properly as an art space. As the building is historically listed, it had certain restrictions. We weren't allowed to put in fixtures of any kind in the interior. That ruled out picture hooks on the walls or in the beams in the ceiling. Although we were grateful to be provided with the space, without being able to fix our art work to the walls or hang it from the ceiling, we were faced with a dilemma.

However, this provided an opportunity for a community call to arms! We put the word out to local businesses and the Construction, Forestry, Mining and Energy Union (CFMEU) came forward and offered to help. They enlisted the help of several firms that were working on various projects in the Pilbara who collectively got on board – Brookfield Multiplex/Cooper and Oxley Joint Venture and

24

Fig. 16.2 Storybook example – "Roebourne Art Group"

16.3 Evaluation

As of 2019, ten Storybooks have been published. Two editions of the Storybook have been produced every 18 months and typically contain 13 stories. The Storybooks are produced in full color, with numerous photographs and "callout" quotes. Although available via the Storybook website (https://www.phaiwa.org.au/indigenous-storybook/), the Storybooks are also produced in hard copy, as the look and feel of the Storybook has been a critical factor of the project's success. In 2016, an extensive process and impact evaluation of the Storybook took place. The evaluation found that between 2011 and 2016:

- 141 authors had contributed to 93 stories,
- 1800 hard copies of the Storybook had been distributed to over 460 media, arts, sport, government, and non-government organizations,
- 10,255 electronic downloads occurred from the PHAIWA website,
- 7 Storybook launches took place, and
  345 people attended a Storybook launch.
- These Storybooks should definitely continue because they are about community people and sharing stories. People love having hard copies to share and show with family and friends. (Survey respondent, author, female, Aboriginal, health professional, 2018)

- It is a great resource for the projects highlighted in the book but also for others that read the book to see the great and varied projects that are happening around the state. (Survey respondent, author, female, Aboriginal, media, 2018)

Storytellers were also invited to complete an evaluation survey (via paper or telephone). Forty storytellers responded to the survey. Overall, it was found that the majority of respondents were happy or extremely happy with the Storybook template (95%), the presentation of the Storybook (98%), the look and feel of the Storybook (98%), the photos (98%), and the Storybook launch (98%). Storytellers indicated that the launch was important and was a positive opportunity for people to come together, meet new people, learn about other projects in the community, and network with key stakeholders.

A great tool to inspire change and innovation in communities. Well done. (Survey respondent, author mentor, female, Aboriginal, health professional, 2018)

People are so impressed with the edition! Each one [story] is such an achievement. This gave us an opportunity to blow the trumpet, building morale and hopefully triggering other good things in the community. What a beautiful occasion the launch was ... and I'm loving the book. The article is a retrospective view that is wonderful to have in our 10th anniversary year. I hope the will is there to allow the Storybook to continue. We felt nurtured by the experience. That's most appreciated! Thanks so much – the concept is a real winner! (Survey respondent, author, female, Aboriginal, artist, 2019)

I really appreciated the opportunity. It was a really good experience from first contact to the launch! (Survey respondent, launch attendee, female, Aboriginal, health professional, 2019)

Overall, 78% of respondents advised that they had forwarded either a hard or an electronic copy of their Storybook to another person, but indicated that the distribution of the book needed to be more extensive so as to encourage community-based innovation, to more widely promote the positive Aboriginal projects/events that are occurring, and to counteract ubiquitous negative media pertaining to Aboriginal Australians.

> I thought the launch was great, however we need to be able to influence 'the other' mainstream services, media, and community to understand Aboriginal people and ways of working with the Aboriginal community. (Survey respondent, female, launch attendee, Aboriginal, Aboriginal Foundation, 2018)

Common feedback from the storytellers was that they felt extremely proud to see their stories in print and thought the Storybooks were a valuable record of their work. Storytellers wanted to share the Storybooks with clients, their community, management, and others more broadly (i.e., other communities and government and non-government organizations), therefore making it a valuable bridge for social transformation between and amongst sectors.

> I loved seeing my story in print, you did a great job of representing who I am and this is something I will always be proud of, show my children, and keep forever. Thank you. (Survey respondent, author, male, Aboriginal, consultant, 2018)

> Brilliant! Thank you. Everyone we have shared the book with has loved it and appreciated the opportunity to hear about what others are doing. It is a book that gets read (not one for the shelf!). There are so many wonderful projects and ideas out there, we don't always get to hear about the good news— especially when it's community projects operating on little budgets doing great work right there on the ground. (Survey respondent, author, female, Aboriginal, Aboriginal Corporation, 2019)

Some storytellers used the Storybooks to generate new interest in their projects or as a tool to successfully secure more funding. Storytellers advised that the Storybooks enabled the replication of successful projects or the creation of new partnerships, and that the sharing of barriers or project problems enabled the development, better design, and increased cost effectiveness of new projects within the community. Respondents also indicated that it was beneficial to have local leaders acknowledged and celebrated via personal narratives, as this increased respect and community cohesiveness. Overall, the Storybooks were found to have an immensely positive impact on Aboriginal people and communities by enhancing connections, communication, self-esteem, positive social identity, and knowledge. The vast majority of respondents felt that the Storybooks should continue to be published (98% agree, 2% unsure).

> These articles assist with the stigma attached in society, changing views and acknowledging achievements. (Survey respondent, partner, female, Aboriginal, health professional, 2018)

> There are lots of untold stories in the community so keep this going! (Survey respondent, launch attendee, female, Aboriginal, teacher, 2019)

16.4 Key Learnings, Outcomes, and Benefits

Through the arts practice of storytelling—which seeks human and social well-being by developing human capacities; personal growth; and social relationships of equality, freedom, and mutual relationship—people are able to flourish (Payne 2011). As suggested via the evaluation feedback, the arts/storytelling process has the power to inspire creativity, invention, self-critique, and self-transcendence (Bauman 1999), and to act as a vehicle to achieve well-being through opportunities for engagement, artistic expression, self-awareness, and skill development (Sen 1992). The storytelling process and the publishing of a high-quality artifact that the storyteller is proud to be associated with (i.e., the Storybook) supports the capacity for authors and their communities to aspire for the future and (via the provision of contact details in each story) to connect with Aboriginal and non-Indigenous members of the community, especially those interested in creating or replicating similar projects/events (Appadurai 2004).

One of the most important things the project team has learned from the Storybooks is that when people are provided with a method of communication that is non-threatening and culturally appropriate, they are comfortable, relaxed, and happy to share their experiences. In addition, when Aboriginal Australians are supported to share their stories, innovation can flourish. We have also learned that the best solutions to remedy local issues come from the community themselves; PHAIWA's role is mostly administrative, with the Aboriginal Steering Committee, Community Elders, and storytellers acting as the innovators and leaders in this project. The ideas for the stories come from the storytellers themselves, and the innovative projects are already happening in communities across Western Australia. The Storybooks provide a forum and opportunity to share these ideas/projects/events that may otherwise go untold or unrecognized. This is why the Storybooks are so important—for now and into the future. As suggested via evaluation feedback, the Storybooks not only provide an outlet for people's voices, they also contribute to a sense of pride, ownership, and mental and social well-being. The Storybooks provide authors with the opportunity to tell their stories in their own words and in a manner that is compatible with the traditional yarning process. The Storybooks are also a creative tool to tap into the valuable yet commonly overlooked social capital resource that exists within many Aboriginal communities and empowers Aboriginal storytellers to tell and write their stories for wider dissemination. This project recognizes that communication needs to be about more than transmitting information and assuming it will be understood and acted upon. This project involves the transformation of health knowledge into key messages that can be readily understood, accepted, and put into action by other Aboriginal communities or practitioners.

As with most projects, a number of challenges were experienced. Some related to literacy levels of some storytellers, as English was often their third or fourth language. This was easily remedied via the help of a translator; however, the translation process often extended the project timeframe. Another challenge that often extended the timeframe of producing an individual Storybook was the length of time needed for storytellers to read, edit, and approve individual stories. Patience was a much-needed attribute in this project. In rare cases, a story was retracted by a storyteller prior to publication due to a change in circumstance in their community or a death within the community.

Overall, the West Australian Indigenous Storybook project bridges a number of public health practice gaps. First, it bridges a gap between geographically dispersed and often remote communities and encourages them to contemplate whether they could replicate the positive projects or activities in the Storybooks. Communities therefore have the opportunity to learn from each other, communicate, offer support, and share knowledge. Second, the Storybook project builds understanding of Aboriginal people, communities, and culture by the non-Indigenous population, who often do not actually know or interact with Aboriginal people or who are only exposed to Aboriginal culture via the media. Third, it provides storytellers, their communities, and their organizations with opportunities to strengthen existing—and create new—partnerships. And fourth, the Storybooks are an advocacy tool that can be used for many purposes, including promoting Aboriginal projects and applying for or extending program funding. For PHAIWA, the Storybooks have resulted in many positive outcomes, especially stronger links with Aboriginal people and their communities.

16.5   Conclusion

The West Australian Indigenous Storybook project is a tool to promote positive narrative. It empowers authors to write about projects, events, and personal stories that they hold dear to their spirits and hearts, using their own words and language. The process is author- and community-led and blends and creates a bridge between Aboriginal and Western storytelling methodologies while taking into account the values, practices, and beliefs of Aboriginal peoples in a way that is respectful and inclusive. The Storybook project values the broad and disparate expertise and understanding that exists in communities and strives to advance and disseminate activities that are of mutual benefit to both Aboriginal and non-Aboriginal people in an effort to enhance the wellness of Aboriginal Australians and diminish negative stereotypes. The Storybooks create a strong and relational means of arts engagement with storytellers, their communities, and the wider non-Indigenous community and provide an ever-expanding, self-sustaining living archive of innovative, successful, constructive, and readily available knowledge, information, and expertise.

Acknowledgement   The authors would like to thank Ms. Sunni Wilson for her assistance in providing some of the data for this Chapter.

References

Appadurai, A. (2004). The capacity to aspire: Culture and the terms of recognition. In V. Rao & V. Walton (Eds.), *Culture and public action* (pp. 59–84). Palo Alto: Stanford University Press.

Australian Bureau of Statistics. (2018). *Aboriginal and Torres Strait Islander peoples*. Retrieved from http://www.abs.gov.au/Aboriginal-and-Torres-Strait-Islander-Peoples

Australian Institute of Health and Welfare. (2014). *Mortality and life expectancy of Indigenous Australians: 2008 to 2012*. Retrieved from https://www.aihw.gov.au/getmedia/b0a6bd57-0ecb-45c6-9830-cf0c0c9ef059/16953.pdf.aspx?inline−true

Balvin, N., & Kashima, Y. (2012). Hidden obstacles to reconciliation in Australia: The persistence of stereotypes. In D. Bretherton & N. Balvin (Eds.), *Peace psychology in Australia*. New York: Springer Science and Business Media.

Barrett, S. (2013). *"This land is me": Indigenous Australian story-telling and ecological knowledge*. Retrieved from https://journals.openedition.org/elohi/592

Bauman, Z. (1999). *Culture as praxis*. London: Sage Publications.

Bretherton, D., & Mellor, D. (2006). Reconciliation between Aboriginal and other Australians: the "stolen generations". *Journal of Social Issues, 62*(1), 81–98.

Cochran, P., Marshall, C., Garcia-Downing, C., Kendall, E., Cook, D., McCubbin, L., et al. (2008). Indigenous ways of knowing: Implications for participatory research and community. *American Journal of Public Health, 98*(1), 22–27.

Datta, R. (2017). *Traditional storytelling: An effective indigenous research methodology and its implications for environmental research*. AlterNative: An International Journal of Indigenous Peoples. Retrieved from http://journals.sagepub.com/doi/10.1177/1177180117741351

Davies, C., Rosenberg, M., Knuiman, M., Ferguson, R., Pikora, T., & Slatter, N. (2012). Defining arts engagement for population-based health research: Art forms, activities and level of engagement. *Arts & Health, 4*(3), 203–216.

Dei, G. (2011). *Indigenous philosophies and critical education: A reader*. New York: Peter Lang.

Dudgeon, P., Wright, M., Paradies, Y., Garvey, D., & Walker, I. (2010). The social, cultural and historical context of Aboriginal and Torres Strait islander Australians. In *Working together: Aboriginal and Torres Strait islander mental health and wellbeing principles and practice* (pp. 25–42). Canberra: Australian Institute of Health and Welfare.

Fletcher, S. (2007). *Communities working for health and wellbeing: Success stories from the aboriginal community controlled health sector in Victoria*. Fitzroy: Victorian Aboriginal Community Controlled Health Organisation and Cooperative Research Centre for Aboriginal Health.

HealthInfoNet. (2011). *The West Australian Indigenous storybook: celebrating and sharing good news stories—the Kimberley and Pilbara edition*. Retrieved from http://healthbulletin.org.au/articles/the-west-australian-indigenous-storybook-celebrating-and-sharing-good-news-stories-the-kimberley-and-pilbara-edition/

Houston, S. (2006). Equity, by what measure? *Health Promotion Journal of Australia, 17*(3), 2006–2009.

Iseke, J. (2013). Indigenous storytelling as research. *Indigenous Storytelling as Research, 6*(4), 559–577.

Kovach, M. (2009). *Indigenous methodologies: Characteristics, conversations, and contexts*. Toronto: University of Toronto Press.

National Aboriginal Health Strategy Working Party (1989). *A national Aboriginal health strategy*. Canberra: National Aboriginal Health Strategy Working Party.

Payne, M. (2011). *Humanistic social work: Core principles in practice*. Chicago: Lyceum Books.

Sen, A. (1992). *Inequality reexamined*. New York: Russell Sage Foundation Clarendon Press.

Simpson, A. (2014). *Mohawk interruptus: Political life across the borders of settler states*. Durham: Duke University Press.

Stoneham, M. J., Goodman, J., & Daube, M. (2014). The portrayal of indigenous health in selected Australian media. *The International Indigenous Policy Journal, 5*(1), 1–13.

Sun, J., & Buys, N. (2015). Addressing the health needs of indigenous Australians through creative engagement: A case study. In S. Clift & P. Camic (Eds.), *Oxford textbook of creative arts, health and wellbeing*. Oxford: Oxford University Press.

Walker, M., Fredericks, B., Mills, K., & Anderson, D. (2014). "Yarning" as a method for community-based health research with indigenous women: The indigenous women's wellness research program. *Health Care for Women International, 35*(10), 1216–1226.

World Health Organization. (1986, November 21). *The Ottawa Charter for health promotion: First international conference on health promotion, Ottawa*. Retrieved from https://www.who.int/healthpromotion/conferences/previous/ottawa/en/

Chapter 17
Silent Silhouettes: A Living Reminder of the Urgent Action Needed to End Gender-based Violence in Trinidad and Tobago

Stephanie Leitch

17.1 Gender-based Violence: A Public Health Priority

Public health has long been regarded as the exclusive domain of health experts to its detriment. However, this capitalist-inspired separation of parts from their whole has rendered efforts in managing public health crises largely ineffective. In the developing world, the widespread absence of dynamic and responsive health care models that incorporate perspectives from across sectors results in the poor distribution of responsibility for health promotion. In Trinidad and Tobago, the disparities in income, the prohibitive cost of private health care, the over-burdened public health care systems, and rising health bills are all critical incentives for an increased interest and investment in public health initiatives. As the editors of this book frame the conversation of this collection (Chap. 1), borrowing from the Ottawa Charter for Health Promotion (1986) and WHO guidelines, health promotion extends beyond the health sector and toward assuring the "healthy lifestyles and well-being" of individuals. This human-centered approach is grounded in the understanding that multi-sectoral involvement is instrumental to the promotion and attainment of national (and global) optimal health.

Locally, while the current health minister has prioritized the need for "healthy living," health promotion is still largely concentrated on the reduction of the national rates of Non-Communicable Diseases (NCDs) (Paul 2016). Given this focus, the minister's main priority has been NCD reduction through the development of the National Strategic Plan for the Prevention and Control of Non-Communicable Diseases (2017–2021) and other programmatic interventions, such as the ban of sugary beverages in schools and the implementation of a Diabetes Wellness Centre (Doughty 2018). Women's health has also been acknowledged as a priority through the implementation of a Directorate of Women's Health in 2015, as well as

S. Leitch (✉)
WOMANTRA, St. Ann's, Port of Spain, Trinidad and Tobago
e-mail: s.leitch@hotmail.com

© The Author(s) 2021
J. H. Corbin et al. (eds.), *Arts and Health Promotion*,
https://doi.org/10.1007/978-3-030-56417-9_17

sustaining the consistent 12-year downward trend in infant and maternal mortality rates, resulting in a 20% reduction (UNICEF 2018). Yet, a concerted effort has not been made to secure the sexual and reproductive health and rights of women and girls, who are made more vulnerable to risky sexual behavior and sexually transmitted infections in violent intimate-partner relationships (Hess et al. 2012). Instead, policy documents such as the Sexual and Reproductive Health Policy and Gender Policy have remained in draft for years, despite the increasing necessity for their implementation. With over 8500 reports of domestic abuse being made by women between 2010 and 2015 in Trinidad and Tobago, comprehensive, systemic reform is urgently needed to reduce the incidents of domestic violence. These policy deficits amidst other forms of state inaction, ultimatey reflect the difference in perceived urgency between the two areas of public health—NCDs versus Gender-Based and Sexual Violence (GBSV).

For both women and girls, GBSV poses a demonstrably significant public health risk that cannot be underestimated. As of 2017, interpersonal violence was the seventh leading cause of death in Trinidad and Tobago, above HIV/AIDS as the tenth (Institute for Health Metrics and Evaluation 2017). When considering the leading causes of premature death, interpersonal violence raises to ranking as the fourth leading cause. Other concerning causes are neonatal disorders (fifth), HIV/AIDS (seventh), and self-harm (tenth) (Institute of Health and Metrics Evaluation 2017). Each of these leading causes of death bears a macabre story of the gendered vulnerabilities of women and girls, masked by its co-morbidity with NCDs and other health complications. With interpersonal violence being positively correlated to many negative health consequences—including the development of neonatal disorders (Bailey 2010), contraction of sexually transmitted infections (STIs), and engagement in self-harm (Boyle et al. 2006)—its ranking as a leading cause of death listed among other diseases that it is often correlated with requires immediate attention and action. Additionally, the specific vulnerability of women, girls, and sexual minorities to gender-based violence and the full gamut of health risks that are associated with it necessitates the development of gender-sensitive health policies, such as the Sexual and Reproductive Health and Gender policies and interagency protocols that are jointly designed, standardized, and implemented, including a minimum standard of care for those affected by gender-based violence.

The national statistics are further compounded by a lack of public awareness and education to successfully empower vulnerable groups to take control of their health. Without the mandatory application of Health and Family Life Education (HFLE) at primary- and secondary-level institutions, as well as making similar curricula accessible to out-of-school youth, young people remain particularly vulnerable to the effects of misinformation about their sexual and reproductive health. Facilitating youth learning of medically accurate and age-appropriate sex education can offer young people knowledge about how to navigate their own sexual and reproductive health, which can reduce rates of gender-based violence and risky sexual behaviors and improve overall sexual and reproductive health (IPPF 2016). Holistic approaches also include the education of adults, including parents and primary caregivers, through facilities such as public health clinics and community centers, which can aid in filling knowledge gaps and can potentially increase health-seeking practices that can be shared and encouraged within households. Finding progressive and creative ways to educate the population and raise awareness about the effects of gendered vulnerabilities is critical to the success of efforts to bolster the national public health profile. Art, then, becomes a natural ally in this project, with a capacity to inspire deep, introspective insight about ourselves, humanity and our planet. It is a catalyst for personal growth, transformation and overall well-being.

17.2   The Organization

WOMANTRA is a linguistic blend of the words "woman" and "mantra." This original portmanteau, which carries deep symbolism, is the brainchild of Trinidadian multimedia artist Michelle Isava. In 2008, Isava was featured at the launch of the public art project "Galvanize" based in Port of Spain, where she performed a ritual of the same name. The performance, grounded in the affirmation of sacred femininity, saw the artist in a stooping position, meditatively drawing seven concentric circles around herself—a number that bears significance in nearly all major religions—propelled by the mantra *"the hole is whole"* blaring from a loudspeaker, much like the adhan or Muslim call to prayer. The embodied message of this performance, which centered the power and completeness of "the feminine," resonated deeply with the project of WOMANTRA, which took shape 3 years later as an intimate celebration of the International Women's Day centenary.

Not unlike the defining consciousness-raising circles of the 1970s, WOMANTRA comprised a small group of young and older women gathered together in an old-fashioned Woodbrook house to share stories, poetry, music, and tantric belly dancing. As the event drew to a close, the commitment was made to stay connected, share photos of the event for our memory banks, and support each other's art and advocacy. In our favor, the WOMANTRA event of 2011 aligned with the burgeoning popularity of the world's most formidable social media site: Facebook. At the point in time when our own nugget of history was being made by a small collective of feminists in Trinidad, history was also being made at a global scale, with Facebook poised to revolutionize the reach and impact of activism everywhere. WOMANTRA began its journey as an online feminist collective through Facebook, with its first members being the women that attended our inaugural event on that fated day—and the rest, as we say, is *herstory*.

As a product of its time and engaged on- and off-line nurturing, WOMANTRA emerged as one of the leading cyber feminist platforms in the Caribbean region, giving voice and much-needed connectivity to an emerging diaspora of social justice activists. By 2014, WOMANTRA began transitioning from the virtual to the "real" world by building on the strength of its online following, and became a registered non-profit as part of a strategic effort to be recognized as a legitimate player in the civil society arena. One of WOMANTRA's first programmatic initiatives was the launch of its originally designed "Sistah2Sistah" mentorship program, designed to address the needs of adolescent girls, including sexuality education. Now, 6 years later in 2020, WOMANTRA has successfully designed a number of campaigns, workshops, and public interventions that address the gendered, social, and health vulnerabilities of women, girls, and sexual minorities, including gender-based and sexual discrimination and violence. More specifically, our current partnerships with local authorities for the design of gender-based violence protocols for first-response agencies has given us a promising pathway to improve service delivery to victims by health care professionals and the police.

According to integrative medicine practitioner, Dr. Rachel Naomi Remen,[1] the creative and healing process arise from a single source. She describes art and healing as a wordless trust of the same mystery, which acts as the foundation of our work and its integrity. As a leader within the new generation of Caribbean feminists, WOMANTRA's commitment to building youth- and queer-led feminist leadership has always had art at its center as a way to translate complex ideas, mobilize communities, and ultimately transform culture.

17.3   Silent Silhouettes

17.3.1   Putting Knowledge into Action

One of the greatest achievements of the feminist and women's movements globally is the successful reframing of domestic violence as a public health issue. Once viewed as a private, family issue—and in the Trinbagonian vernacular as "man and woman business"—domestic and intimate partner violence is now rightfully recognized internationally as a public health priority, in urgent need of attention, action, and resources from the international community (Chibber and Krishnan 2011; Krantz 2005). Another important piece in the evolution of our understanding about how violence against women functions is its pervasiveness and global applicability, constituting a wider system of violence with key indicators and outcomes known as gender-based violence. Yet, even with this reckoning, gender-based violence remains a global epidemic (Sprechmann 2014; WHO 2013), with regional violence rates in many countries surpassing the global average (Le Franc et al. 2008).

A regional study on interpersonal violence revealed that more than 50% of Trinbagonian women and girls aged 15–30 reported experiencing physical violence (53%), being sexually coerced (54%), or exposed to other types of violence (65%) as initiated by strangers, acquaintances, or in intimate partner relationships (Le Franc et al. 2008). These alarming statistics illuminate the stark level of gender inequalities that expose women to the most pernicious effects of the violent attitudes that form part of a continuum of traditional, culturally sanctioned, and harmful gender-based practices. In the 2006 Multiple Indicator Cluster Survey, 7% of

---

[1] http://journeyofhearts.org/kirstimd/create_grief.htm

women aged 15–49 believed that "wife-beating" was justifiable in at least one of five instances identified, the most common being "when she neglects the children." This research, which focused primarily on attitudes toward violence, established a co-relation between women's educational achievement, social status, and wealth to their ability to reject harmful ideas about spousal abuse (Pemberton and Joseph 2018).

It can be extrapolated from the above findings that there are complex intersections of physical and psychological implications for gender-based violence and that a multifaceted approach is needed to develop a robust national response. Any such strategic response should include gender-aware approaches that challenge traditional gender roles and unpack harmful stereotypes; are sensitive to socio-economic conditions and perceived class, as well as gender-based violence's differential impact on various populations; and garner the psycho-social support needed for survivors still living in violent situations. Further, while the state may sponsor a domestic violence hotline or provide the infrastructure to house battered women, collaborations must also be cultivated with the advocates who do the lion's share of the heavy lifting to increase sensitivity around victim support; provide nuanced situation analyses; use human rights mechanisms to inform policy making and reform; and provide services and education that are not accessible by the average citizen and are even less so by those with marginalized identities, including people living with HIV, people living with disabilities, and LGBT+ people.

In the developing world, the shared experience of insufficient funding and state support for civil society actors poses significant challenges to those who typically work on-the-ground to provide critical services for victim support but are themselves in need of institutional, capacity, and financial strengthening (Delisle et al. 2005). These constraints are exacerbated by a lack of human resources, since many organizations cannot afford full-time staff or to pay for the expertise of external consultants when needed. Added to this is the strain that workers experience when engaging in psychologically and emotionally demanding work, often leading to burnout that remains unaddressed due to insufficient or nonexistent de-briefing mechanisms (Chen and Gorski 2015; Craiovan 2015) and which ultimately compromises their capacity to continue serving others without causing harm to themselves. This environment effectively reduces non-profit actors' ability to provide sustained care for survivors, in spite of the expertise and sophisticated solutions they often bring to the table. Despite these truths, the incremental changes that are achieved through the commitment of dedicated individuals to fill the gaps of state-led interventions contribute to a cumulative impact that is essential to changing the lives of those most affected by gender-based violence.

Developing countries—particularly Small Island Developing States (SIDS) like Trinidad and Tobago—either do not have the capacity to or infrequently collect the specific data required by international agencies for generating analyses on the health profile of the region (Caribbean Development Bank 2016; Nicholls 2015). Data on SIDS is even further compromised by the geographic classification of the region, which includes Central and South American countries, irrespective of their distinct demographic differences from the Caribbean subregion. This lack of available data has a significant impact on the (sub)region's capacity to implement evidence-driven decision making at the state level, particularly in specialized areas that rely on indicators that are standardized at the global level. Instead, local researchers, including civil society actors, rely on key insights derived from myriad secondary data sets that offer an overall view of the situation, requiring sustained efforts and innovative data collection techniques. These sources can include hospital records, police and judicial reports and statistics, or newspaper articles. In other circumstances, recognizing the value of anecdotal data can be a sufficient motivator for engaging change work. The fact that the average woman has either experienced, witnessed, or knows someone who is a survivor of gender-based violence gives weight to the grounded epistemology of *who feels it knows it*.

For WOMANTRA, the challenge was to create a campaign that bridged the fictive gap between evidence and ethos, with the specific aim of raising awareness around gender-based violence in a way that was compassionate and moving. With the majority of interventions focused on survivors, the "Silent Silhouettes" campaign commemorates an obvious but often overlooked group of women—those who have been made to pay the ultimate price of their lives to gender-based violence. As a practical component of the installation, being able to accurately reflect the number of femicides annually is a key feature of the campaign's credibility and impact. But on a more personal level, the WOMANTRA team's capacity to intimately engage with the brutal violence meted out to these women and to create something meaningful in the midst of such tragedy is at the core of the campaign's ability to honor their memory.

In the early stages of developing the campaign, we asked ourselves a series of questions, which ultimately guided our continued commitment to the intervention: *How do we remember the women who are gone? What actions can we take that respect the wishes and needs of families who are left to grieve? What can we do for all of the women confronted with these stories every day in the newspaper and in our communities?* Through brainstorming and exploring these questions, Silent Silhouettes became the most resonant answer as it offered a cathartic space to learn, heal, and remember together in the symbolic presence of the women and girls lost.

17.3.2 Project Description

Silent Silhouettes is closely patterned after the U.S.-based Silent Witness (n.d.) campaign, initiated by a coalition of artists, writers, and women's rights organizers in Minnesota following the murder of 27 women. This original installation was intended to commemorate the women whose lives ended violently at the hands of a husband, ex-husband, partner, or family member and to promote an end to domestic violence through community-based exhibits and performance in 50 states across the United States and 23 countries globally.

Much like the Silent Witness, the Silent Silhouette is a free-standing, life-sized wooden figure, each with a fastened breastplate bearing some details of the woman or girl whose memory it honors. As part of the project's original design, the silhouettes are each painted black and cut to a size that generally reflects the victims' ages, using a generic female form for the categories of girl child, adolescent, and adult female (see Fig. 17.1). Typically displayed in a well-trafficked or public area, the silhouettes represent the undeniable loss of life, which is both unsettling and relatable, stimulating onlookers to stop, read, and share personal stories about domestic abuse and to remember the victims.

In preparation for the installation, team members are briefed on what to expect, since the audience (particularly women who enter the space) are likely to ask questions not only about the women and girls represented in the installation but also about resources for victims—inquiries that are often framed for the benefit of a friend or someone else they know. Other women more openly share their experiences with violence and require the attention of capable persons who can listen compassionately and without judgement. Within this context, all volunteer "voices" that accompany the installation assist with telling the victims' stories and with distributing relevant literature from partner organizations and service providers that offer viewers information about how to identify toxic patterns or unhealthy relationships and how to access various health services, including STI screening and counseling.

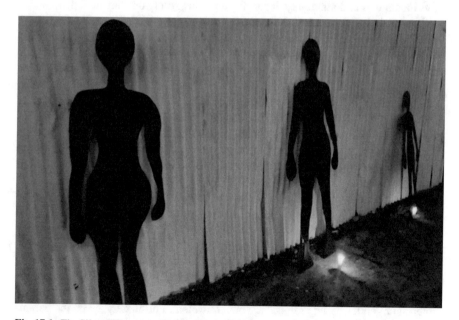

Fig. 17.1 The Silent Silhouettes displayed at the She Look Fah Dat: A #LifeinLeggings Discussion, hosted by WOMANTRA and I am One on Human Rights Day 2016

17.3.3   Approach

In the Trinidad landscape, Silent Silhouettes has become a feature of the local "16 days of activism" activities. To ensure that the installation accurately reflects the incidents of femicide, WOMANTRA collaborates with the Crime and Problem Analysis (CAPA) branch of the Trinidad and Tobago Police Service, which is responsible for the dissemination of official statistics on crime. Traditionally, the installation is first featured on November 25, which is the International Day for the Elimination of Violence Against Women as well as the first day of the "16 days of activism." Given the specificity of this campaign, data is requested outside the generic calendar year for all femicide-related murder from November 25 of the previous to the current year. This creates a tricky timeframe between the issuing of a formal request for statistics, the receipt of those statistics, and the accurate reflection of those statistics in the installation. Through trial and error, WOMANTRA worked out that if the request is received by CAPA in the first week of November, it takes approximately 2–3 weeks to receive a response, leaving only be a few days (give or take) in which the team has to monitor the media closely, in the event of any additional murders of women or girls that need to be recorded and included in the installation.

In previous years, police statistics were further cross-referenced with media reports of domestic-violence-related murders. The intention behind engaging with news media was to deliberately depart from relying solely on statistical data, which can bear little impact against the powerful effect of national desensitization. With the constant flood of loss and death covered in stories of murders, kidnappings, and disappearances, citizens are no longer moved by *just* numbers. Also, considering the massive death toll—generally staying above 400 murders per annum (Crime Statistics 2019; Trinidad and Tobago Police Service 2019)—the seemingly "meager" number of 20-something femicides is often met with indifference. By focusing on capturing the humanness of the victims, as opposed to bluntly stating the cause-of-death descriptions provided by the police (like stabbed, shot, or beaten), we were able to construct a humanizing narrative of each woman and girl, including where she lived, whether children and a grieving family were left behind, and her relationship to her killer.

Another benefit of this approach was that it served as a verification process for official data, given the state of police underreporting. According to Trinidad and Tobago's recently completed National Prevalence Study on domestic violence (Pemberton and Joseph 2018), a shockingly low 5% of women affected by intimate partner violence disclose these incidents to the police. Within this context, the media may serve as a more reliable source of data for domestic-violence reporting than the police. This may be especially true for instances in which definitions of domestic violence or gender-based violence are not equivalent. Fortunately, given the parameters of this project, data sets provided by the police when compared with media reporting were closely aligned on each occasion. There are, at times, other related incidents that the media is able to cover that are not reflected in the police data, which can impact the project's goal of painting a full picture of the problem of gender-based violence and its impact on the local population.

Our dual methodology, for example, allows us to include Trinidadian women who live in foreign countries, as well as members of our growing migrant population. In November 2018, for example, our installation included femicide victim Jenny Koonoolai-Jagdeo, a Trinidadian woman whose murder made headline news after she was tragically killed by her Trinidad-born ex-boyfriend in Florida. In the same month, another woman of Trinidadian parentage, Erica Renaud, was killed by her Trinidadian partner in their Brooklyn home. The fact that these murders happened outside the jurisdiction of our local borders didn't make their stories any less worthy of our observance, and so they too were memorialized.

17.3.4   Process

The simple design of Silent Silhouettes required only a few materials, including plywood, nails, and paint, as well as the human labor needed for construction. Given WOMANTRA's non-profit status, the small team of volunteers that produce the installation each year find creative ways to raise the capital needed through donations or in-kind contributions. Throughout the project's lifespan, WOMANTRA has received support from various donors, including the University of the West Indies' Student Guild, UNIFEM, and the United Nations Population Fund. In the years when funding was not available, the more traditional tactics of penning sponsorship letters to community hardware stores and requesting free shuttle services for the silhouettes by transport companies located in and around event locations proved to be an effective alternative. Despite the added elbow grease needed for this door-to-door approach, the value of the contributions made by community-based suppliers should not be underestimated. Not only is it an effective way to avoid accruing large capital costs, but it also results in developing meaningful relationships with community members, who can take ownership of the project and become invested in its outcome through an organic engagement.

The second phase—construction of the silhouettes—required equal amounts of physical and emotional labor. The process of creating a life-sized template for the silhouette design invariably meant needing to draw the outline of a human figure onto tracing paper, much like the chalk outline drawn around murder victims. This exercise, which in many ways mimicked a re-enactment of what police officers might do upon finding a murder victim's body, compelled those who participated in this activity to confront the deaths of these women and girls in a visceral way. Art has always been a powerful excavation tool for the artist, used to process one's own experiences and attempt to make sense of them. Similarly, for a project like Silent Silhouettes, even though volunteers may not approach the work consciously looking to or expecting to be moved emotionally, the process often raises complex feelings for participants and brings them to the surface. In a country where gender-based violence has touched almost the entire population, the repetition of drawing, sawing, and painting each silhouette the dark color of mourning becomes its own ritual in memory that is connected to a *herstory* that goes way beyond the activity itself.

Over the years the organization has pursued strategic partnerships, seeking to secure the sustainability of the project beyond financial contributions. In 2016, in one of our most recent collaborations, WOMANTRA partnered with the United Nations Population Fund to produce the Silent Silhouettes campaign. As the official coordinator of the agency's "Youth Advisory Group," consisting of young leaders from various groups around the country, we were able to facilitate their direct participation in all aspects of project development, including the design and promotion of a social media campaign as well as the construction of the silhouettes. One of our volunteers, from the Caribbean Youth Environment Network (CYEN-TT), shared a reflection on her experience:

> The task was physically straining. Sawing and lifting heavy pieces of wood, and having my body slowly outlined with chalk, led me to reflect deeply on these Silent Silhouettes. The silence was deafening and emotionally jolting. Constructing these representations of lost lives transcended the physical experience and created a space to contemplate. It felt as though I could feel the pain of my sisters, young and old. I questioned worth and value and love, and what these women and girls must have gone through. Recreating these stories in this way undoubtedly led to a newer and more gravely empathetic outlook on domestic violence.

In the 2020 installation of Silent Silhouettes, we hope to partner with the Volunteer Center of Trinidad and Tobago, or other youth-centered groups, to continue facilitating and encouraging young people's participation in the campaign, which we consider to be a crucial aspect of the change work in which the idea and production of this installation is grounded (Fig. 17.2).

17.3.5   Impact

Similar to the Silent Witness campaign, Silent Silhouettes has incorporated performance art as part of its strategy to enhance the overall impact of the intervention, particularly on the audience's capacity to connect with the issue on a deeper level. Before WOMANTRA was given its name by artist Michelle Isava, we collaborated to produce the first Silent Silhouettes installation in 2008. In her performance entitled "The Intercession," Isava presents a dramatic body count of 18 murder victims, delivering dead flowers to each one of them as a symbol of the broken promises made by their loved ones. This performance was filmed in two locations and later made into a short film, which to our credit was selected the following year to be featured at the Trinidad & Tobago Film Festival. What began as an experimental project between friends more than a decade ago is now WOMANTRA's flagship campaign, born out of a need to unpack the shared experience of being a woman, which is far too often marred by violence.

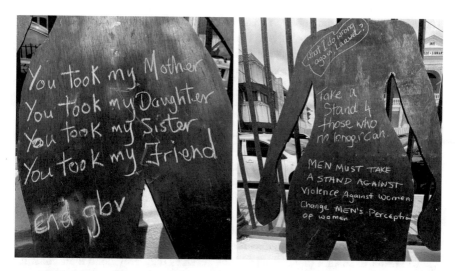

Fig. 17.2 Silhouettes with chalk messages from participants in the solidarity action, 'Orange Day: Remembrance for Victims of Gender-based Violence' in January 2020 (Port of Spain, Trinidad)

Since then, the Silent Silhouettes have been displayed in various contexts across the country, among the most notable being the Commonwealth People's Forum in 2009 and #SheLookFuhDat: A Life in Leggings Discussion in 2016—stretching over almost a decade of the campaign's evolution and history. Local women's rights and state-led organizations have also requested the inclusion of the installation at their own "16 days of activism" events, including at the annual gender-based violence fair led by the Gender and Child Affairs Division of the Office of the Prime Minister and the Equal Opportunity Commission. And so, while the mobility and reach of the installation has not significantly increased over the years, the Silent Silhouettes' presence has been recognized at critical junctures in the movement to end gender-based violence.

Viewers' reactions, however, remain the most powerful impact of the campaign. The imagery conjured by these shadowy figures, standing in formation like a small army, paradoxically lend strength and legitimacy to their shared experience. Despite the decision not to include the names of victims out of respect for their families, it's always striking that passersby, particularly women, were able to recall details of the victims that were not included in the installation. In some instances, their information came from media reports, while for others their own relationship to the victim allowed them to fill in the gaps of their story. It became clear that the majority of women who viewed the installation were in tune with these deaths in a way that validated the space we were creating through Silent Silhouettes—a space for women to talk about their own experiences and those of other women, and to collectively debrief about the state of violence against women, for which we shared a deep concern. One experience that stood out to us over the years was watching a young man who said a silent prayer for the victims, touching each silhouette on its forehead.

These types of engagements demonstrated that a wide audience of women, men, survivors, relatives, and others who came into contact with the installation had a unique opportunity to connect with the presence of the women and girls who are gone and to express what that loss meant for them.

17.3.6 Challenges

Despite the relatively low expenditures needed for the Silent Silhouettes project, producing the installation requires a significant effort, typically executed by a small team of volunteers. The coordination of this effort has not always been possible, given WOMANTRA's constraints as a small non-profit with no paid or full-time staff. Not unlike many of the organizations functioning within the civil society landscape, NGOs often juggle the management of multiple projects in tandem with paid work in order to sustain themselves and the services they provide to their constituencies. But given that necessity is the mother of invention, WOMANTRA was able to continue producing Silent Silhouettes in a way that was sustainable through the introduction of a poster campaign (see Fig. 17.3) that is shared on WOMANTRA's digital platforms. The execution of this alternative design requires much of the same groundwork, including research, collection of statistics, and preparation of select narratives, which are presented as a virtual compilation of stylized posters and

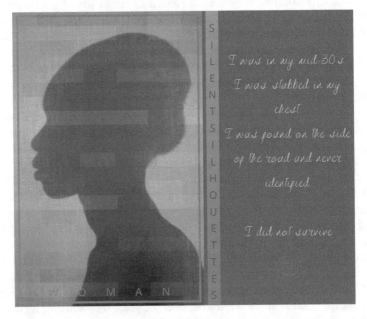

Fig. 17.3 Silent Silhouette poster campaign featured during the 16 days of activism on WOMANTRA's social media platforms

infographics. While it is difficult to measure the impact of these two variations against each other given the very different audiences and modes of engagement with the work, the continuity of the project in its attempt to honor the victims of femicide remains the organization's priority.

Another unique challenge was finding ways to maintain our commitment to keeping the focus on women and girl victims of gender-based violence while responding to men's concerns about inclusion. The reality that women and girls are disproportionately affected by gender-based violence—and more specifically are the overwhelming majority of domestic-violence-related murder victims—didn't seem to be the precipitating impetus for feedback by the majority of male viewers of the installation. As the 2018 National Women's Health Survey confirms, one in three women are affected by intimate partner violence, which is consistent with the global average. Between 2006 to 2011, male victims accounted for only 32.8% of homicides by an intimate partner or family member (Hosein 2018). Despite these statistics, each time the installation has been shown, men have inquired about their absence in the space, asking why there are no male deaths reflected in the installation. The fundamental issue created by this articulation is that it divests attention away from the women and girls being honored in that moment and whose lives were almost exclusively taken by men. It also illuminates a "bigger picture" question about why, in this space, men are inclined to focus on their own representation. We were again faced with a series of questions, including: *How can safe spaces for men be created such that these dialogues can take place? And on whom does this responsibility fall?* Finding ways to compassionately respond to these questions while remaining committed to the purpose of the work is complicated and nuanced. As a feminist organization, we triumph when we are able to continue engaging in advocacy around the rights and vulnerabilities of marginalized genders and against pushback that attempts to decenter or delegitimatize those experiences.

17.4   Conclusion

The approach to managing public health has been evolving all over the world. The divergence away from focusing only on the aspects of public health that are addressed through the health sector, to incorporate intersectional health concerns, has required increased stakeholder engagement outside the traditional frameworks, including a recognition of the role of arts advocacy. With this shift, organizations that engage in health advocacy or provide services for key populations can highlight risk factors and other implications not typically addressed within the health care system. As stated in Chap. 21 of this volume, the impact of health promotion initiatives often produce a mixture of results, both wanted and unwanted, and so understanding the particular context and audience is critical to any results-based intervention. For WOMANTRA, this has meant raising awareness about the fatal effects of gender-based violence and the specific vulnerabilities of women and girls. By featuring the Silent Silhouettes in public spaces, viewers are able to viscerally connect with victims and bear witness to the ultimate consequence of gender-based violence, which strikes a chord with so many onlookers, as it is filtered through the backdrop of shared experience.

When it comes to gender-based violence, a lot of emphasis is put on breaking the silence, but significantly less considered are the interconnected social and structural systems that keep women silent—some of which have been explored in this chapter. The Silent Silhouettes, though a small contribution, provide a solemn reminder to us all of the work still required to bring justice to these women and girls and the urgent need to end gender-based violence. May their memory live on.

References

Bailey, B. (2010). Partner violence during pregnancy: Prevalence, effects, screening, and management. *International Journal of Women's Health, 2,* 183. https://doi.org/10.2147/ijwh.s8632.

Boyle, A., Jones, P., & Lloyd, S. (2006). The association between domestic violence and self harm in emergency medicine patients. *Emergency Medicine Journal, 23,* 604–607. https://doi.org/10.1136/emj.2005.031260.

Caribbean Development Bank (CDB). (2016). Lack of comprehensive data on gender-based violence in the region. In *Lack of comprehensive data on gender-based violence in the region.* Caribbean Development Bank. https://www.caribank.org/newsroom/news-and-events/lack-comprehensive-data-gender-based-violence-region

Chen, C. W., & Gorski, P. C. (2015). Burnout in social justice and human rights activists: Symptoms, causes and implications. *Journal of Human Rights Practice, 7,* 366–390. https://doi.org/10.1093/jhuman/huv011.

Chibber, K. S., & Krishnan, S. (2011). Confronting intimate partner violence: A global health priority. *Journal of Medicine: A Journal of Translational and Personalized Medicine, 78,* 449–457. https://doi.org/10.1002/msj.20259.

Craiovan, P. M. (2015). Burnout, depression and quality of life among the Romanian employees working in non-governmental organizations. *Procedia—Social and Behavioral Sciences, 187,* 234–238. https://doi.org/10.1016/j.sbspro.2015.03.044.

Crime Statistics. (2019). Retrieved from https://www.ttcrime.com/crime-statistics/

Delisle, H., Roberts, J. H., Munro, M., Jones, L., & Gyorkos, T. (2005). The role of NGOs in global health research for development. *Health Research Policy and Systems.* https://doi.org/10.1186/1478-4505-3-3.

Doughty, M. (2018, October 7). NCRHA opens diabetes wellness centre. Trinidad & Tobago Newsday. https://newsday.co.tt/2018/10/07/ncrha-opens-diabetes-wellness-centre/

Hess, K. L., Javanbakht, M., Brown, J. M., Weiss, R. E., Hsu, P., & Gorbach, P. M. (2012). Intimate partner violence and sexually transmitted infections among young adult women. *Sexually Transmitted Diseases, 39,* 366–371.

Hosein, G. J. (2018). Gender based violence in Trinidad & Tobago: A qualitative study. UN WOMEN.

Institute for Health Metrics and Evaluation. (2017, September 20). http://www.healthdata.org/trinidad-and-tobago. Accessed 17 May 2019.

International Planned Parenthood Federation. (2016). Everyone's right to know: Delivering comprehensive sexuality education for all young people. https://www.ippf.org/sites/default/files/2016-05/ippf_cse_report_eng_web.pdf accessed 2 June 2020

Krantz, G. (2005). Violence against women. *Journal of Epidemiology & Community Health, 59,* 818–821. https://doi.org/10.1136/jech.2004.022756.

Le Franc, E., Samms-Vaughan, M., Hambleton, I., & Fox, K. (2008). Interpersonal violence in three Caribbean countries: Barbados, Jamaica, and Trinidad and Tobago. *Revista Panamericana de Salud Pública.* https://doi.org/10.1590/s1020-49892008001200005.

Nicholls, A. (2015) Securing better statistical data for better Caribbean lives: Reflecting on the data problem in the Caribbean. *Caribbean Trade Law and Development.* https://caribbeantradelaw.com/2015/10/17/securing-better-data-for-better-caribbean-lives/

Ottawa Charter for Health Promotion. (1986). Health. *Promotion International, 1*(4), 405–405. https://doi.org/10.1093/heapro/1.4.405.

Paul, A. (2016, July 26). Minister on cutting healthcare costs: Healthy living is the answer. *Trinidad Guardian.* http://www.guardian.co.tt/article-6.2.356393.9a645f79ad

Pemberton, C., & Joseph, J. (2018). National women's health survey for Trinidad and Tobago: Dataset. https://doi.org/10.18235/0001013.

Silent Witness. (n.d.). About Silent Witness national initiative. Retrieved from http://www.silentwitness.net/about-us.html

Sprechmann, S. (2014). Gender-based violence: A global epidemic requiring committed and effective action. *Care Insights.* https://insights.careinternational.org.uk/development-blog/gender-based-violence-a-global-epidemic-requiring-committed-and-effective-action

Trinidad & Tobago Police Service. (2019). Comparison by year. Retrieved from http://ttps.gov.tt/Statistics/Comparison-By-Year

UNICEF. (2018). Trinidad and Tobago (TTO)—Demographics, health & infant mortality. UNICEF DATA. https://data.unicef.org/country/tto/?fbclid=IwAR1-RcKVXsVFHKpEWF1gWyzgB-Gpp4GtVJaHNka5z1VJx7OYxK_ExYWvgwUc. Accessed 25 June 2019.

World Health Organization (WHO). (2013). Violence against women: a 'global health problem of epidemic proportions.' Retrieved from https://www.who.int/mediacentre/news/releases/2013/violence_against_women_20130620/en/. Accessed 25 May 2019.

Chapter 18
Movimiento Ventana: An Alternative Proposal to Mental Health in Nicaragua

Andrea Deleo, Roberta Romero, and Enmanuelle A. Zelaya

18.1 Introduction

Mental health is recognized as a fundamental part of health and is considered a basic global priority for the overall well-being of individuals, societies, and countries (WHO 2013), and is identified as one of the targets in the UN Sustainable Development Goals (SDGs) from 2015 to 2030. Despite this, resources and funding for this area of health represent a budget of less than 1% in most countries, including Nicaragua. In addition, Nicaragua does not have policy or legislation on the subject (PAHO 2013), and most of the services are centralized in the Psychosocial Care Teaching Hospital "José Dolores Fletes Valles." These factors leave an overwhelming treatment gap and help maintain an asylum model of treatment that contradicts the worldwide resolutions to develop programs for community-based care (PAHO 2013).

Nicaragua is one of the poorest countries in the Western Hemisphere and its population is prone to developing psychosocial problems due to multiple traumatic events that have occurred in its history (wars and armed revolutions, corruption, poverty, natural disasters, etc.). This results in a psychologically vulnerable population and is combined with risk factors such as substance abuse, commercial and/or sexual exploitation, high rates of violence, high rates of femicide, teenage pregnancy, illiteracy, and severe mental disorders.

At the moment, Nicaragua is immersed in a socio-political and human rights crisis that began in April 2018 with a series of social protests that were violently repressed by the authorities and pro-government armed groups. The evidence shows that the overall response of the government to these protests failed to meet

Translation by Audrey Sharp

A. Deleo (✉) · R. Romero · E. A. Zelaya
Movimiento Ventana, Managua, Nicaragua
e-mail: movimiento.ventana@gmail.com

© The Author(s) 2021
J. H. Corbin et al. (eds.), *Arts and Health Promotion*,
https://doi.org/10.1007/978-3-030-56417-9_18

applicable standards of the management of assemblies, in violation of international human rights law. Other human rights violations documented include disproportionate use of force by the police that sometimes resulted in extrajudicial killings; enforced disappearances; obstructions to access to medical care; widespread arbitrary or illegal detentions; prevalent ill-treatment and instances of torture and sexual violence in detention centers; and violations of freedom of peaceful assembly and expression, including the criminalization of social leaders, human rights defenders, journalists, and protesters considered critical of the government (United Nations Human Rights 2018).

This crisis has implied a setback in terms of democracy, destabilizing the territory and leaving by the end of 2018 more than 300 deaths, 2000 persons injured, and approximately 740 political prisoners (Amnesty International 2018; United Nations Human Rights 2019). The situation has affected all social spheres, forcing thousands to migrate or live in exile, polarizing Nicaraguan society, and extending poverty levels (FUNIDES 2018). This has forced us to suspend activities at Movimiento Ventana due to levels of insecurity in the country and repression of any form of organization outside the government. When the crisis comes to an end, we will have the challenge as a country to re-establish democracy and respect for human rights, and also the opportunity to heal the psychosocial traumas we have carried through our history and build a healthier society. As a social movement, we hope to be part of these processes to heal old and new traumas.

18.2 Movimiento Ventana and its Beginnings

Movimiento Ventana traces its beginnings back to 2011, when four students in their last year of high school were developing a monographic project relating to schizophrenia in the Psychosocial Hospital in Managua, Nicaragua. Entering the hospital meant being confronted by a reality hidden behind the walls of the institution; it inevitably gave a very disconcerting first impression to experience firsthand the facility's scarcities, enclosed rooms, limited access to basic health resources, and the use of drugs as the primary means to inhibit undesirable behavior. This striking reality motivated the students to organize a way to improve the conditions in which people with mental disorders were living. This gave way to the first activity in the Psychosocial Hospital at the end of November 2011, where users, students, and a few volunteers used art-based elements to create a common space.

Then, in 2012, the students began to organize structured visits that facilitated Art Therapy techniques as a means to guide interactions in the activities. Since then, the visits have taken place every fifteen days, or two Saturdays a month. Over time, other techniques such as laughter therapy and psychodrama have been used, and beginning in 2016, we started to implement Biodanza as an additional work modality.

18.2.1 Why Movimiento Ventana?

The name Movimiento Ventana (see Fig. 18.1 for the its logo) is in honor of Alfonso Cortés (1893–1969). Cortés, a famous Nicaraguan poet that belonged to the post-modernist movement, is considered to be one of *the three greats*, after Rubén Darío. Cortés wrote *Ventana (Window)* and other literary works in a psychotic state, and although he was recognized for his art, he spent many years of his life locked away in a room in his home and later on in the same psychiatric hospital that we visit today. Because of his mental disorder, Cortés was a victim to the same stigma of society that persists today. The poetic and symbolic background of this poet and his work made him the perfect frame for what we wanted to accomplish with this movement: to open a window for the people living in this hospital.

Movimiento Ventana's activities have improved over the years, learning empirically through the practice of merging the activities with a complementary theoretical knowledge. It is in that way that we've moved from an assistive perspective (based merely on the intention to help) to a perspective geared toward recovering and restitution of rights.

From its beginning until now, the movement has functioned in a completely self-run manner—that is to say, without relying on any permanent financial support from an organization or institution. Its survival has been based on the symbolic contribution of volunteers and donors coming from within our own networks. Today, Movimiento Ventana relies on a core team of volunteers that manage each visit to the hospital. The team is made up of twelve people with diverse degrees and is divided into five work groups—finances, communication, volunteer work, training, and human development—with each group responsible for different tasks. The volunteers dedicate their time, knowledge, and abilities to the creation and

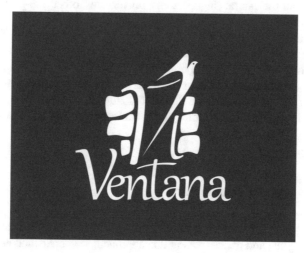

Fig. 18.1 Movimiento Ventana logo

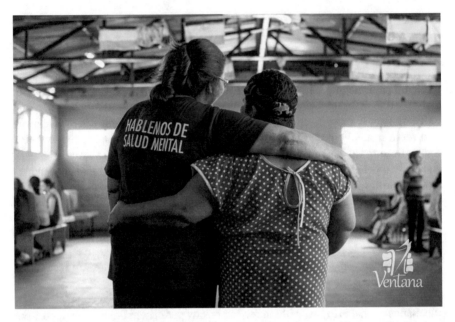

Fig. 18.7 "Let's talk about mental health" Movimiento Ventana motto. (Photo credit: Cristiana Castellón)

development of Movimiento Ventana. In this way, we stand out not just as an organized movement, but as a movement built in a collective.

Currently, Movimiento Ventana is defined as a social movement that works to promote mental health and reduce stigma against people living with mental disorders. This is achieved through formative mental health spaces placed in various spots throughout the capital (high schools, universities, other non-profits, etc.) and through social volunteering at the Psychosocial Hospital where alternative therapeutic activities (Biodanza and Art Therapy) are implemented with users. Volunteering is kept open for the various activities in an effort to address the topic of mental health with the general public without any fear or stigma, so that we can begin to talk about mental health as a part of the human experience and recognize that it is a part of ourselves that we should look after as much as we do our physical health. This is why our main motto at Movimiento Ventana is: "Let's talk about mental health" (Fig. 18.7.).

18.3   Conceptual Framework

Movimiento Ventana's work is developed around a focus on mental health promotion, human rights, and gender. Using this approach, we understand people as bio-psycho-social beings and recognize that mental health is a question of welfare that goes well beyond the absence of illnesses (WHO 2013). As well, we revisit how health and illness are intimately related with the intersectionality between social constructs such as sex, gender, race, ethnicity, age, religion, and economic status (Bauer 2014). Furthermore, we recognize that within this work, there is a convergence of certain power dynamics and varying social and scientific understandings of what it means to be crazy (Foucault 1990; Goffman 1970). This marked stigma that exists in the population—and within the very same mental health professionals— helps to form a pertinent barrier to addressing the social integration of people living with mental illnesses (Arnaiz and Uriarte 2006). Thus, we are looking for new ways to tackle mental disorders, moving away from the closed-minded, institutional model built around illness and instead moving toward a community-comprehensive, open-minded, and complex model built around fortitude, capacity, and rights recovery (Rodríguez et al. 2009).

For this approach, we use the *personal recovery model* as a theoretical-conceptual basis, a relatively new term based on the subjective processes of self-improvement in spite of an illness (Rebolleda and Florit 2010). The World Health Organization set forth this concept of personal recovery, understood from the perspective of a person living with mental illness, in their Mental Health Plan 2013–2020:

> Gaining and retaining hope, understanding of one's abilities and disabilities, engagement in an active life, personal autonomy, social identity, meaning and purpose in life and a positive sense of self. Recovery is not synonymous with cure. Recovery refers to both internal conditions experienced by persons who describe themselves as being in recovery—hope, healing, empowerment and connection—and external conditions that facilitate recovery—implementation of human rights, a positive culture of healing, and recovery-oriented services (WHO 2013, p. 43).

According to this model, the term "public health services user" replaces the term "patients" (Rebolleda and Florit 2010), with the understanding that the use of the word "patient" denotes a position of passive, dependent, and stigmatizing inequality. Instead, the word "user" refers to an individual in search of professional support, with strengths and weaknesses, with rights, and with a capacity to form an opinion on their own active journey toward recovery.

Lastly, we are reclaiming alternative models of mental health that leverage art and expression as a means to strengthen well-being and as a therapeutic tool to work and develop areas where traditional therapies are limiting. As mentioned in Chap. 1 in this volume, art can be a tool to address complex health promotion issues, and also act as a bridge connecting people to one another in their humanity.

The British Association of Art Therapists (1969) defines Art Therapy as a form of psychotherapy that uses art media as its primary mode of expression and communication. In the same sense, Menéndez and Olmo (2010) define Art Therapy as a psychotherapeutic modality that utilizes artistic language and the creative process to express personal contexts and life experiences, create meaning, and work on psychological conflicts. Research on the use of Art Therapy with people living with mental disorders highlights the benefits achieved from this technique. Vallejo (2011), Menéndez and Olmo (2010), and Ceballo et al. (2012) found, at a psychological level, improved levels of self-esteem, self-affirmation, and self-awareness;

recognition and expression of emotions; and a reduction in psychiatric symptoms with an improved orientation toward reality. At a group level, they found positive therapeutic results in the development of social interaction, social abilities, altruistic behavior, and companionship.

On the other hand, the epistemological origin and practice of Biodanza (which literally means "dance of life") dates back to 1965; its founder, Rolando Toro, developed and incorporated this technique in a psychiatric hospital in Chile, using dance as a form of therapy to help "humanize psychiatry" (Toro and Terrén 2011). From that point on, he discovered the influence that music, body movement, and exercise has on people, and his techniques have continued to spread across the globe. After nearly half a century since its creation, Biodanza is defined as an affective system of integration, organic renovation, and relearning of the original functions of life (Toro and Terrén 2011). Based on experiences prompted by dance, music, singing, and group settings, it has constituted itself as a complementary approach with its own paradigm.

In Biodanza, there exists five areas of growth, called "lines of experience," which summarize the five universal functions common to everybody: vitality, sexuality, creativity, affectivity, and transcendence. The results found in Biodanza-related research reflect that people, after participating in Biodanza sessions, showed signs of being more motivated, relaxed, and supported while demonstrating a better grasp of their feelings, an improved expression of basic emotions, a lowering of their defenses, reinforcement of positive emotions, increased creativity and spontaneity, better posture, higher rates of visual contact, and development in their social abilities (Castro and Rossi 1996; Granada and Sáez 2005).

Art Therapy and Biodanza, due to its methodological essence, provides elements necessary to creating a safe, therapeutic environment and an equal, homogenous understanding. These elements foster the user's empowerment, and its application at a group level provides for more dynamic methods and a development in diverse areas such as affectivity, self-esteem, self-understanding, expression, creativity, psychomotricity, social abilities, verbal communication abilities, and behavioral control.

18.4 A Look into Movimiento Ventana's Activities

The social volunteer activities within the Psychosocial Hospital are Movimiento Ventana's primary mission, as they allow us to influence both the users and the general population that attends. It is because of this that a major part of our efforts revolves around these activities, and the ways in which we develop such activities have adapted and improved over time.

18.4.1 Activity Coordination

To start, the core team meets to plan the activities and design the central therapy that will take place at each visit, be it Art Therapy, Biodanza, or an alternative recreational activity that might coincide with a special celebration (including the Day of Love and Friendship, Mother's Day, International Mental Health Day, etc.). Weeks before each visit, all of the logistical details are prepared in order to implement the activities, such as putting out a call-to-action on social media, coordinating transportation, and compiling recreational materials and snacks. For this, Movimiento Ventana works with a methodology called support networks, where a few organizations and individuals provide materials for the activities either on a permanent or sporadic basis. Our primary support network has been Saint Teresa's Academy (an institution that has helped us since the beginning), who provides for the transportation of volunteers for each visit. We also depend on the collaboration of a few young volunteers and entrepreneurs who provide food for each visit. One of the best examples of this method has been working with approximately 20 fruit vendors at the Israel Lewites Market. Each vendor donates as much fruit as they can and together create a big fruit salad to be shared at the activity. This provides a crucial nutritional supplement that the hospital users would typically go without, while at the same time creating a space to talk about the importance of mental health among the market workers.

The other main preparation point mentioned earlier is the call-to-action, which mostly happens through a Facebook event and by word-of-mouth, but also is spurred by visiting university classrooms or speaking to specific groups of people, such as psychology students.

18.4.2 Activity Execution

The visits take place for four to five hours throughout the morning. Each one begins with a gathering at a central point in the capital, where volunteers and the core team are picked up and brought to the Psychosocial Hospital via private transportation. The volunteers that participate are almost entirely young people who live in the capital and are predominantly between the ages of 18 and 25 years old; there is on occasion a more experienced professional that joins.

The activities typically begin by working with the volunteers to lower their defenses, reduce anxiety, and create a trusting environment. In this space, we also provide orientation, clear up any doubts, and communicate hospital rules (such as not taking any photos or videos), while also striving to foster a space of openness, trust, respect, and safety.

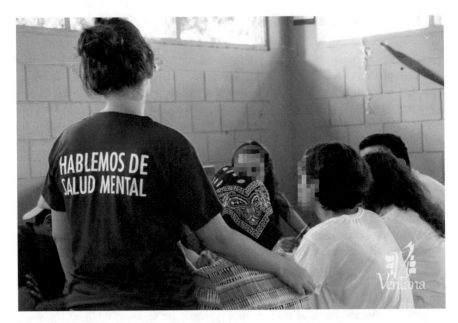

Fig. 18.2 Educational segment at the beginning of the activities. (Photo credit: Cristiana Castellón)

Next, an educational activity takes place where volunteers dialogue about a theme relating to mental health (Fig. 18.2). This educational segment is very important to the visit because it makes our volunteers more aware by sharing important information in a simple and practical way. Some of the questions tackled include: *What are the myths and realities surrounding mental disorders? What is stigma?* Other basic topics relating to personal experience with mental health are explored, such as: *What is self-esteem? What is resilience? What factors can affect your mental well-being?*

After preparing the volunteers, we continue on with the main activity for the day. The users start to arrive and we are met immediately with joy, especially from those who have attended an activity before. Then, depending on the day, the session of Art Therapy or Biodanza begins. There are typically around 30 users, with an equal mixture of men and woman, and the ideal scenario is that there is at least one volunteer for every two users; this provides for the best interaction and allows volunteers to support the users throughout the session. After the main activity finishes, the volunteers, users, and nursing staff share a snack together. It is an emotional closing space between the volunteers and the users. Afterward, the users say goodbye to the group and return to their pavilions.

The visit culminates in a segment of feedback and empathetic listening with the volunteers, led by the core team. This is the key moment for them to share about their experience, navigate certain lessons, and absorb what they've learned that day.

18.4.3   Art Therapy and Biodanza

As both Art Therapy and Biodanza are central elements of each visit, art and creativity are always at the center of each session; however, each element has its own distinctive features.

In the case of Art Therapy (Fig. 18.3), the sessions can last as long as an hour or an hour and a half and are not implemented from a specialized clinical psychotherapy approach, but rather are employed in a group format under a free and nondirective methodology. Although the process is completely therapeutic, it does not possess the rigorousness of a theoretical, methodological, and practical structure that more formal sessions within a psychotherapy process would have. The focus instead is geared toward stimulating creativity and integrability while at the same time promoting self-expression, a relationship with both the internal and the external, an emotional connection, and empowerment. To facilitate this, different artistic materials are provided, and the volunteers and users collaborate as a group to create projects. These activities leave a lot of space for verbal interaction and other spontaneous activities such as dancing and singing.

On the other hand, Biodanza (Fig. 18.4) relies on a specialized facilitator that guides the sessions to develop the five lines of experience suggested by the technique. The sessions last between 45 minutes and an hour, in which the facilitator reproduces previously selected music specifically for the line of experience being worked on that day, along with the related movements and exercises. On many occasions, the Biodanza sessions turn into accompaniment sessions, where the volunteers model the facilitator's instructions to the users, accompany them, and set the pace. This is due to the fact that the users often possess rigid psychomotricity and a

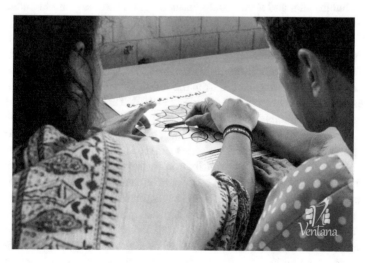

Fig. 18.3 Development of an Art Therapy activity in the Psychosocial Hospital. (Photo credit: América Solórzano)

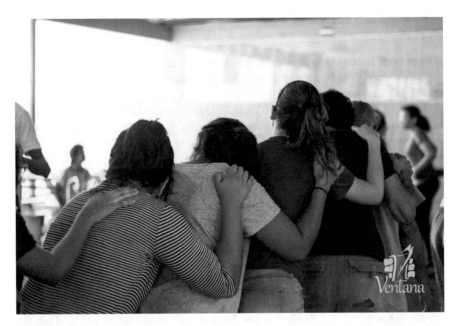

Fig. 18.4 Use of movement and body expression in Biodanza activity. (Photo credit: Gina Solórzano)

limited attention span, and this is why the volunteers' participation is fundamental to the success of the conciliatory experience.

Both techniques, by nature of their practice, create an opportunity to create connections, laugh, hug, and speak, and—in their applied forms—can facilitate established trust, human contact, and a mutual agreement. Additionally, the visits help to build a perception of people facing mental health challenges as individuals with qualities, strengths, and deficiencies like anyone else, where their mental disorder is more a variable than a condition.

Some of the results we gathered from the activities' work was found from exploratory research done by Deleo and Gutiérrez (2016). The authors identified the perceptions the participants have of Movimiento Ventana's activities through five in-depth interviews of hospital users, two focal groups within Movimiento Ventana's volunteers, and observations from a series of Art Therapy and Biodanza activities within the hospital. One major contribution to this research was centered on the perception of the users, reclaiming a point of view typically forgotten by science and rescuing the protagonist role of people with mental disorders during the recovery process. Among its biggest findings is the emphasis on how the activities are seen as a space for expressing oneself, getting to know oneself, sharing, enjoying, and using Art Therapy and Biodanza as a means to group interaction. For the users, these aspects were highlighted as principal within the activities, yet they provided little therapeutic attribution to the techniques. Conversely, for the volunteers, the activities were related to personal growth and in contrast to the users, they expressed consciousness of the therapeutic contribution of the activities.

Despite the users not directly recognizing the activities as therapy, within discourse, the authors found aspects that alluded to a state of improved well-being as a result of their participation in the activities. Among these, they found changes in their affective experience, an increase in their recognition of emotions, the development of skills for the adequate management of behaviors, greater control of their actions, and an increase in the initiative to participate in activities. They also found changes in social relations, considering that the volunteer work was postulated as a support network for users. Specifically, in each technique, they found that Art Therapy favors the development of verbal expression and an evolution in language, while Biodanza facilitates the significant improvement of body movements and greater fluidity, as well as an increase in contact capacity and reciprocity.

On the other hand, Tchaikovsky (2017) systemized Movimiento Ventana's experiences between 2011 and 2016. For this, she applied in-depth interviews from different actors: four hospital users, two members of the nursing staff, the general director of the Psychosocial Hospital, and the Biodanza specialist that facilitates sessions. She also applied a focal group with the core team of Movimiento Ventana. In her study, Tchaikovsky highlights Movimiento Ventana's evolution throughout the years, specifically noting its departure from an assistive approach and its move toward a comprehensive vision that promotes and enables the empowerment of users. The author emphasizes as a key factor the volunteers' perception of the users, which transformed over time from "patients" to "friends," allowing for affective reciprocity and engendering a greater commitment and motivation to the cause.

Finally, she finds that Movimiento Ventana's activities provide a solution to the negative symptoms of the illness, having a direct and positive influence on affective weakness, emotional distance, apathy, lack of initiative, and more. Many of these are symptoms that are resistant to pharmacological treatment and, with increasing intensity, can determine the longevity of the disorder.

18.5   The Volunteers' Experience

For the volunteers, the visits provide a unique space for awareness, learning, dialogue, and a reflection on mental health and the reality of what it's like to live with a mental disorder. By participating and interacting with the users (Fig. 18.5), the volunteers have the opportunity to confront and question these ideas, prejudices, and stigmas that society has taught them about mental illness.

Volunteers experience varied emotions on these visits; some volunteers connect with the users' energy, enthusiasm, and willingness to share, while others better understand the environment and social limitations being placed on the users. Others also ask themselves, "How is it possible that nobody is talking about this?" Or they simply feel guilty for having long thought that people with mental disorders were violent or crazy, for example.

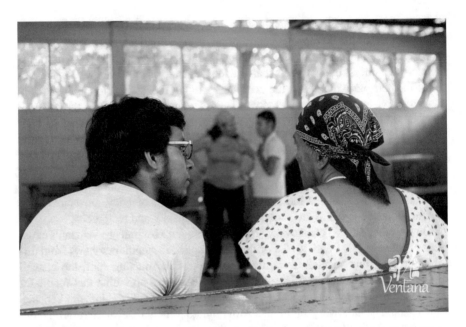

Fig. 18.5 Conversation between volunteer and user in an activity. (Photo credit: Cristiana Castellón)

The volunteers' experience with the users is crucial for diminishing negative assessments of them; it takes away the perception that users are dangerous or unpredictable, which the stereotype on mental illness often implies, and thus mitigates the insecurity and fear that might stand in the way of them meeting or getting to know someone living with a mental disorder (Arriba-Rossetto et al. 2008). In this way, as stated in Chap. 21 in this volume, arts-based activities allow to deepen connections with others by creating a shared experience of new knowledge or by increasing empathy for others' lived experiences.

Likewise, we look to create a natural and comfortable space, where the volunteers can identify with the personal experiences of others and feel safe sharing about their own mental health without feeling judged and can trust, count on the support of others and can realize the importance of mental health (Fig. 18.6).

18.6 Successes and Challenges

Among the successes achieved at Ventana is the completion of nearly 7 years of work and being one of the first groups to focus exclusively on the topic of mental health in Nicaragua. Through these years, we have been able to address the topic of mental health with more than 1000 volunteers and carry out approximately 112 hospital visits to the Psychosocial Hospital. We have developed a strategy to reduce

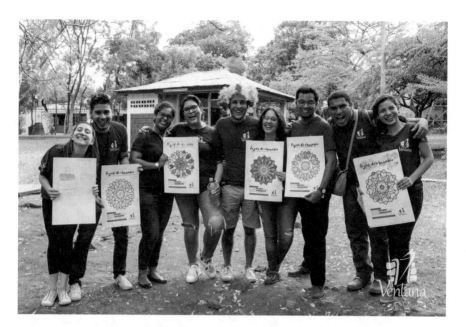

Fig. 18.6 Group photo at the end of an Art Therapy activity. (Photo credit: América Solórzano)

mental health stigma that combines first-hand experience with simple and practical information, components that have been identified as key to promoting social change (Arnaiz and Uriarte 2006). And we have successfully implemented art-based activities such as Art Therapy and Biodanza in a group and non-directive format that results in an effective and cost-efficient accompaniment to the recovery and promotion of mental health with users.

Among the challenges faced have been the lack of theoretical knowledge of mental health matters on part of some team members, not being legally registered as a social organization or NGO, and the scarce systemization and record-keeping of successful activities over the years. These facets limit measuring achievements, the development of new activities as an organized movement, and the possibility of obtaining long-term financing.

In addition, another challenge has been coexisting within a hospital that maintains a model of asylum-prison care and working with institutionalized users that have lost most of their community roles and connections, present severe motor and cognitive limitations, and are treated almost exclusively with high levels of psychiatric drugs. These have proven to be large barriers to Ventana's stated goals of recovery and promotion of mental health, while at the same time threaten users' human rights.

As staff and professionals, we also continue to battle our own stigmas and question our roles of power within this system. It is a constant challenge not to fall into discriminatory, exclusionary, relief, or caretaking practices when working with mental health users.

Another important point is that, as we mentioned at the beginning of the chapter, in April 2018 we have been forced to suspend all activities due to a high level of government repression. The fact that the Psychosocial Hospital is a public psychiatric institution that depends on government support and requests has meant that our volunteer work has been interrupted indefinitely. This has created an uncertain future for the movement and poses a great challenge, but also an opportunity to rethink new strategies for the mental health field in Nicaragua.

Our work over the years has taught us the importance of the systemization of work and ongoing training for the project team. Equally, it has highlighted the possibilities that the use of art can open up in creating new forms of treatment and community integration that are removed from the asylum model, as well as the need to continue to encourage the empowerment and participation of people living with mental disorders and health care practices that are in line with these principles. As is the claim of people living with mental health challenges around the globe, "Nothing about us without us!"

18.7   Conclusion

Around the world, there are a number of examples of social organizations working to improve mental health care, enhance living conditions, and reduce stigma toward people with mental disorders. Many of these, including Movimiento Ventana, use art in its diverse modalities (theater, music, dance, plastic arts, writing, radio production, etc.) both for its therapeutic benefits and for the opportunities it provides for social participation and group empowerment. Examples of such artistic approaches include the "Radio La Colifata," "Radio Vilardevoz," "Abracadabra Creatividad," and the "Frente de Artistas del Borda," (Mad in América Hispanohablante 2017) to name just a few. These experiences in the field of creativity and mental health show how collectivity and the recognition of rights can generate a social and political impact in the creation of laws and public policies of countries, and can open pathways for freedom, autonomy, and decision-making in the processes of recovery and in the overall lives of people living with mental disorders.

In this way, art now becomes a tool and a bridge for transformation at the individual, community, and social levels that attempts to traverse the real and symbolic walls of the insane asylum, or "manicomio," generating links toward the community and reverting the codifying effects of the insane asylum practices—thus enabling the users to position themselves as active subjects of their decisions and of the transformation of their own reality by the path of artistic experience (Bang 2016). Similarly, its practical implementation enables generating the opposite of insane asylum practices; that is to say, it allows for going from the loss of subjectivity, stigmatization, and confinement of people to the creation and re-creation of subjective productions within group-based and communal bonds (Gutiérrez et al. 2018).

The use of art through the alternatives therapies of Art Therapy and Biodanza has allowed us to have a direct and positive impact on the users, at both individual and social levels, in areas such as a growth in their recognition of emotions, development of verbal expression, greater control of their actions, improvement and greater fluidity of body movements, an increase in capacity of contact and reciprocity, and a decrease in the negative symptoms of their illness. As well, the use of art techniques fosters social participation and a more active role of users in the activities (Deleo & Gutiérrez 2016; Tchaikovsky 2017). In this way, Art Therapy and Biodanza have proven to be effective techniques when working with people living with mental disorders and show that, when applied in a group format, they are a more cost-effective and comprehensive development approach (Menéndez and Olmo 2010). Parallel to this, the space in the activities allows us to work with the community to transform the social image of what is understood by "madness" and "being crazy," promote the importance of mental health, and contribute to building a society more inclusive of psychosocial diversity.

Beyond the specific techniques, human connections, mental health service users' empowerment and the creation of more horizontal spaces are fundamental and shed light on a possible path toward recovery. We recognize that when working with users facing mental health challenges, it is important to not only take into account the techniques that are applied but also to consider the way in which this specific population is approached (Deleo and Gutiérrez 2016), namely one of respect and recognition for human rights and fundamental freedoms (Fig. 18.7).

References

Amnesty International. (2018). Instilling terror: from lethal force to persecution in Nicaragua. https://www.amnesty.org/en/documents/amr43/9213/2018/en/. Accessed 3 Dec 2018.

Arnaiz, A., & Uriarte, J. J. (2006). Estigma y enfermedad mental. Norte de salud mental. http://documentacion.aen.es/pdf/revista-norte/volumen-vi/revista-26/049-estigma-y-enfermedad-mental.pdf. Accessed 20 Oct 2018.

Arriba-Rossetto, A., Seoane-Pesqueira, G., Senra-Rivera, C. (2008). Papel de la experiencia en la aceptación vs. rechazo del paciente con esquizofrenia. Revista Latinoamericana de Psicología. https://www.researchgate.net/publication/26576290_Papel_de_la_experiencia_en_la_aceptacion_vs_rechazo_del_paciente_con_esquizofrenia. Accessed 10 Oct 2018.

Bang, C. (2016). *Creatividad y salud mental comunitaria: tejiendo redes desde la participación y la creación colectiva*. Argentina: Buenos Aires.

Bauer, G. (2014). Incorporating intersectionality theory into population health research methodology: Challenges and the potential to advance health equity. Social, Science & Medicine. https://www.researchgate.net/publication/261407967_Incorporating_intersectionality_theory_into_population_health_research_methodology_Challenges_and_the_potential_to_advance_health_equity. Accessed 18 Oct 2018.

British Association of Art Therapists. (1969). What is art therapy? *The BAAT Register.* https://www.baat.org/About-Art-Therapy. Accessed 10 Oct 2018.

Castro, M., & Rossi, M. (1996). Influencia de la biodanza en el proceso terapéutico. Dissertation: University of San Carlos, Guatemala.

Ceballo, Y., Vasconcelos, J., Ferreira, A. (2012). Efectos de un programa de arteterapia sobre la sintomatología clínica de pacientes con esquizofrenia. Dissertation: Central University of Venezuela.

Deleo, A., & Gutiérrez, Y. (2016). Arteterapia y biodanza en el Hospital Psicosocial. Un análisis desde las y los participantes. Dissertation: Universidad Centroamericana UCA. http://reposito-rio.uca.edu.ni/4836/. Accessed 20 Sep 2018.

Foucault, M. (1990). *Technologies of the self.* Barcelona: Paidós Ibérica.

Fundación Nicaragüense para el desarrollo económico y social. (2018). Economic impact of social conflicts in Nicaragua 2018. FUNIDES register. http://funides.com/noticias/436-economic-impact-of-social-conflicts-in-nicaragua-2/. Accessed 10 Oct 2018.

Goffman, E. (1970). *Stigma: Notes on the management of spoiled identity.* New York: Simon & Schuster. https://sociologiaycultura.files.wordpress.com/2014/02/goffman-estigma.pdf. Accessed 10 Oct 2018.

Granda, A., & Sáez, R. (2005). Efectos de la biodanza en las habilidades sociales básicas de los pacientes esquizofrénicos. *Revista de Psicología, 7,* 25–31.

Gutiérrez, L., Scocozza, S., Garavetti, R., Gonzalez, A., Oliveto, C. D. (2018). Arte y salud mental. Recomendaciones para la red integrada de salud mental con base en la comunidad. Irección Nacional de Salud Mental y Adicciones. http://www.msal.gob.ar/images/stories/bes/graficos/0000001358cnt-2018-10_arte-y-salud-mental.pdf. Accessed 10 Oct 2018.

Mad in América Hispanohablante (2017). Radios locas: Redacción Mad in América Hispanohablante. https://madinamerica-hispanohablante.org/radios-locas-redaccion-mad-in-america-hispanohablante/. Accessed 26 Mar 2019.

Menéndez, C., & Del Olmo Romero-Nieva, F. (2010). Arteterapia o intervención terapéutica desde el arte en rehabilitación psicosocial. *Informaciones Psiquiátricas, 201*(3), 367–380.

Pan American Health Organization. (2013). WHO-AIMS: report on mental health systems in Latin America and the Caribbean. https://www.paho.org/hq/dmdocuments/2013/ENG-WHOAIMSREG-(For-Web-Apr-2013).pdf. Accessed 10 Oct 2018.

Rebolleda, C., & Florit, A. (2010). Del concepto de rehabilitación al de recuperación. *Informaciones Psiquiátricas.* http://www.informacionespsiquiatricas.com/anteriores/201_inf%20psiq.pdf. Accessed 13 Oct 2018.

Rodríguez, J., Kohn, R., Aguilar-Gaxiola, S. (2009). Epidemiología de los trastornos mentales en América Latina y el Caribe. Pan American Health Organization. http://iris.paho.org/xmlui/bitstream/handle/123456789/740/9789275316320.pdf. Accessed 14 Oct 2018.

Tchaikovsky, N. (2017). Sistematización de experiencias del Movimiento Ventana, realizadas en el Hospital Psicosocial "José Dolores Fletes Valle" durante el periodo comprendido 2011–2016. Dissertation: Universidad Centroamericana UCA.

Toro, V., & Terrén, R. (2011). El placer de ser humano. Revista Argentina de Biodanza: una poética del encuentro humano, (1).

United Nations Human Rights. (2018). Human rights violations and abuses in the context of protests in Nicaragua, 18 April–18 August 2018. Office of the United Nations High Commissioner for Human Rights (OHCHR). https://www.ohchr.org/Documents/Countries/NI/HumanRightsViolationsNicaraguaApr_Aug2018_EN.pdf. Accessed 5 Oct 2018.

United Nations Human Rights. (2019). Seguimiento a la situación de derechos humanos en Nicaragua, Boletín Mensual N.5 - Enero 2019. Office of the United Nations High Commissioner for Human Rights (OHCHR). http://www.oacnudh.org/wp-content/uploads/2019/02/Nicaragua-Boletin-Mensual-Enero-2019.pdf. Accessed 15 Feb 2019.

Vallejo, P. (2011). Arte terapia en Trastornos Mentales Severos: efectos terapéuticos derivados de una intervención grupal no directiva, desde el discurso de sus participantes, usuarios de servicios de salud ambulatorios. Dissertation: University of Chile. http://repositorio.uchile.cl/handle/2250/106322. Accessed 10 Jan 2018.

World Health Organization. (2013). Mental health action plan 2013–2020. *The WHO Register.* https://apps.who.int/iris/bitstream/handle/10665/89966/9789241506021_eng.pdf;jsessionid=8A1818837783220915F4E4B0CBA7DB45?sequence=1. Accessed 20 Oct 2018.

Chapter 19
Using Art to Bridge Research and Policy: An Initiative of the United States National Academy of Medicine

Charlee Alexander, Kyra Cappelucci, and Laura DeStefano

19.1   Introduction

The National Academy of Medicine (NAM) (formerly the Institute of Medicine) was established in 1970. Its mission is to improve health for all by advancing science; accelerating health equity; and providing independent, authoritative, and trusted advice nationally and globally. The NAM is one of three academies that make up the National Academies of Sciences, Engineering, and Medicine (the National Academies) in the United States. Together, the National Academies are private, non-profit institutions that work outside of government to provide objective advice on matters of science, technology, and health. To achieve its mission, the NAM engages in a number of activities, including assembling volunteer study committees comprising some of the world's foremost scientists, scholars, policy makers, and health professionals to address some of society's toughest challenges. The NAM also hosts numerous conferences, workshops, symposia, forums, roundtables, and other gatherings that attract the finest minds in academia and the public and private sectors. The NAM's vision is a healthier future for everyone and prides itself on being:

- An independent, evidence-based scientific advisor.
- A national academy with global scope.
- Committed to catalyzing action and achieving impact.
- Collaborative and interdisciplinary.
- An honorific society for exceptional leaders.

Over the past 2 years, the NAM has piloted a new strategy to engage with stakeholders at the individual and community levels through three nationwide calls for

C. Alexander (✉) · K. Cappelucci · L. DeStefano
National Academy of Medicine, Washington, DC, USA
e-mail: CAlexander@trinitywallstreet.org; Kyra.Cappelucci@ama-assn.org;
ldestefano@nas.edu

© The Author(s) 2021
J. H. Corbin et al. (eds.), *Arts and Health Promotion*,
https://doi.org/10.1007/978-3-030-56417-9_19

art—two related to the concept of health equity, and one related to clinician well-being. The arts offer an essential medium through which people can shape their identities, express their experiences, learn more effectively, and view society more wholly. Art stretches the imagination and connects people to one another and to the world around them. Research shows that the arts can enhance teaching and learning in school settings (Ernest and Nemirovsky 2015; Gullat 2008) and can improve learning outcomes and readiness for employment (National Academies of Sciences, Engineering, and Medicine 2017). The arts can also help people communicate complex ideas more effectively (Pollack and Korol 2013) and can offer an outlet for authentic community engagement. Drawing on these insights, the NAM designed a participatory art approach as a way to foster meaningful communication around the concepts of health equity and clinician well-being, promote inclusivity, elevate underrepresented voices, and more fully understand the challenges and lived experiences of people in diverse communities.

These calls for art were a departure from the NAM's more traditional methods of connecting with key stakeholders. Results from this approach included the collection of invaluable insights from communities, young people, and clinicians around the nation (which the NAM has used to inform the development of its programs), as well as the establishment of productive new connections between the NAM and other organizations. Elements of the approach have also been replicated by other organizations, and the calls for art have served to connect external organizations to one another. Included in this chapter is a description of the NAM's calls for art, the outcomes from those calls, lessons learned, and insights for organizations interested in pursuing a similar path.

19.2   Visualize Health Equity

The NAM's first call for art in the fall of 2017—*Visualize Health Equity*—originated from the NAM Culture of Health Program. This program aims to advance health equity in the United States by furthering the knowledge base, bridging science to action, strengthening community assets, influencing policy reform, and making health a shared value. Health equity is the state in which everyone has the opportunity to attain full health potential and no one is disadvantaged from achieving this potential because of social position or any other socially defined circumstance. Promoting health equity means creating the conditions in which individuals and communities have what they need to enjoy full, healthy lives (National Academies of Sciences, Engineering, and Medicine 2017).

Community voice is an important component of the program, and the goal of this community art project was to encourage more thought and discussion about health equity and the social determinants of health (SDOH) by soliciting and elevating insights directly from people in diverse communities across the United States. SDOH are conditions in the environments in which people are born, live, learn, work, play, worship, and age that affect a wide range of health, functioning, and quality-of-life outcomes and risks (Healthypeople.gov 2019). The hope was that through a creative lens, the NAM could better understand what people across the country see as the most important health challenges and opportunities facing their communities. With this call for art, the NAM aimed to initiate conversations centered on the need for more equitable policies so that everyone has an equal chance to thrive. The NAM also leveraged its position as a trusted national convener and advisor to share insights gleaned from the lived experiences of participating artists with policy makers, academics, and organizational leaders. The images and excerpts below are taken from artwork and statements submitted by artists who contributed to *Visualize Health Equity* (Figs. 19.1, 19.2, 19.3, and 19.4). Each excerpt provides insight into how artists and communities think about health equity and its importance to their lives.

Listen to Filipino and Mexican farmworkers laugh together over lunch—a right afforded to them under labor laws that, after years of struggle, protect historically excluded agricultural and domestic workers. Observe racially and culturally diverse friends meeting in neighborhoods created by federal housing policies that encourage and support, rather than obstruct and undermine, neighborhood integration. Listen to children of all backgrounds swim together because their community supports each of them and a public pool that welcomes everyone...These are the signs of health. These are the signs of equity. (Connie Cagampang-Heller, *Imagine Belonging*, Berkeley, CA)

There is something magical that happens when people can see and hear themselves in their communities. There is a building of agency and sustainable change when people have ownership over the spaces that they occupy and when they see themselves all around them. Creating through a lens of equity will not always be easy. It will take work, require outside-of-the-box thinking and may not always be the most lucrative position, but it is worth it to at least attempt to use our creativity as artists to leave this world a better place for others because we were in it. (*Visualize Health Equity* submission)

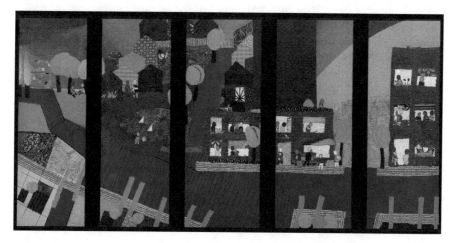

Fig. 19.1 *Imagine Belonging*, © Connie Cagampang Heller, Berkeley, CA; reproduced with permission from the artist from http://nam.edu/visualizehealthequity/#/.

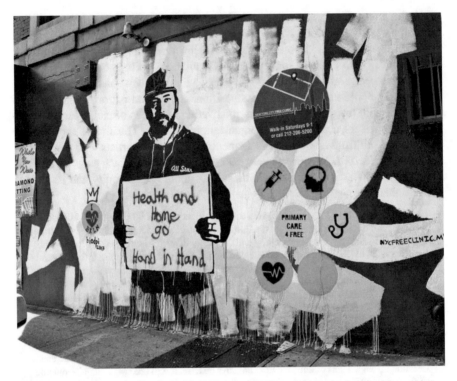

Fig. 19.2 *A Picture of Health*, © John Colavito, New York, NY; Reproduced with permission from the artist from http://nam.edu/visualizehealthequity/#/. All rights reserved

Visualize Health Equity relied on a simple prompt: "What does health equity look, sound, and feel like to you?" (See Box 19.1 for full text of the call for art.) The NAM distributed the call in June 2017 via listserv announcements, social media, and direct outreach to organizations interested in health equity and communities engaged with the program. Community members from a broad span of geographic locations in the United States were a key audience for this project, as the NAM aimed to shed light on experiences and challenges faced by communities around the nation in achieving health equity. Interested participants had 6 weeks to prepare a submission. Altogether, the NAM received 120 submissions for this inaugural call for art. Submissions came from 29 different states in the United States, Puerto Rico, and Ontario, Canada. People from a broad span of ages, races, genders, socioeconomic status, and abilities submitted pieces highlighting topics including food insecurity, immigration, LGBTQ health and well-being, homelessness, and addiction, among others. Submissions covered a range of media, from drawings and paintings to sculptures and slam poetry.

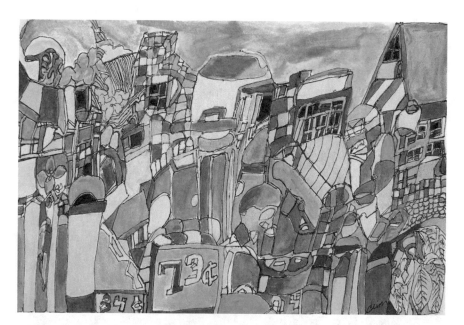

Fig. 19.3 *Neighborhood Community*, © Egbert "Clem" Evans, Washington, D.C.; Reproduced with permission from the artist from http://nam.edu/visualizehealthequity/#/.

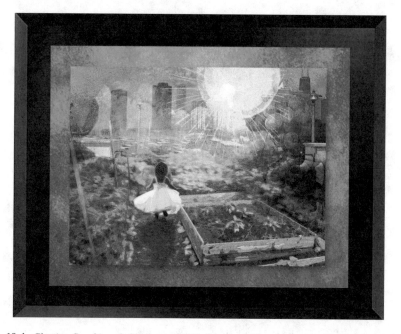

Fig. 19.4 *Chasing Sunshine*, © Stephanie Kohli, Weston, WI; reproduced with permission from the artist from http://nam.edu/visualizehealthequity/#/.

Box 19.1 *Visualize Health Equity* **Call for Art**
The National Academy of Medicine (NAM), a non-profit research organization in Washington, DC, is calling on artists to Visualize Health Equity for a nationwide community art project.

Show us what health equity would look like to you—whether it's access to healthy food or safe neighborhoods, good education or a living wage, clean drinking water or affordable housing, connection to cultural heritage or lack of discrimination, or any other opportunity that helps you live your healthiest life. This project is part of the NAM's Culture of Health Program, sponsored by the Robert Wood Johnson Foundation, which is working to identify strategies that support equitable good health for everyone living in the United States. Artwork submitted for this project will help us understand what people across the country see as the most important health challenges and opportunities facing their communities. The insights we gain will be shared with a national audience and used to inform future directions of the Culture of Health Program.

Guidelines:

- Visual and nonvisual art, such as music and creative writing, are welcome. Accepted mediums include drawings, paintings, photographs, mixed media, murals, collage, sculpture, film, poetry, digital art, performance art, and more. Please provide clear photographs of all visual artwork, from multiple angles or showing close-up detail as appropriate. Creative writing should be submitted in PDF format, and performance art or music should be submitted in video format. File size limit: 50 MB.
- You may submit previously existing artwork, such as a community art installation, as long as you are the original artist or have formal permission from the artist to submit their work for this project.
- All entries must be accompanied by a completed submission form, which includes a brief written explanation of how your artwork relates to health equity.
- By submitting your artwork for this project, you are granting non-exclusive lifetime permission for the NAM to display, publish, and share your artwork in digital and print formats. This includes the written explanation you submit with your work. Full credit will always be given to the artist, and copyright will remain with the artist. Artwork submitted for this project will not be reproduced for purchase or profit.
- Individuals and groups may participate. Limit three submissions per person/group.
- Artists under the age of 18 must have permission from a parent or guardian to participate.
- Non-English-language submissions are encouraged.
- The NAM reserves the right not to display, publish, or share submissions that are not responsive to the prompt or contain inappropriate language or themes.

SOURCE: National Academy of Medicine (2017)

A panel of reviewers drawn from the Culture of Health Program advisory committee, a 20-member body providing strategic guidance for the program, evaluated entries for creativity and responsiveness to the prompt. Together, this group reviewed the submissions using the following criteria:

1. Responsiveness to prompt
2. Uniqueness of insight
3. Visual impact
4. Overall impression

Reviewers used the overall scores to choose 30 submissions to include as part of an in-person gallery at the NAM and identified four artists to present their work to expert attendees during a NAM convening. All 120 submissions are displayed in a permanent digital gallery accessible from the NAM's website: http://nam.edu/visualizehealthequity/#.

Following the launch of the in-person art show and digital gallery, the NAM received numerous inquiries about future calls for art and displaying the submissions at conferences, events, and gallery spaces. In response, NAM developed a free, ten-piece traveling art gallery to promote better understanding of the social determinants of health, illustrate how communities are driving health equity, and encourage communities and organizations to undertake similar initiatives Within the first few weeks of announcing the traveling gallery, the first several months were booked. The traveling gallery has been hosted at six conferences since November 2018, including the South by Southwest (SXSW) Conference and Festival in Austin, Texas, and the annual conference of the American Public Health Association in San Diego, California. Several organizations are scheduled to host the art show throughout 2019. Many others have adopted the NAM's prompt to develop their own calls for art. Information on the traveling exhibit is available at http://nam.edu/visualize-healthequity/#/traveling-gallery.

Audiences who have viewed the traveling and digital galleries are quick to relate to the experiences represented through the artwork. Many viewers were inquisitive about the term "health equity" and how it relates to their lives. Anecdotal feedback suggests that after viewing the artwork, viewers are able to more clearly explain what health equity means for them and their communities. Viewers find the artwork relatable and can easily see their own lives reflected back to them. Viewing the artwork is often an emotional experience for attendees, with many viewers eager to share insights from their own experiences evoked by the artists' work. At one national conference in late 2018, a viewer commented: "This is my life. This is everything I've been trying to explain to anyone who would listen over the past two decades. I feel validated today."

In early 2019, the NAM launched an additional call for art on the topic of health equity. The new call asked "young leaders" aged 5–26 to imagine a world in which everyone has an equal opportunity to live a healthy life. This call for art aimed to help young people develop a deeper understanding of health equity and to elevate their lived experiences. Please visit the project website for additional details: https://nam.edu/programs/culture-of-health/young-leaders-visualize-health-equity/. The call for art ended in March 2019 and an online gallery launched in fall 2019.

19.3   Expressions of Clinician Well-Being

Bolstered by the success of *Visualize Health Equity*, in 2018 the NAM launched a second call for art, this time as part of the Action Collaborative on Clinician Well-Being and Resilience (the Collaborative). The Collaborative aims to improve the well-being of health care professionals by partnering with organizations to raise visibility of clinician anxiety, burnout, depression, stress, and suicide; improve understanding of the factors affecting clinician well-being; and advance evidence-based, multidisciplinary solutions to improve patient care by caring for the care-giver. For this call, the NAM asked stakeholders to submit artwork that expresses what clinician well-being looks, feels, and sounds like to them (see Box 19.2 for full text of the call for art). The ultimate goal was to promote greater awareness and understanding of barriers to the well-being of health professionals, trainees, and students—and of solutions that promise a brighter future.

By raising awareness and elevating the experiences of clinicians, patients, and clinicians' loved ones, the NAM hoped to incite purposeful dialogue on this critical issue and begin to decrease stigma. To engender this dialogue, the call for art was designed to create a supportive environment that promotes social connection and fosters new relationships, as discussed by Urke and colleagues in Chap. 1. There were several key audiences identified for this project. First and foremost, the NAM aimed to hear directly from practicing health professionals about their experiences with burnout and challenges to their overall well-being. Additionally, the NAM sought submissions from patients, because clinician well-being largely affects qual-ity of care and outcomes. By sharing insights directly from clinicians and patients, the NAM strived to extract emotions and stories that would invite an open dialogue about burnout between clinicians and health system leaders and would shed light on an issue of national importance. The images below are taken from artwork submit-ted by artists who contributed to *Expressions of Clinician Well-Being* (Figs. 19.5, 19.6, 19.7, and 19.8).

The NAM distributed the call for art via listserv announcements, social media, and direct outreach to clinician well-being stakeholders such as medical schools, residency programs, hospitals and health centers, professional societies, and mem-bership organizations. The NAM also engaged arts-focused organizations from around the country. The NAM received over 350 submissions from clinicians and their loved ones, patients, organizations, and other interested stakeholders. Topics of the artwork spanned the well-being of women physicians, the resilience journey from burnout to well-being, joy in practice, self-preservation, and empathy, among others. Submissions included poetry, paintings, music, videos, creative writing, and more. The excerpts below are taken from several artist statements from *Expressions of Clinician Well-Being*. Each excerpt accompanies a piece of art and provides insight into how the experiences of these artists help them to conceptualize clinician well-being.

> This song speaks to clinician resilience and the journey from burnout to well-being. In the first verse, I compare my experience in Iraq as a medic to the gang violence here on

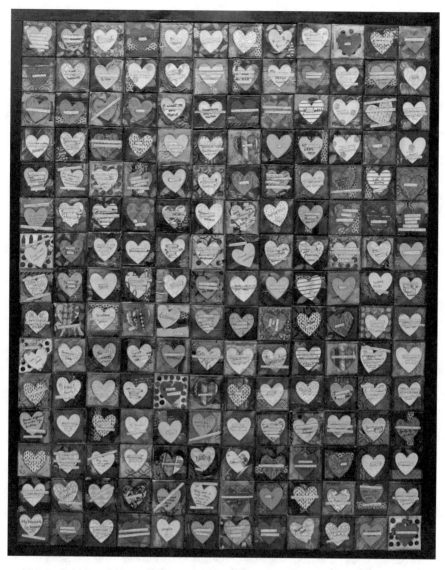

Fig. 19.5 *Hearts in Medicine*, Residents, fellows, and faculty of the University of Arizona College of Medicine—Phoenix Graduate Medical Education Programs, Phoenix, AZ; reproduced with permission from © Cheryl O'Malley from http://nam.edu/expressclinicianwellbeing/#/.

American soil. In the second verse, a patient addicted to heroin evokes my father's death by a heroin overdose when I was nineteen years old. Entailed in these verses are the emotions that emergency physicians manage every day and the difficulty of debriefing after crises in a busy emergency department. In verse three, I awaken, burned out, and I discuss my transformation from burnout to well-being. (*Expressions of Clinician Well-Being* submission)

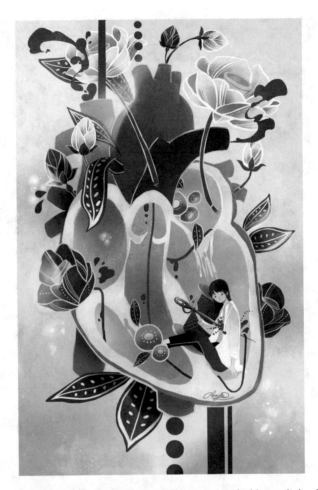

Fig. 19.6 *The Red Thread*, © Sonia Lai, Fremont, CA; reproduced with permission from the artist from http://nam.edu/expressclinicianwellbeing/#/.

Dental professionals are mindful of patients' anxiety mostly caused from pain associated with receiving treatment and financial stress related to out-of-pocket costs. The stereotype of dentists being "monsters," rather than heroes, in the health care realm can affect self-worth and self-image. Over time, patient dissatisfaction, pressures of running a successful practice, and paying back high student loans can all lead to clinician burnout, depression, isolation, clinical errors, and decline of overall health. This poem addresses such struggles, but also reminds the reader to self-reflect and draw strength from all the good that comes from the privilege of serving and treating patients. (*Expressions of Clinician Well-Being* submission)

We choose medicine as a profession in order to help other human beings. It is the connection between practitioner and patient that becomes the foundation of the healing relationship and it is exactly that bond which has inherent in it both the possibility of clinician and patient well-being and the risk of burnout. Too often we think of the doctor-patient relationship as a one-way street. The truth is that we receive as much from our patients as we give to them. (*Expressions of Clinician Well-Being* submission)

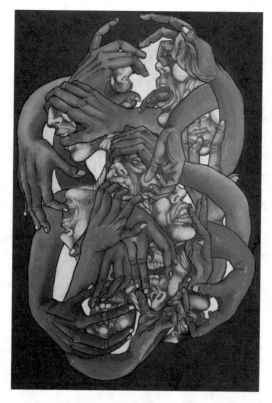

Fig. 19.7 *Resilience*, © Cheyanne Silver, Forest Park, IL; Reproduced with permission from the artist from http://nam.edu/expressclinicianwellbeing/#/.

Box 19.2 *Expressions of Clinician Well-Being* **Call for Art**

Supporting clinician well-being requires sustained attention and action at organizational, state, and national levels, as well as investment in research and information-sharing to advance evidence-based solutions. More broadly, sustained change requires diverse, collective action and the experiences and voices of many.

Use any art form to show us what clinician burnout, clinician resilience, and/or well-being means to you. Whether it's a depiction of how you de-stress from a busy day, how you feel when taking care of patients, or a picture of your favorite clinician, show us—what does clinician well-being look, feel, and sound like to you? Everyone has a stake in this issue—what's yours?

The well-being of our clinicians impacts everyone. This art show will promote greater awareness and understanding of barriers to clinician well-being—and of solutions that promise a brighter future.

(continued)

Box 19.2 (continued)

Participation Guidelines
[Same as Box 19.1].
Need Inspiration?
Below are questions to help spark your creativity! These questions are provided as examples only; your submission does not necessarily need to answer one of them.

- If you had the opportunity, how would you express your gratitude to a clinician who provided excellent care to you or a loved one?
- Who has made a difference in your care? How did that clinician make you feel?
- What was your "turning point" in clinician well-being? When did you first start thinking about clinician burnout and well-being? Was there an experience before that turning point that made you think about well-being? How has your life changed since then?
- How do you feel on your worst days versus your best days? What factors affect this?
- How do you support your loved one(s) in taking steps toward achieving a state of well-being?
- How have your loved one's experience(s) with burnout and well-being affected you?
- How does your organization/team/work unit create an atmosphere that supports well-being?
- Why does clinician well-being matter to you? Why should it matter to others?

SOURCE: National Academy of Medicine (2018)

A panel of reviewers drawn from participants of the Action Collaborative on Clinician Well-Being and Resilience evaluated entries for creativity and responsiveness to the prompt, using the same criteria from *Visualize Health Equity*. Reviewers used the overall scores to choose 30 submissions to include at an in-person gallery at the NAM and identified three artists to present their work to expert attendees during a NAM convening. One hundred of the submissions are displayed in a permanent digital gallery accessible from the NAM's website: http://nam.edu/express-clinicianwellbeing/#/. This digital collection has been shared broadly with clinicians from around the country through social media and at national medical and health conferences. The Collaborative also asked each of its 190+ network organizations to share the digital collection with their constituents in an effort to broaden and promote a national dialogue among clinicians and health system leaders on the importance of enacting change to support well-being and prevent burnout.

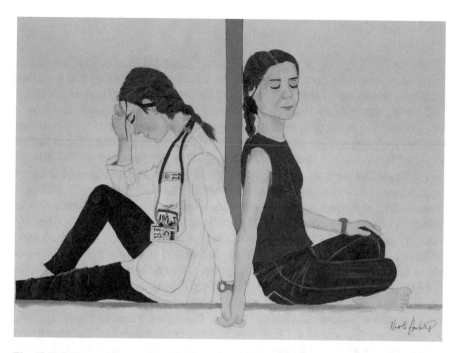

Fig. 19.8 *Self-Preservation*, © Nicole Hawkins, Norfolk, VA; Reproduced with permission from the artist from http://nam.edu/expressclinicianwellbeing/#/. All rights reserved

Similar to *Visualize Health Equity*, the NAM created a free, traveling gallery of *Expressions of Clinician Well-Being* . Viewers of both the traveling and digital galleries are quick to note the validation they feel when viewing the artwork. At one national conference a clinician commented that those who have suffered from burnout for decades may feel as though the artwork gives them "permission to emerge from the shadows" on an issue that has been silenced through stigma for so long. Viewers of the traveling gallery empathize with the artists and their fellow viewers, expressing relief that clinician burnout is finally being discussed openly. Patients who view the artwork often express shock and curiosity; during a NAM convening, a patient noted that he "had no idea clinicians were suffering this way." *Expressions of Clinician Well-Being* makes clinician burnout and suicide a more visible issue and may help viewers understand and engage with their health care providers on a more personal level.

The gallery has traveled to more than 20 external conferences and events. Additionally, several organizations have hosted their own art show using the NAM's prompt. Artwork from the show has been used for several temporary galleries at universities and hospitals around the country. For additional details, please visit http://nam.edu/expressclinicianwellbeing/#/traveling-gallery.

19.4 Conclusion

While the NAM is still an institution primarily grounded in advancing science to improve health, these calls for art represent a new way of thinking and engaging with the communities it seeks to serve. In addition to continuing to convene experts and elevate the evidence base, the NAM recognizes the important role that artistic expression can play in fully understanding the lived experiences of people so that policies and programs are responsive to their actual needs, a concept that is further explored by Corbin and colleagues in Chap. 20. The submissions gathered through this strategic and purposeful effort deepen our collective understanding of the lived experiences of those living in the United States and the global community. We heard from an Iraq war veteran-turned-emergency room doctor how his experiences in war are similar to the crises he deals with daily in the emergency room (*Rise Up Now*, Expressions of Clinician Well-Being). A young student from St. Louis, Missouri, shared her insights on how a single highway effectively ensures the separation of affluence and poverty, deepening disparities and inequities (*Delmar Divide No More*, Visualize Health Equity). A California artist used a stitched collage to illustrate the importance of racially and culturally diverse communities in strengthening overall well-being and health (*Imagine Belonging*, Visualize Health Equity). A medical student shared the hardships she has faced because of her gender and how fellow physicians sometimes feel smothered and trapped by the myriad outside influences that inhibit their ability to provide the best patient care (*Resilience*, Expressions of Clinician Well-Being). Future calls for art might include a follow up mechanism to understand what effects the art shows have on participants in terms of new knowledge, ideas, or behavior.

The snapshots provided here barely scratch the surface of the robust perspectives collected through the art projects, but they provide important insights that are necessary for the academic community, policy makers, and others in understanding the lived realities of so many people. By understanding these realities more fully, stakeholders can more strategically direct their action and resources. Art has offered a way for the NAM to foster new relationships, raise awareness of critical issues, and engage stakeholders in meaningful dialogue around issues that greatly affect the health and well-being of all.

References

Ernest, J. B., & Nemirovsky, R. (2015). Arguments for integrating the arts: Artistic engagement in an undergraduate foundations of geometry course. *Primus, 26*(4), 356–370. https://doi.org/10.1080/10511970.2015.1123784.

Gullatt, D. E. (2008). Enhancing student learning through arts integration: Implications for the profession. *The High School Journal, 91*(4), 12–25.

HealthyPeople.gov. (2019). Social determinants of health. https://www.healthypeople.gov/2020/topics-objectives/topic/social-determinants-of-health. Accessed 25 Feb 2019.

National Academies of Sciences, Engineering, and Medicine. (2017). *Communities in action: pathways to health equity*. Washington, DC: The National Academies Press. https://doi.org/10.17226/24624.

National Academy of Medicine. (2017). Visualize health equity: A community art project. http://nam.edu/visualizehealthequity/#/. Accessed 25 Feb 25 2019.

National Academy of Medicine. (2018). Expressions of clinician well-being: an art exhibition. https://nam.edu/expressions-of-clinician-well-being-an-art-exhibition/. Accessed 25 Feb 2019.

Pollack, A. E., & Korol, D. L. (2013). The use of haiku to convey complex concepts in neuroscience. *Journal of Undergraduate Neuroscience Education, 12*(1), A42–A48.

Chapter 20
Art and Innovation at International Health Promotion Conferences

Christa Ayele, J. Hope Corbin, Emily Alden Hennessy, Mariana Sanmartino, and Helga Bjørnøy Urke

20.1 (Re)Thinking the Dynamics of International Conferences

The first international scientific conferences were held in the mid-1800s; since then around 170,000 conferences have followed, and they now occupy a ubiquitous presence in all scientific fields (SciConf 2019). SciConf, a research group in Sweden formed to study conferences, suggests that they are worthy of critical inquiry. The group poses questions such as: "What happens at scientific conferences? How have they exchanged knowledge and shaped expertise? What forms of sociability have

C. Ayele
International Union for Health Promotion and Education's Student and Early Career Network, Philadelphia, PA, USA
e-mail: christaamayele@gmail.com

J. H. Corbin
Department of Health and Community Studies, Western Washington University, Bellingham, WA, USA
e-mail: hope.corbin@wwu.edu

E. A. Hennessy
Department of Psychology, Institute for Collaboration on Health, Intervention & Policy, University of Connecticut, Storrs, CT, USA
e-mail: ehennessy@mgh.harvard.edu

M. Sanmartino
Grupo de Didáctica de las Ciencias, IFLYSIB, CONICET – UNLP. Grupo ¿De qué hablamos cuando hablamos de Chagas?, La Plata, Buenos Aires, Argentina
e-mail: mariana.sanmartino@conicet.gov.ar

H. B. Urke (✉)
Department of Health Promotion and Development, Faculty of Psychology, University of Bergen, Bergen, Norway
e-mail: helga.urke@uib.no

© The Author(s) 2021
J. H. Corbin et al. (eds.), *Arts and Health Promotion*,
https://doi.org/10.1007/978-3-030-56417-9_20

developed in these meetings, what rituals have been performed? How have scientific conferences embodied social hierarchies and international relations? How have they informed policies on relevant subjects?" (SciConf 2019). This recognition of conferences as important formal structures that embody social hierarchies and conform to accepted practices is important to examine, particularly in a field like health promotion, which is concerned with participation, collaboration, and equity (for more background on this issue, see Chap. 1, this volume).

Most traditional scientific conferences, including in the health promotion field, have a fairly predictable structure to their scientific programs. The central daily feature is usually one or two keynote speakers that each give a lecture on a topic of their expertise. These lectures typically range from 20–45 minutes, and sometimes there will be time for questions in the end. Parallel panel sessions are another common component of traditional scientific conferences, where a number of researchers present work on related topics. Usually three to five presenters are allocated 10–15 minutes to present, and again, there may be a bit of time at the end for questions from the audience depending on the speakers' adherence to their time guidelines and the militancy of the session chair/timekeeper. Poster presentations are another popular session type that typically involve a room of hanging posters that are each attended by their author, which should enable conference participants to engage in conversation with poster authors about their research (although this exchange does not always take place). Other conference activities include roundtable discussions, symposia, and workshops, which may or may not involve deeper engagement than the session types described above.

From a pedagogical perspective, the conference structure described above adheres almost entirely to Freire's "banking" concept of education (Freire 1970). That is, the presenter—whether speaking at a keynote, panel session, or poster presentation—is the "expert" who is "depositing" knowledge, while the audience is relegated to "receiving, filing and storing the deposits" (Freire 1970, p. 53). This vertical education approach and non-dialogic dynamic is a feature of traditional Western/Northern education systems (Tikly 2004). Boaventura de Sousa Santos (2016) describes the ubiquity of this educational approach in the notion of the *monoculture of knowledge*, which describes how hegemonic, modern notions of science and high culture are turned into the only criteria upon which all others' ways of thinking and creative expressions are judged (de Sousa Santos 2016). As a result, approaches not recognized by this monoculture are essentially ignored or assumed non-existent. Chilisa (2005) brings the limitations of these models—and indeed the dominance of the Western/Northern way of knowing—into stark light in the arena of health promotion by acknowledging that the knowledge and health promotion programs produced in this manner risk the lives of people in the Global South because of a lack of cultural relevance and honest engagement with multiple ways of knowing (for more background on this issue, see Chap. 21, this volume).

The scientific conference serves as a forum in which new ideas can be presented to a knowledgeable and critical audience and where findings and methods can be debated and discussed and networks can be built for future collaborations (Simkhada et al. 2013). However, when much of the conference program is characterized by a presenter and his/her/their audience engaging in one-way communication, several of these aims have limited potential of being fulfilled through the formal program.

The informal program (coffee breaks, lunchtime, social events) can, of course, be a more suitable arena for the interaction. However, there may be undiscovered/unexplored potential for more fruitful interaction in the formal agenda.

Luckily, more and more examples of scientific events that seek to break with this classic scheme can be found, promoting spaces of more authentic exchange and less "scientificism" (Varsavsky 1969). Such is the case, for example, in the events promoted by the Latin American and Caribbean Network for the Popularization of Science and Technology (RedPoP) or the so-called *unconferences,* which are meetings that place less emphasis on formal speeches and presentations and devote more time and focus to discussions and connections between researchers/participants, applying a range of participatory methods for the exchange of knowledge (Zimmer et al. 2011). In order for academic conferences to fulfill their potential as true spaces of collaboration, critical reflection, exchange, and ultimately liberatory educational experiences (Tikly 2004), we argue that innovations are required that transcend formal structures, language barriers, and rigid ways of knowing.

20.2   The Contribution of Arts-based Approaches

Arts-based approaches have been used as vehicles for understanding in various contexts. Graham (1995) argued that art is a medium that can be used for education to "develop the mind and promote understanding" (p. 28). For example, while teaching adult nursing students, Nguyen et al. (2016) found that students who used art to dialog were able to communicate experiences that words would not adequately convey. Furthermore, they argued that art inspired "emotion, personal awareness, and exploration" (Nguyen et al. 2016, p. 408). Fox et al. (2016) utilized themes from the popular fictional story "Alice in Wonderland" to facilitate discussions concerning the challenges and strategies of professional collaboration. These authors found that their method introduced participants to new pathways of learning as well as inspired self-awareness and confidence on personal levels (Fox et al. 2016). These personal outcomes were a result of the arts-based approach but also worked to support shared interactions and the insights with others.

Arts-based approaches are naturally multidimensional; in contrast to conventional methods of understanding, in these approaches, validation exists beyond the dichotomy of right or wrong. Eernstman et al. (2012) explains that within art several paths of understanding can be explored, and that the need to make a decision based on correctness is not as dire as with other subjects. The space that art creates for multiple truths to coexist is, arguably, one of the most significant characteristics of utilizing an arts-based approach. For these reasons, we consider such approaches to be a fertile arena to promote an Ecology of Knowledges—an alternative to address the monoculture of modern science (de Sousa Santos 2012; Chap. 12, this volume). The ecology of knowledges assumes that all interactions between human beings and nature involve multiple manifestations of knowledge (de Sousa Santos 2012). Within this framework, and from the critical view that we have been proposing, we argue that for a field like health promotion, arts-based conference presentations should be intentionally incorporated, as they could respect and invite reflection on different forms of knowledge, thus better reflecting the participatory and social justice intentions of health promotion (WHO 1986; Chap. 1, this volume).

In this chapter, we provide an example of how the Student and Early Career Network of the International Union for Health Promotion and Education (ISECN) found an innovative and dialogical way of breaking with the classic model of the scientific conference by incorporating art in multiple sessions at international health promotion conferences.

20.3 The International Union for Health Promotion and Education's (IUHPE) Student and Early Career Network (ISECN) and Their Conference Sessions

The ISECN was founded in 2006 to create a space for students and early career professionals interested in pursuing a community within the larger IUHPE global network. The purpose of ISECN, while constantly evolving, is to unify great minds, bridge research interests, and inspire action that positively influences the world (Corbin et al. 2012). Global networks, as such, encourage the cross-cultural partnerships that continuously diversify our knowledge base. To deepen connections within the network and to contribute to the field of health promotion, ISECN from its inception worked to plan conference sessions at the IUHPE's conferences. The use of art as a medium for communication for an ISECN conference session was first raised during the planning for the ISECN's participation in the 5th IUHPE regional Latin-American conference in Mexico City in 2012.

The decision to include art-based presentations began as an entirely pragmatic decision. In planning for this conference in Mexico, we were faced with a practical problem: how can a group of people who all speak different languages successfully organize and conduct a session for a largely Spanish-speaking audience, without the possibility for simultaneous translation? And, how could we do so in a way that resulted in synergy among conference attendees (see Chap. 21, this volume)? The answer to these questions resulted in the inspiring and foundational idea that became the title of our first session on arts and health promotion: "How to speak about health without words?"

20.3.1 Speaking About Health Without Words: Mexico City, Mexico, 2012

The session (90-minutes) incorporated three key strands: arts-based research and practice projects being conducted by ISECN members, original artistic contributions created particularly for the session by ISECN members, and finally an interactive mural activity facilitated by professional artists from Mexico City.

Table 20.1 Arts-based research and practice presented in Mexico City, Mexico

Title/Topic	Art Form	Author/Presenter	Country
Mental Health Problems & Substance Abuse Among Women	Photos taken by women in a photovoice project	Hilary McGregor	Canada
Child-led Households and Children with Caretaker Responsibilities due to HIV/AIDS in Africa	Reproductions of photography and drawings made by children	Morten Skoval	Kenya
Combination of Contributions from Art and Science to Communicate About Chagas Disease	Projections of painting from series CHAGAS by artist Néstor Favre-Mossier	Mariana Sanmartino	Argentina
Illustrating Chagas Disease	Projections of drawings illustrated by Mexican children	Janine Ramsey and Alba Valdez Tah	Mexico

The first 45 minutes of the session were set up as a "gallery walk" with art pieces displayed around the room. We played songs with health promotion themes and allowed participants to wander the room looking at the various presentations. The presentations of research and practice initiatives (see Table 20.1) consisted of a photovoice project on the topic of mental health and substance use in Canada, photography and drawings created by children with caretaker responsibilities in child-headed households in Kenya, and paintings on the topic of Chagas disease produced by both a professional artist (from Argentina) and by children (from Mexico).

During the gallery walk, participants also had the opportunity to view and listen to materials created by ISECN members for this session to answer the following question: "What helps me be healthy?" The visual displays consisted of drawings and paintings that were collected from children ranging in age from 3–12 years. ISECN members went to local schools in Puerto Rico, Norway, Argentina, and the U.S. and asked children to reflect on the aforementioned question with drawings or paintings. The illustrations were placed all over the venue for participants to enjoy and consider.

Before the conference, ISECN members were asked to record sounds in answer to that same question (Fig. 20.1), through which we obtained sounds such as a smoothie being slurped through a straw, the deep breathing of someone exercising, and children singing. These sounds were artfully combined and edited by Alejandro Valencia-Tobón (Colombia), and during the session, a computer was set up at a table in the middle of the room with headphones to allow participants to listen to the compilation. Pads of blank sticky notes were provided, and participants were asked to reflect on what they were hearing using a word or phrase in their language.

The final 45 minutes of the session were devoted to the co-creation of a mural. Prior to the meeting, ISECN members connected with a local artist group, Cultura Colectiva, to create a mural depicting ideas directly related to the prompt of the session. The concept for the mural was to create a garden with all of the participants contributing a plant, flower, animal, or some other element. The activity was meant to be accessible for people of all artistic levels. By providing many materials, participants had the ability to paint or collage or draw—whatever felt most comfortable

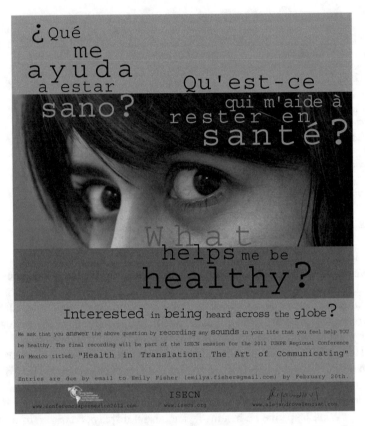

to them (Fig. 20.2). Everyone was working at the same time, and there was conversation, laughter, and joy as participants were able to bring aspects of themselves to the conference space (e.g., aesthetics, tactile engagement, creation) that are almost never given space or voice in a typical session.

The results of this session in Mexico were overwhelmingly positive; it was very well attended and those who came seemed engaged with the various materials. Many people remarked that it was a refreshing break from traditional conference formats. We observed that opting out of using words as the dominant form of communication allowed attendees to connect with others and with global research through visuals, different sensations, and emotions.

20.3.2   Art as a Tool and a Bridge: Curitiba, Brazil, 2016

The second arts-based session organized by ISECN was presented at the 22nd IUHPE World Conference in 2016 held in Curitiba, Brazil. Again, a team of ISECN members—a combination of a few who had worked on the conference in Mexico

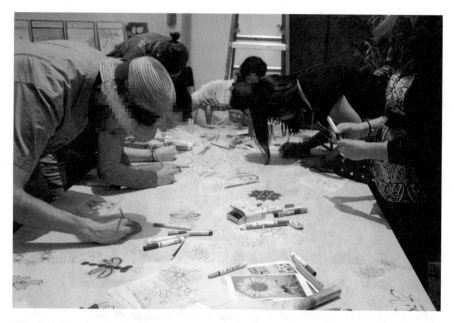

Fig. 20.2 Attendees working on the mural in Mexico City, Mexico

and a few new members—proposed a sub-plenary session, titled "Art as a Tool and Bridge for Health Promotion," which was approved by the IUHPE global scientific committee. Having already gained momentum and experience in utilizing art, we approached the conference in Brazil with excitement and more confidence.

Following the successful model in Mexico, this session again included a gallery walk and a creative activity. As new ISECN members were involved, new arts-based health promotion projects were represented. Visual art pieces were presented along all the walls of the conference room, and session attendees could navigate the space as they wished (Fig. 20.3). Presenters stood by their work and were able to interact with participants and answer questions. This approach encouraged attendees to engage (with presenters and other attendees) through conversation, prioritizing comprehension and dialogue as opposed to the speaker-audience dynamic normalized in conference culture. The gallery included various forms of art including poetry, photography, video, music, and a variety of illustrations (see Table 20.2).

The interactive portion of the session was more informal than the activity in Mexico. We provided diverse raw materials for art projects and provided the following prompt: "Tools help us to build and create. Bridges allow us to go where we could otherwise not go. Before you begin to create, take a moment to close your eyes and think about the tools and bridges that facilitate health promotion." Participants could draw, paint, use mixed media, or create collages (Fig. 20.4). There was then an area to display and view the art created within the session.

Another powerful aspect of the session was the presence of live music. We connected with Brazilian colleagues prior to the conference and arranged to have Kauey Alves Atanascovick Uchoas da Silva sing and play guitar during the entirety of the

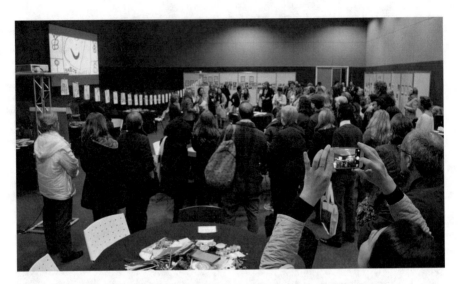

Fig. 20.3 ISECN leadership and presenters welcoming attendees in Curitiba, Brazil

Table 20.2 Arts-based research and practice presented in Curitiba, Brazil

Title/Topic	Art Form	Author	Country
El Camino de Promoción de Salud: Health & Wellness as a Pilgrimage	Various visual art media	Erika Bro	USA
Photovoice as a Health Promotion and Empowerment Tool	Photos taken by Syrian refugee youth in a photovoice study	Ozge Karadag Caman	Turkey
Grafitti: Street Voices for Health Promotion	Graffiti photographic survey	Bianca Palmeri	Brazil
Using Art as a Teaching Tool in the University Classroom	Various forms of illustrations	Hope Corbin & Western Washington University Students	USA
Lines and Colors to Rethink the Complexity of Chagas Disease	Watercolors of the Argentine illustrator Carlos Julio Sánchez	Mariana Sanmartino	Argentina
Spiritual Health Through Poetry	Poetry	Sara Zarei	Iran
How to Speak About Health Without Words	Video elaborated with images taken in Mexico session in 2012	ISECN Edited by Alejandro Valencia-Tobón (Colombia)	Mexico

session. This music created atmosphere and contributed to the general vibe in the room, which was one of openness and inspiration.

The results were, again, astonishing. Both attendees and presenters described the session as passionate, powerful, and transformative. The session also attracted the interest of an academic press who contacted us prior to the session and encouraged us to submit a proposal, laying the groundwork for the volume you now hold in your hands (or see on your screen). Indeed, the projects presented in Chaps. 3 and 10 of this volume were presented as part of this sub-plenary session.

20.3.3   Creative and Participatory Approaches to Promote Planetary Health and Sustainable Development: Rotorua, New Zealand, 2019

At the 23rd IUHPE World Conference, held in 2019 in Rotorua (New Zealand) and themed "Promoting Planetary Health and Sustainable Development," ISECN led a sub-plenary titled "Creative and Participatory Approaches to Promote Planetary Health and Sustainable Development." As with the previous conferences, the session consisted of a gallery walk showcasing the arts-based presentations followed by an interactive and creation-focused activity. There were diverse arts-based presentations by ISECN members, and invited colleagues shared the creative ways health promotion work was being conducted globally (see Table 20.3).

The interactive portion of the session combined elements from the Mexico and Brazil conferences. We created a "tree" design and invited participants to use pastels to color in the "leaves." We asked attendees to think about the connection between human and planetary health in their drawings. Similar to the mural during the interactive session in Brazil, the individual "leaves" enabled people to introduce their own themes and to work on them for as little or as long as they liked, while the overall impact of combining these individual contributions into a larger image was

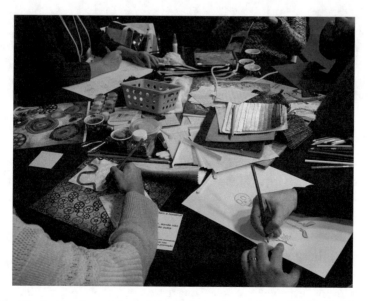

Fig. 20.4   Attendees creating art pieces during the interactive session in Curitiba, Brazil

Table 20.3 Arts-based research and practice presented in Rotorua, New Zealand

Title/Topic	Art	Author	Country
Advocacy Efforts Using Alternate Media to Address Air Pollution in Delhi, India	Illustrations & PowerPoint presentation	Sridevi Adivi	United Arab Emirates
Small-scale Evaluation as a Participatory Action Research	Interactive poster	Anna Mary Cooper-Ryan	United Kingdom
Arts-based Mental Health Promotion Workshop for Indigenous Youth	Photography	Sahar Fahnian	Canada
Unlocking Love Film Series: Low-budget Entertainment Education (EE) Films for Changing Norms Related to Gender-based Violence (GBV) in Timor-Leste	Film	Ba Futuru's Domin Nakloke (Organization)	Timor Liste
Student Creativity in a School Food Intervention in Denmark	Mixed art activities, including visual arts and cooking	Dorte Ruge	Denmark
What Do You See as the Future of Health Promotion?	Video	ISECN Network	Global

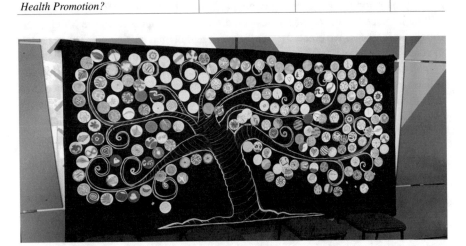

Fig. 20.5 The final product created by session participants at the IUHPE World Conference in Rotorua, New Zealand

reminiscent of the "garden" mural created in Mexico. The resulting tree (Fig. 20.5) was on display in the foyer of the conference hall for the days following the sub-plenary session and evoked much conversation.

20.4 Challenges

While the overall experience of organizing these sessions was overwhelmingly positive, there were a few challenges that we faced, especially as we were implementing a new format within a long-established scientific conference protocol.

20.4.1   Advocating for Sessions

The first challenge had to do with presenting the rationale for the session format in a way that conference program reviewers could understand; this involved careful explanation of the actual session logistics and needs as well as why such an approach would add value to the conference. Because the sessions are very different from typical conference sessions, and the typical conference submission portals do not allow for the deviations that we were proposing, we had to provide extra information and detail outside of the formal submission opportunity and even answer specific questions from the scientific review committee. At times it was difficult for individuals on the scientific committee to understand the idea, and this required additional work on our end to ensure the sessions happened and that we were given appropriate space. In more recent years, we were fortunate to have internal advocacy efforts because some committee members had experienced the Mexico session and could attest to its value for future conferences.

20.4.2   Room Requirements and Extensive Set-up

Given the need to hang images, posters, and other materials, our sessions had unique space requirements. We needed, for example, to be able to use blue tape or pins or blue tack to post the various exhibits on the walls. We had to get special permission for these, at times. Set-up also required a significant amount of additional supplies and time. We would often have to talk with the conference organizers about when we would be able to access the room, requesting that the session be scheduled for the first morning slot or immediately following lunch. We had to organize a crew of volunteers to get the room ready for the session and to help with breakdown after the session. Depending on the interactive project, we also had to find funding for art supplies and find ways to bring these supplies and any pre-made projects to the conference location.

20.4.3   Attendance Complications

From an equity perspective, we sought to include anyone with relevant work regardless of their ability to appear in person at the conference because our members often lacked funding to attend the conference. For some conferences, bursaries were available; for others, there were no funds. For these and other reasons, many of our presenters had to send their materials, and we presented them on their behalf. In New Zealand, however, a last-minute change by the organizers required that unregistered participants have their names removed from the program, which led to a few ISECN members withdrawing their contributions.

20.5 Brief Reflections

For centuries, art has been used as a vehicle to express meaning and articulate ideas. The act of doing so is not only effective but also an act of activism within learning. Richardson and Ricketts (2017) reviewed the use of art at an education conference and argued that it moved participants "…away from traditional vertical hierarchies of knowledge dissemination towards more lateral exchanges and emergent learning structures" (p. 168). These new "exchanges" and "structures" (Richardson and Ricketts 2017) disrupted traditional flows of knowledge sharing and introduced new paths of understanding to the human mind. While challenging the power dynamics and norms within education is significant, the use of art simultaneously enhances the meaning of the content being explored.

The purpose of attending conferences, especially global conferences, is to network with professionals, share ideas and knowledge, and connect to evolve the field. The idea is to leave with more than you came with. Art is a potential bridge for this purpose while, simultaneously, working to dismantle the hierarchy of formal education and the monoculture of scientific knowledge (de Sousa Santos 2012). Arts-based activities can facilitate the equalizing of knowledge and world-views by relinquishing notions of "right" and "wrong" and by creating space for a diversity of ideas and artistic expression (Williams 2002).

By engaging in artistic expression, participants are able to share their knowledge as well as reflect on the creation of others. Participants can choose to share their perspectives or allow for others to reflect through their own process (Williams 2002). Art purposefully demolishes the boundaries of verbal communication while enhancing meaning and showcasing the diverse answers individuals can have to the same question. From our experience, the level of relevance this has to the purpose of international conferences is astounding. Whether the goal is to transcend language barriers, enhance shared meaning, or bring fun to learning, art is a powerful strategy. However, disrupting conference norms in this way, while powerful, takes additional effort and strategizing. Thus, we hope that sharing our multiple experiences in this process will enable others to both understand the value of this work and to improve the ability to plan accordingly.

Acknowledgements The authors would like to recognize the contributions of the following conference session organizers: Erika Bro, Mackenzie Foster, Sharon Ortiz, Bianca Palmeri, Sara Rodgers, Kauey Alves Atanascovick Uchoas da Silva, and Ankur Singh. **We would also like to thank Erma Manoncourt, Suzanne Jackson, Ann Pederson, and Robyn Perlstein for their encouragement, support, and help setting up and taking down.**

References

Chilisa, B. (2005). Educational research within postcolonial Africa: A critique of HIV/AIDS research in Botswana. *International Journal of Qualitative Studies in Education, 18*(6), 659–684. https://doi.org/10.1080/09518390500298170.

Corbin, J. H., Fisher, E. A., & Bull, T. (2012). The International Union for Health Promotion and Education (IUHPE) Student and Early Career Network (ISECN): A case illustrating three strategies for maximizing synergy in professional collaboration. *Global Health Promotion.* https://doi.org/10.1177/1757975912441232.

de Sousa Santos, B. (2012). Public sphere and epistemologies of the South. *Africa Development, XXXVII*(1), 43–67.

de Sousa Santos, B. (2016). *Epistemologies of the South: Justice against epistemicide.* New York: Routledge.

Eernstman, N., Van Boeckel, J., Sacks, S., & Myers, M. (2012). Inviting the unforeseen: A dialogue about art, learning and sustainability. In *Learning for sustainability in times of accelerating change* (pp. 201–212). Wageningen: Wageningen Academic Publishers.

Fox, A., Gillis, D., Anderson, B., & Lordly, D. (2016). Stronger together: Use of storytelling at a dietetics conference to promote professional collaboration. *Canadian Journal of Dietetic Practice and Research, 78*(1), 32–36. https://doi.org/10.3148/cjdpr-2016-027.

Freire, P. (1970). *Pedagogy of the oppressed.* New York: Herder and Herder.

Graham, G. (1995). Learning from art. *The British Journal of Aesthetics, 35*(1), 26–37.

Nguyen, M., Miranda, J., Lapum, J., & Donald, F. (2016). Arts-based learning: A new approach to nursing education using andragogy. *Journal of Nursing Education, 55*(7), 407–410. https://doi.org/10.3928/01484834-20160615-10.

Richardson, P., & Ricketts, K. (2017). Review of "arts-based contemplative practices in education": 2017 Canadian Society for Studies in Education ARTS Pre-conference. *Art/Research International: A Transdisciplinary Journal, 2*(2), 168–175. https://doi.org/10.18432/R2S91K.

SciConf. (2019). The Scientific Conference—Department of History of Science and Ideas—Uppsala University, Sweden. https://www.idehist.uu.se/forskning/forskningsprojekt/the-scientific-conference/. Accessed 18 Feb 2020.

Simkhada, P., Teijlingen, E. V., Hundley, V., & Simkhada, B. D. (2013). Writing an abstract for a scientific conference. *Kathmandu University Medical Journal, 11*(3), 262–265. https://doi.org/10.3126/kumj.v11i3.12518.

Tikly, L. (2004). Education and the new imperialism. *Comparative Education, 40*(2), 173–198. https://doi.org/10.1080/0305006042000231347.

Varsavsky, O. (1969). Ciencia, política y cientificismo. Capital Intelectual S. A.

Williams, B. (2002). Using collage art work as a common medium for communication in interprofessional workshops. *Journal of Interprofessional Care, 16*(1), 53–58. https://doi.org/10.1080/13561820220104168.

World Health Organization. (1986). The Ottawa Charter for Health Promotion. https://www.who.int/healthpromotion/conferences/previous/ottawa/en/. Accessed 20 Feb 2020.

Zimmer, B., Carson, C. E., & Horn, L. R. (2011). Among the new words. *American Speech, 86*(3), 355–376. https://doi.org/10.1215/00031283-1503937.

Part V
Conclusion

Chapter 21
Arts, Health Promotion, and Social Justice: Synergy in Motion

J. Hope Corbin, Mariana Sanmartino, Helga Bjørnøy Urke, and Emily Alden Hennessy

21.1 Introduction

This volume, *Arts and Health Promotion: Tools and Bridges for Practice, Research, and Social Transformation*, has presented 19 chapters illustrating how the arts have been incorporated into a variety of health promotion programs, research projects, and social mobilization initiatives. In this final chapter, drawing from examples shared throughout the book and using the Bergen Model of Collaborative Functioning, we propose a way of understanding how art increases synergy in the pursuit of health promotion goals. We argue that art can increase synergy by facilitating deeper engagement with one's self and with others, as well as by supporting the process of making sense of context. In line with reaching the goals of health promotion delineated in the Ottawa Charter (see Chap. 1, this volume), we also argue that art promotes social justice by amplifying voice, leveraging power, and

J. H. Corbin (✉)
Department of Health and Community Studies, Western Washington University, Bellingham, WA, USA
e-mail: hope.corbin@wwu.edu

M. Sanmartino
Grupo de Didáctica de las Ciencias, IFLYSIB, CONICET – UNLP. Grupo ¿De qué hablamos cuando hablamos de Chagas?, La Plata, Buenos Aires, Argentina
e-mail: mariana.sanmartino@conicet.gov.ar

H. B. Urke
Department of Health Promotion and Development, Faculty of Psychology, University of Bergen, Bergen, Norway
e-mail: helga.urke@uib.no

E. A. Hennessy
Department of Psychology, Institute for Collaboration on Health, Intervention & Policy, University of Connecticut, Storrs, CT, USA
e-mail: ehennessy@mgh.harvard.edu

© The Author(s) 2021
J. H. Corbin et al. (eds.), *Arts and Health Promotion*,
https://doi.org/10.1007/978-3-030-56417-9_21

honoring multiple ways of knowing. We conclude by highlighting implications for the field of health promotion and suggesting lines of further research.

21.2   Art and Synergy

The Bergen Model of Collaborative Functioning (BMCF) has been employed as an analytical tool for understanding interactions in health promotion programs and initiatives (Corbin et al. 2016). The model depicts inputs, throughputs, and outputs and describes pathways for how collaborative processes interact to produce additive results, synergy, or antagony (see Fig. 21.1). Health promotion initiatives can be mapped according to the BMCF as they all center around a mission (the problem they are trying to solve or the purpose of the initiative); they all involve people (partner resources) including the participants, the health promotion professionals, and ideally other community stakeholders; and very often, they involve financial or other material resources. The processes of leadership, communication, role/procedures, and input interaction vary from arrangement to arrangement but will have an impact whatever those dynamics might be (Corbin et al. 2016). Lastly, all health promotion initiatives have results of some kind, whether people do what they would have done anyway without being impacted by the project (additive); whether there

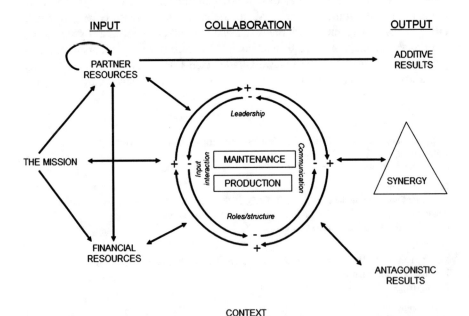

Fig. 21.1 Bergen Model of Collaborative Functioning. (Reproduced from Corbin et al. (2016). Figure 1. https://doi.org/10.1093/heapro/daw061, licensed under the terms of the Creative Commons Attribution Non-Commercial License (http://creativecommons.org/licenses/by-nc/4.0/))

is little, no, or a negative impact from the initiative (antagony); or whether the results of the collaboration are multiplicative—equaling more than the sum of its parts (synergy) (Corbin and Mittelmark 2008). In the best-case scenario, initiatives would only produce synergy, but in real-world scenarios, there are often mixes of these three outputs at different stages of collaborations.

Using the BMCF as a framework for analyzing the projects and experiences described in this book, we argue that arts-based initiatives may deepen and increase the interaction between the production tasks of the project (the arts-based activity), the partners (participants' engagement with themselves), communication (participants' engagement with other participants, their community, existing artwork, and audiences), and the context (both by using art to make better sense of their experiences, and/or using art to have an impact on the context). In the chapters of this volume, participants, practitioners, and researchers often describe these interactions in terms associated with the concept of synergy; yet, there are also some experiences of antagonistic results given the nature of this work.

21.2.1 Partners: Art and Increased Engagement with the Self

A number of chapters in this volume describe health promotion initiatives integrating art at the level of the individual as processes that enabled participants to deeply engage with their own experiences and beliefs. In many cases, participants and authors note synergy by suggesting that the engagement would not have been possible without the unique dynamics created by introducing art-based elements.

Katisi, Jefferies, and Sebako (Chap. 2) describe the combination of drawings, therapy, and group discussions to uncover the young people's unprocessed trauma surrounding their parent's deaths, in synergistic terms:

> Drawing, as employed in this context, appears to work well when used in conjunction with written and verbal narratives. **It appears to achieve what other types of approaches could miss...** such as when the children felt unable or unwilling to bring up issues in group or individual sessions but were able to draw them. (Katisi, Jefferies, and Sebako, Chap. 2, p. 34, emphasis added)

The authors argue that the interaction with drawing encouraged the young people to dig deeper into their experiences and emotions, enabling them to uncover more than would have been possible if they were only provided traditional processing tools.

Another example of this deeper engagement with the self is the CuidarNos project in Puerto Rico (Ramírez et al., Chap. 6), which organized workshops employing a number of diverse artistic and sensory experiences to support the processing of personal and vicarious trauma among intimate partner violence (IPV) service providers in the wake of Hurricane Maria:

> Participating in Encuentro CuidarNOS **gave a space to breathe** and unwind at times when it had been difficult to get it out, and maybe I had not allowed that space. Sometimes, trying to follow the hectic pace of everyday life, it becomes difficult for us to take a space to disconnect, recognize ourselves and allow ourselves to feel and let go. **Having this space**

through CuidarNOS was wonderful with an incredible healing power. (Ramírez et al., Chap. 6, p. 97, emphasis added)

This second example highlights the unique space art activities can create—space to "breathe and unwind"…space to "feel and let go." This space allowed for deeper engagement with the self, described as "recognizing ourselves," which the participant experienced as healing.

21.2.2   Communication: Art and Increased Engagement with Others

As art has the potential to deepen connections to one's experiences and emotions, multiple chapters in this volume demonstrate how arts-based activities can also deepen connections with others by creating a shared experience of new knowledge or by increasing empathy for others' lived experiences. Again we see the language of synergy used to describe these processes.

Marx and Regan (Chap. 8) describe the connections between participants and the resulting communication tool, a documentary produced during a youth participatory action research (YPAR) project with trans/gender non-conforming (TNGC) youth in the U.S., in the following terms:

> In many ways, this project represents a fulfilment of the promise of YPAR and documentary film. **It represents a valuable source of data that would otherwise not be available**—a rich text that captures TGNC youth's experiences unmediated, direct from the source. In many respects, this was possibly only because the project was participatory in nature and organized and completed by the youth themselves; their own connection to the material and to the art form enabled the project's success… The project also **afforded students an opportunity to connect more deeply around a shared purpose**. (Marx and Regan, Chap. 8, p. 132, emphasis added)

Ruge (Chap. 4), reflecting on a project involving schoolchildren, teachers, and staff in a school-based nutrition initiative in Denmark, describes the complex interactions and collaborations the art projects inspired:

> …(T)he combination of teachers' didactic work with professional art and student creativity supported improved relations and the **development of a shared ownership** among students. (Ruge, Chap. 4, p. 54, emphasis added)

Art can also deepen connections by providing spaces for people to have fun and create aesthetically pleasing works of art. A participant engaged in creating ceramic tiles for display at a home care center in Scotland explains:

> It was SO much fun! Chatting with residents and seeing their creativity! Working with the children, at first everyone was unsure what to do but really everyone put so much in. (Barton, Chap. 5, p. 78)

Arts-based health promotion can create bridges of connection not just among participants within projects but also between groups of people who have marked differences in their understanding and experiences, thus enabling them to gain insight from new perspectives. Leitch (Chap. 17) demonstrates the potential for arts-based initiatives to promote connection and empathy and to provide windows to better understand others, specifically regarding the experience of gender-based violence in Trinidad and Tobago and the importance of preventing such violence:

> The task was physically straining. Sawing and lifting heavy pieces of wood, and having my body slowly outlined with chalk, led me to reflect deeply on these Silent Silhouettes. The silence was deafening and emotionally jolting. **Constructing these representations of lost lives transcended the physical experience and created a space to contemplate.** It felt as though **I could feel the pain of my sisters**, young and old. I questioned worth and value and love, and what these women and girls must have gone through. Recreating these stories in this way undoubtedly led to a newer and more gravely empathetic outlook on domestic violence. (Leitch, Chap. 17, p. 288, emphasis added).

Similarly, describing the historical use of community theater in Japan, Sandhu, Jimba, Hirose, and Yui (Chap. 7) describe how theater deepens the experience of empathy among people:

> …(D)rama is an enduring and powerful intervention for changing people's mindsets. In particular, drama has unique characteristics whereby the relationship between the audience and the characters creates empathy. Empathy brings us the emotional experiences of the characters on stage as if the action of the play were happening to us. (Sandhu, Jimba, Hirose, and Yui, Chap. 7, p. 116)

21.2.3 Context: Art for Meaning-Making

The theory of Salutogenesis offers a way of understanding people's resilience in coping with life's stressors. One concept that is central to that theory is Sense of Coherence (SoC). SoC refers to an individual's ability to make sense out of life events and has been associated with increased resilience to stressors (Mittelmark 2017). Art offers a novel medium for contemplating life events, one which leans toward story and sense-making. Some of the initiatives described in this book report on how the process of telling stories through art or using art as a framework for interpreting experiences contributes to participants' ability to make meaning from their experiences in health-promoting ways.

Zarei (Chap. 3) describes the use of the ancient poetry of Rumi to support Iranian women following divorce. One participant reflected how Rumi's poetry enabled her to see that there are lessons to be learned and positive actions to take, even in the face of difficult experiences:

> Honestly, I was never sure I could stand on my feet again after I got divorced. I had a lot of problems (after the divorce). Now I found that divorce has taught me a lesson. So I would rather accept all outcomes from divorce—loneliness, stigma, and even rejection—because in Rumi's poems I realized that even a misery is the basis for self-development and growth. (Zarei, Chap. 3, p. 48)

21.2.4 Antagony: Deep Engagement Can Also Go Awry

Of course, health promotion initiatives that incorporate art do not always have synergistic impacts. Indeed, especially when dealing with sensitive topics and populations, this deeper engagement can trigger negative memories or emotions and might result in antagony. As a result, those using art in this work must attend to preparing for ways to manage these potential negative processes or outcomes. The home care initiative in Scotland discussed how the project resulted in some distressing feelings:

> While there was much joy and laughter throughout the project, one resident found that taking part triggered memories that were upsetting. The female resident initially spent a happy, creative two hours during the first workshop; however, when she returned on the second day, she was despondent, lamenting about her lack of inspiration. (Barton, Chap. 5, p. 78)

However, in this case, as family members joined the process, there was an opportunity to repair the distress and build connections:

> When a family member arrived later, she was able to put this reaction into context as the resident had, in the past, baked beautiful wedding cakes, and this experience brought back memories as she grieved for her younger self. The resident did, however, return to a later workshop to paint her two tiles—a butterfly for the tree and a bird for her bedroom door. (Barton, Chap. 5, p. 78)

In addition, if participants in arts-based initiatives are encouraged to share their personal experiences and have high hopes of improved conditions, but those in leadership are not willing/able to make substantial changes, the project can produce antagony for both groups in conflict. Thus, leaders of these initiatives and their partners must be realistic about what outcomes can be expected from these projects.

Another consideration, as conveyed in the chapter on art-based conference sessions (Ayele et al., Chap. 20), is that planning, organizing, setting up, and taking down art works and supplies may require more time and flexibility than more traditional health promotion approaches.

Figure 21.2 depicts the relationships described above. The "partners"—which may be the participants, researchers, community members, or other stakeholders—engage in art activities (the production tasks of these initiatives) and connect more deeply with themselves and one another, as indicated by the circular arrow from partners to partners and by the arrow to communication. Art also impacts the context in a bi-directional way by helping participants to make sense of their contextualized experiences and by impacting context through sharing, activism, and wider dissemination. The arrow to synergy indicates the potential for arts-based practices, by increasing these interactions, to contribute more than what the initiative could have achieved without their inclusion. Finally, the dotted line to antagony reminds health promoters of the possibility that such deep engagement or time-consuming processes could produce unintended or negative consequences, especially with unrealistic expectations or unwilling partners.

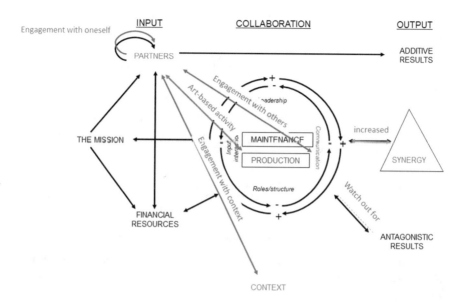

Fig. 21.2 The Bergen Model of Collaborative Functioning (BMCF) depicting dynamic relationships in art initiatives. (Adapted from Corbin et al. (2016). Figure 1. Some modifications were made. https://doi.org/10.1093/heapro/daw061, licensed under the terms of the Creative Commons Attribution Non-Commercial License (http://creativecommons.org/licenses/by-nc/4.0/))

21.3 Art, Health Promotion, and Social Justice

Above, we described how the chapters in this volume led us to understand art as a way of deepening engagement and increasing synergy in health promotion work. Our second conclusion relates to art's ability to work toward the health promotion goal of social justice. As referenced in Chap. 1, Bell and Desai (2011) argue that art has a critical role to play in the move towards achieving social justice. Based on the many contributions in this volume, we also propose that art can work to address social injustices when included in health promotion initiatives. There are at least three ways art promotes justice in health promotion initiatives: by amplifying marginalized or silenced voices, by leveraging power, and by honoring multiple ways of knowing in the knowledge production process.

21.3.1 Art Amplifies Voices for Social Justice

The social processes of oppression work to routinely silence the voices of marginalized people and communities (Spivak 1988) by rendering them nonexistent. Ways of thinking that do not fit into the dominant discourse of Western ways of knowing or colonial narratives are discounted, silenced, and suppressed (Chandanabhumma and Narasimhan 2019; de Sousa Santos 2016; Chilisa 2005). We argue, however, that art has the ability to speak directly to—and can even be used in the fight against—those social processes of oppression.

The Western Australian Indigenous Storybooks project (Stoneham, Davies, and Christopher, Chap. 16) is an art-based activity that provided a medium for Indigenous communities in Western Australia (and elsewhere) to connect, reclaim, and revitalize what had become a negative narrative about Indigenous peoples. The Storybooks project enabled community members themselves to write about positive stories of Aboriginal Australian individual and community life:

> The Storybooks provide a forum and opportunity to share these ideas/projects/events that may otherwise go untold or unrecognized... As suggested via evaluation feedback, the Storybooks not only provide an outlet for people's voices, they also contribute to a sense of pride, ownership, and mental and social well-being. The Storybooks provide authors with the opportunity to tell their stories in their own words and in a manner that is compatible with the traditional yarning process. (Stoneham, Davies, and Christopher, Chap. 16, p. 275)

This project worked to amplify community voice for the greater community. When voices are amplified and directed toward powerful stakeholders, we see it as leveraging.

21.3.2   Art Leverages Power for Social Justice

Arts-based activities can leverage and/or create an exchange of power in both practice and in research. In the LOMA project in Denmark, schoolchildren had the ability to contribute to organizational thinking about nutrition within their school (Ruge, Chap. 4). Likewise, Marx and Regan (Chap. 8) describe how the participatory methods of arts-based research also can transfer power:

> This participatory video may also open space for societal transformation as it offers a way of allowing research subjects to direct the audience's gaze and control the audience's understanding of the subjects' experiences (Kindon 2003). This radical restructuring of the research process not only transfers power to those who may otherwise be powerless within a traditional research paradigm, but it also enables the types of discussions that may give rise to material changes in the lives of TGNC youth. (Marx and Regan, Chap. 8, p. 137)

Photovoice exhibitions can leverage power in a way that language oftentimes cannot. By presenting unflinching visuals, which have been provided by individuals within their own context, photovoice products transcend layers of social stratification. In Chap. 10, Caman describes how photos provided a direct conduit that served to elevate and amplify the stories of displaced Syrian youth in Turkey to policy makers:

> Photovoice was often a language bridge for young people, who experienced forced migration from a neighboring country with a different language and a different alphabet... photovoice might also have helped to create a channel for young people to talk about their migration-related traumas or challenges... Photovoice also acted as a bridge to policy makers and other stakeholders, who had the power to create system-level changes. By seeing the

> photos and reading the quotations, they might have felt something viscerally that moved them, through empathy, to change certain policies and/or practices. (Caman, Chap. 10, p. 175)

While arts-based practice and research methods can amplify and leverage voices, these efforts also provide an important perspective for building our understanding of health promotion when they provide the basis for knowledge production.

21.3.3 Art Honors Multiple Ways of Knowing to Promote Social Justice in Knowledge Production

A key issue in health promotion work is that interventions[1] are often developed outside the communities where they are implemented. This can lead to disconnections between what health promotion professionals think communities need and what they actually need (Chandanabhumma and Narasimhan 2019). Chilisa (2005) argues for the importance of honoring Indigenous worldviews of disease processes as vital to ethical health promotion and painstakingly documents the ways in which HIV-prevention efforts in Botswana failed because of a lack of connection between Northern conceptions of disease and local ways of knowing. An important feature of arts-based interventions is that they often allow for participant expression and multi-way communication of understanding health issues that are usually lacking in "traditional" health education approaches.

Amieva et al. (Chap. 12), reflecting on their work using literary and other arts-based methods, describe how art enables diverse stakeholders to engage in thinking about and contributing to a more robust understanding of Chagas disease:

> We are sure that both arts and education, in a broad and inclusive sense, are key elements to shorten the distance between formal and non-formal knowledge and build alternatives that impact and transform reality. For this reason, we promote joint work among researchers, teachers, students, and the community in general at all educational levels (school as well as technical and professional training levels) and in all possible contexts (rural/urban, formal/informal, where there are/are not vector insects, etc.) with the purpose of engaging a greater number and diversity of voices talking about Chagas (Carrillo et al. 2018). (Amieva et al., Chap. 12, p. 213)

Arts-based research methods provide a clear pathway for translating marginalized and/or Indigenous or local knowledge into published scholarship. In the case presented by Madsen et al. (Chap. 11), poetic analysis was used to highlight the absence of stories of recovery from mental health concerns in the Aboriginal communities. This case is an example of using this form of art to work around "culturally toxic stories":

---

[1] This term is used purposefully here to denote the problematic nature of "intervention" as a health promotion approach as this way of thinking reflects a top-down imposition of "experts' agendas" on communities.

This term describes the way settler or colonizing stories do harm to Indigenous storytelling practices, culture, and community stories in an ongoing way. A key quote from one of the storytellers and co-researchers that shaped the direction for the research project captures it well: "It's about the way they tell their stories about us. It's about the way we then have to tell our stories within their stories. No wonder you go womba (mad/crazy)" (Saunders 2016, p. 16). (Madsen et al., Chap. 11, p. 190)

21.4   Final Reflections

This volume has provided numerous examples of how arts-based activities have been incorporated into a variety of health promotion initiatives. In Chap. 1 these initiatives are presented in the frame of the five action areas outlined in the Ottawa Charter for Health Promotion. Further, the projects, experiences, and reflections have demonstrated how art supports the key values of health promotion: art is inherently interactive and thus encourages deep engagement and participation; art inspires connection, collaboration, and synergy; art empowers by serving as a conduit and lever to power; and art promotes social justice by honoring multiple ways of knowing and amplifying marginalized and historically silenced voices to counteract hegemony.

In this chapter, using the Bergen Model of Collaborative Functioning (Corbin et al. 2016), we put forward a way – among others – of theorizing how arts-based initiatives might contribute added value to health promotion research and practice. We argue that by increasing engagement within and among participants and with context, these initiatives are able to achieve more. We begin to trace these pathways by aligning the experiences described in this book's chapters to an existing health promotion model in the hope that other researchers might pick up this line of thinking and use a process model framework to assess and evaluate arts-based initiatives. Much more research is needed to build our understanding of not just *if* arts-based initiatives produce synergy but *how* and *why*. Ultimately, we hope these efforts will build our understanding and knowledge base in a way that both connects with existing theory and also encourages co-creation of knowledge in partnership with communities and their members.

In addition to thinking of art as a way to increase synergy, we also argue that it can contribute to the promotion of social justice and reduce inequities in health. As described in the introductory chapter of this book (Chap. 1), the field of health promotion is fundamentally concerned with social justice. The Declaration of Alma-Ata for universal primary health care was a response to the recognition that good health is not experienced equitably (Corbin 2005). The prerequisites of health (WHO 1986) and later the social determinants of health (CSDH 2008) support our understanding of health inequities and how health is experienced by different communities across a social gradient. What is less often discussed are the historical processes that have led to the experience of this inequity and how we might, as scholars and practitioners, begin to redress these inequities (Spencer et al. 2019).

By incorporating the arts, we do not limit ideas to Northern/Western and other traditional hierarchies of power. Of course, it is essential to be attentive to the inherent risk of falling into a naive position that assumes that just because an initiative has art, then surely it is "healthy," democratic, and respectful of a diversity of ways of knowing. Indeed, art is difficult to decouple from its colonial significance, which like other knowledge traditions insists on a hegemonic view that the more "Western" an art form, the more legitimate it is— reflexivity, questioning and critical thinking are crucial in any initiative that seeks to incorporate art as a liberatory practice (Chalmers, 2019). In actuality, what imparts these characteristics to an initiative is the theoretical foundation and ideologies upon which it is based, as well as engaged and reflective practitioners/researchers/activists. In other words, the use of art itself does not guarantee social justice; however, if the use of art is taken up with the intention of social justice, a spirit of collaboration, with the leadership of diverse communities and a decolonial perspective (Chandanabhumma and Narasimhan 2019) – much is possible.

Finally, our goal with this book was to produce a collection of arts-based projects that enable other health promoters, artists, researchers, practitioners, and communities around the world to have access to tangible ideas for how to incorporate art into their own work, projects, and everyday life. We hope that you, dear reader, may go forth and put these ideas into action.

References

Bell, L. A., & Desai, D. (2011). Imagining Otherwise: Connecting the Arts and Social Justice to Envision and Act for Change: Special Issue Introduction. *Equity and Excellence in Education, 44*(3), 287–295. https://doi.org/10.1080/10665684.2011.591672.

Carrillo, C., Sanmartino, M., Mordeglia, C. (2018). Education, communication, and lots of creativity: a good combination to face complex problems like Chagas. *Social Innovation Journal, 45.* https://www.socialinnovationsjournal.org/75-disruptive-innovations/2775-education-communication-and-lots-of-creativity-a-goodcombination-to-face-complex-problems-like-chagas. Accessed 4 November 2018.

Chalmers, F. G. (2019). Cultural colonialism and art education: Eurocentric and racist roots of art education. In D. Garnet & A. Sinner (Eds). *Art, culture, and pedagogy: Revisiting the work of F. Graeme Chalmers* (pp. 37–46). https://doi.org/10.1163/9789004390096_005.

Chandanabhumma, P. P., & Narasimhan, S. (2019). Towards health equity and social justice: An applied framework of decolonization in health promotion. *Health Promotion International,* daz053. Advance online publication. https://doi.org/10.1093/heapro/daz053.

Chilisa, B. (2005). Educational research within postcolonial Africa: A critique of HIV/AIDS research in Botswana. *International Journal of Qualitative Studies in Education, 18*(6), 659–684. https://doi.org/10.1080/09518390500298170.

Corbin, J. H. (2005). Health for all by the year 2000: A retrospective look at the ambitious public health initiative. *Promotion & Education, 12*(2), 77–81. https://doi.org/10.1177/175797590501200204.

Corbin, J. H., & Mittelmark, M. B. (2008). Partnership lessons from the global programme for health promotion effectiveness: A case study. *Health Promotion International, 23*(4), 365–371. https://doi.org/10.1093/heapro/dan029.

Corbin, J. H., Jones, J., & Barry, M. M. (2016). What makes intersectoral partnerships for health promotion work? A review of the international literature. *Health Promotion International, 3*(1), 6 daw061. https://doi.org/10.1093/heapro/daw061.

CSDH (Ed.). (2008). *Closing the gap in a generation: Health equity through action on the social determinants of health: Commission on social determinants of health final report.* Geneva: World Health Organization, Commission on Social Determinants of Health.

de Sousa Santos, B. (2016). *Epistemologies of the south: Justice against epistemicide.* New York: Routledge.

Kindon, S. (2003). Participatory video in geographic research: a feminist practice of looking? *Area, 35*(2), 142–153. https://doi.org/10.1111/1475-4762.00236.

Mittelmark, M. B. (2017). Introduction to the handbook of salutogenesis. In *The handbook of salutogenesis* (pp. 3–5). New York: Springer.

Saunders, V.-L. (2016). "...": using a non-bracketed narrative to story recovery in Aboriginal mental health care. PhD thesis: James Cook University.

Spencer, G., Corbin, J. H., & Miedema, E. (2019). Sustainable development goals for health promotion: A critical frame analysis. *Health Promotion International, 34*(4), 847–858. https://doi.org/10.1093/heapro/day036.

Spivak, G. C. (1988). *Can the subaltern speak?* Basingstoke: Macmillan.

World Health Organization. (1986). *The Ottawa charter for health promotion.* https://www.who.int/healthpromotion/conferences/previous/ottawa/en/. Accessed 20 February 2020.

Index

A

Aboriginal
  Australians, 268–270, 274, 275
  health, 269
  mental health care, 190
  Steering Committee, 270, 271
Abuse, 20, 32–34, 36, 280, 283, 285, 295, 333
Academic community, 251, 326
Action areas
  build healthy public policy, 9, 10
  create supportive environments, 8
  develop personal skills, 7, 8
  reorient health services, 9
  strengthen community action, 6, 7
Active characters analysis, 210
Activism, 281, 286, 289, 290
Advocacy, 7, 10, 115, 165–177, 187, 227, 269, 276, 281, 291, 338, 339
Aedes aegypti, 251, 252, 255–257, 259–261
Affective sexual health (ASH)
  artistic expressions, 236
  co-creation processes, 235
  Diverxualitat program (*see* Diverxualitat program)
  health promotion approach, 235
  immigrant populations, 235
Aging, 69, 70
"*Allachburn Art Project*", 72
Alternative therapies, 298, 299, 309
Alzheimer's disease, 70
Alzheimer's Society, 70
American Art Therapy Association, 91
American Psychological Association, 88
Animation videos, 242, 243
Arbovirus, 251, 252, 255, 257
The "Around Me" program, 239

Art-based presentations
  advocating, sessions, 339
  attendance complications, 339
  conventional methods, 331
  ecology of knowledges, 331
  education, 331
  ISECN
    Curitiba, Brazil (2016), 334, 336, 337
    Mexico City, Mexico (2012), 332–335
    Rotorua, New Zealand (2019), 337, 338
    students/early career professionals, 332
    (*see also* Scientific conferences)
  self-awareness, 331
  set-up, 339
  space requirements, 339
Art-based research (ABR)
  ABR projects, 193
  farming and reforming arts, 180, 181
  health promotion, 194
  HIV prevention, PNG, 185–187
  IMPACT Community Choir, 183–185
  IT ALL BEGINS WITH LOVE, 181, 182
  poetic inquiry, 187–192
Art in Healthcare (AiH), 72, 74, 77
Artistic expressions, 236, 245, 249
Artists, 5, 10, 57, 58, 63, 77, 181, 182, 192, 203, 227, 228, 236, 242, 246, 284, 315, 318–320, 324, 325, 332, 355
Artivism, 10
Art-making, 217, 218
Art medium, 103
Arts-based health care providers, 116
Arts-based initiatives
  care home setting, 67
  health promotion, 87

© The Author(s) 2021
J. H. Corbin et al. (eds.), *Arts and Health Promotion*,
https://doi.org/10.1007/978-3-030-56417-9

Arts-based interventions
  community challenges, 104
  fields, 103
  health promotion, 117
  impacts, 104
  practices, 104
  programs, 104
  recreational, 104
Arts-based methods
  communication promotions, 141
  features, 142
  health promotion, 141, 142
  knowledge translation, 142
  participatory, 143
  performing arts, 142
  SHINE (see Project SHINE)
  student participants, 143
  tools, 142
Arts-based research (ABR)
  documentary film, 136
  forms, 180
  health promotion, 179, 180
  impacts, 180
  intricacies and contradictions, 126
  project design, 130
ArtScience
  approach, 253–255
  education strategies, 252
  goals, 252
  health education activities, 262
  health promotion, 252, 262
  interdisciplinary concept, 252
  workshops, 252, 255–257, 259, 261
Arts-focused organizations, 320
Arts-infused practice, 217
Arts-related programs, 104
Arts therapy, 68, 224, 296, 299, 300,
        302–305, 307

B
Balekane EARTH, 35
  in Botswana, 22
  data analysis, 23
  home communities, 22
  individual-focused narrative therapy, 22
  method, 22, 23
  therapy sessions, 22
Bergen Model of Collaborative Functioning
        (BMCF), 127
  arts-based initiatives
    antagony, 350
    communication, 348, 349

    context, 349
    partners, 347
    health promotion programs and
        initiatives, 346
    mission, 346
    synergy, 347
Biodanza, 300, 302–305, 307
Biomedical dimension, 200
Boal, Augusto, 6, 111, 112, 116, 228
Botswana's Ministry of Local Government, 23
Brazilian education system, 251
British Association of Art Therapists
        (BAAT), 68

C
Capitalism, 105
Care Home Family (CHF), 72
Caregiver suicide, 28–32
Caribbean Youth Environment Network
        (CYEN-TT), 288
Cave drawings, 68
Chagas
  artistic languages, 201
  biomedical dimension, 199
  definition, 197
  educational and social contexts, 201
  epidemiological dimension, 200
  kaleidoscopic puzzle, 199, 200
  literary productions, 204
  literary texts, 205
  political dimension, 201
  socio-cultural dimension, 200
  socio-environmental health issue, 198
Child labor, 170
CienciArte, 253, 254
CI-research (Collective Impact research), 228
Clay, 9, 73, 77, 78, 257
Clinical initiatives, 224
Clinician burnout, 322–325
Clinician resilience, 320, 323, 324
Clinician well-being, 320, 322–325
Cognitive injustice, 213
Cognitive Justice, 203
Collaborative documentary filmmaking, 126
Collective Encounters, 70
Collective Impact (CI), 228
Collective kaleidoscope, 213
Colonialism, 4, 105, 202, 203, 351, 355
Communities of practice, 59
Community arts (CA)
  ABR, 218, 219
  CA approaches, 228

CI-oriented research, 228
definition, 217
ecological analysis
    dynamic social context, 219
    macro-level, 223
    meso-level, 223
    micro-level, 223
economic benefits, 227
goals and epistemologies
    articulating/uncovering process, 225
    empirical methods, 224
    mapping mechanism, 226
    scaling up, 224, 225
    theory-based evaluations and
        frameworks, 224
health-promoting impacts, 217, 218
initiatives, 217
investigators and practitioners, 224
limitations, 229
literature review, 218, 219
participatory practice, 218
practices, 219, 228
programs, 223
reductionism, 227
tension, 227
youth, 223
Community-based interventions, 248, 249
Community-Based Participatory Action
        Research (CBPAR)
methodology, 176
participants, 166
photovoice, 166
qualitative study, 174
traditional, 175
vulnerable/disadvantaged groups, 177
Community-based participatory research
        (CBPR), 126, 142, 149, 156, 157,
        159, 160
Community-based practice, 225
Community-driven mitigation strategies, 155
Community empowerment, 248
Community Engaged Research Core,
        128, 133
Community engagement, 314
Community health agents, 246–248
Community Intersectoral Management
        Council, 261
Community involvement, 174
Community leaders, 33
Community members, 34
Community-needs assessments, 87
Community-researcher partnerships, 155
Community's farmers, 106
Community voice, 314

Comprehensibility, 20, 23, 35, 36
Conceptual structure of dimensions, 209
Conceptualization, 212, 223
Coordinadora Paz para la Mujer (CPM),
        87–91, 98
Coping strategies, 43, 48, 49
Cosmovisions, 200
COVID-19, 4
Creative expression, 217, 219, 223
Creative/transformational approach, 227
Crime and Problem Analysis (CAPA), 286
Cross-cultural context, 192
Cross-disciplinary research, 192
Cultural guide/mentor advisor, 193
Culturally toxic stories, 190
Cultural production process, 227

D
Dance, 7, 9, 94, 95, 157–159, 300, 308
Dance movement therapy (DMT), 95
Danish schools, 53
Deep learning, 57, 63, 64
Deficit discourses, 191
Dementia, 70
Democratic rights, 105
Dengue, 251, 252, 255, 257, 259
Developing personal skills, 43
Dialogical education, 57, 59, 64
Dichotomies, 213
Disaster, 86, 99
Disaster behavioral health training, 100
Disaster-related scenarios, 89
Diverxualitat Espictools, 240–244
Diverxualitat program
    ASH, 240
    Catalonia, 240
    co-creation, 236, 240
    Espictools, 240–242, 244
    Espictools-Actua health
        promotion program
    community actions, 240, 246
    train to act, 244–246
    use, expressive arts, 240
Diverxual workshop, 242, 244
Divorce
    definition, 41
    factors, 42
    Iran, 41, 42
    Iranian women post-divorce
        contexts, 42
        developing personal skills, 43
        sexual well-being, 43
        social/cultural context, 41

Documentary film
  aim, 136
  HBO-produced, 126
  limited release, 132
  making aspects, 129
  medium, 137
  moments, 136
  participants, 136
  participatory, 126
  post-production, 137
  research notes, 126
  research team, 128
  social justice and belief, 132
  transformative potential, 137
  YPAR, 127, 130, 132
Domestic and family violence (DFV), 181
Domestic violence, 282, 284, 286
Drama, 8, 34, 68, 104, 105, 107, 110–116,
    142, 349
Drawing
  health and well-being, 19
  sensory motor skills, 19

E
Early marriage and adolescent
    pregnancies, 170
Ecological approach, 88
Ecological concepts, 223
Ecology of Knowledge, 202, 203, 252, 253,
    262, 331
Educational levels, 213
Educational tools
  actions and implementation, 238
  art and culture, 236
  created tools, 237, 238
  Espictools-Actua programs, 238, 239
El baño (the bath), 92
El Yunque, 92
Empathy, 116
Empowerment, 156, 167
Encuentro CuidarNOS
  administrators and supervisors, 98
  art and movement, 98
  CPM, 90, 91
  creative dynamic, 91
  design purpose, 89
  element, 89
  experience opportunity, 98
  integrated intervention, 89
  participants experiences, 97, 98
  participants' profiles, 90
  phases
    emotive memory, 92
    expression, 94

    harmonization, 92
    kinesthetic dynamics, 94, 95
    la brega, 95
    love networks, 95
    sensitization, 92
  Purple Caravan, 90, 91
  purpose, 90, 95
  safe space, 100
  service providers, 100
  state of emergency, 90
Environment-occupant-health framework
    (E-O-H), 68
Epidemiological dimensions, 200
Epistemologies of the South, 202, 213
Espictools-Actua health promotion program
  co-creation, 246
  community actions, 240, 246, 247
  educational tools, 238, 239
  train to act, 244–246
  use, expressive arts, 240
Evidence-based practice, 224
Evidence-informed policy making, 226
Existentialism, 44, 49

F
Farmer's arts, 106, 107, 110
Floating reading, 206
Focus groups, 23, 25, 26, 60, 79, 154, 160,
    169, 183, 184, 186, 187, 225,
    237, 242
Forced migration, 165
Freire, Paulo, 6, 57, 151, 228, 253, 262, 330

G
Galactic guardian (Game), 95
Gallery walk, 333, 335
Gay, lesbian and bisexual (GLB), 125
Gender-Based and Sexual Violence
    (GBSV), 280
Gender-based violence, 87, 88
  art, 281
  GBSV, 280
  health policies, 280
  health promotion, 279
  holistic approaches, 280
  national statistics, 280
  NCDs, 279
  physical and psychological
    implications, 283
  public health, 279
  STIs, 280
  WOMANTRA, 291
  women and girl victims, 291

women's health, 279
  youth learning, 280
Generalized resistance resources (GRR), 21
Gender Policy, 280
Geographical distribution, 209
Ghosts and dead, 27–29
Gold standards, 224

H

Harmonization, 92
Healing, 68, 87, 89, 91, 97–99
Healing Built Environment (HBE), 68
Health
  and arts, 3
  community-based experiences, 4
  concept, 3
  context and social determinants, 4
  individual characteristics, 4
  social dimension, 5
Health and Family Life Education
        (HFLE), 280
Health awareness, 251
Healthcare buildings, 68
Health care communication, 252
Health equity
  call for art, 319
  community voice, 314
  in-person art, 319
  lived experiences, 315, 319, 326
  NAM, 315, 316
  NAM's Culture of Health Program,
        318, 319
  neighborhood community, 317
  picture of health, 316
  SDOH, 314
  viewing the artwork, 319
Health promotion, 71
  action areas, 5–10
  and arts, 3
  community-based experiences, 4
  definition, 87
  discipline, 3
  field of knowledge, 252
  field of practice, 252
  immigrant populations, 235
  international health care, 235
  NCDs, 279
  Ottawa Charter, 5
  physical, mental and social well-being, 3
  role, 87
Health promotion action areas
  build/building healthy public policy,
        9, 10
  create/creating supportive environments, 8

develop/developing personal skills, 7, 8
  reorient/reorienting health services, 9
  strengthen community action, 6, 7
Health-related endeavors, 217
Healthy Maasai community, 147
HEPARJoc, 241–243, 246, 247
HIV/AIDS, 20
HIV prevention, PNG
  big man/big meri, 186
  ever-present risk, 185
  male circumcision, 186
  qualitative research methods, 186
  storyboarding, 186
  transmission, 186
Holistic methodological response, 190
Hurricane María
  CPM, 87–89
  economic crisis, 86, 99
  Encuentro, 91
  Puerto Rico, 86, 92
  Relief Fund, 91
  sense of vulnerability, 100
  traumatic experiences, 88
Hygiene-related illnesses, 154

I

Immigrant populations, 235, 236, 241, 242
IMPACT Community Choir, 183, 192
  cognitive abilities, 183
  community service organization, 183
  participatory manner, 183
  participatory research methods, 184
  performances, 184
  photovoice's gold standard, 184
  self-esteems, 184
  social connectedness, 183
"Index of Wellbeing in Later Life", 69
Indigenous
  listening "Dadirri", 189
  peoples, 187
  poetics, 189
Individual-focused narrative therapy, 22
Inductive mneumonic questioning
        technique, 151
Inquilinx (the tenant), 94
Institute of Health Equity, 67
Institutional Review Board, 133, 135
Intergenerational trauma, 4
International Organization for Migration
        (IOM), 165
International Union for Health Promotion and
        Education's (IUHPE), 332, 335,
        337, 338
Intimate partner violence (IPV), 347

Iranian women post-divorce
  contexts, 42
  developing personal skills, 43
  experiences, 48
  feelings and perceptions, 48
  goal setting, 49
  initiative, 46
  lived experiences, 47, 48
  Logotherapy approach, 48
  sexual well-being, 43
IT ALL BEGINS WITH LOVE, 181, 182,
    192, 193
IUHPE Student and Early Career Network
    (ISECN), 332–338

J
Japanese farming communities, 107, 108
Japanese society/community arts
  community theater stages, 105
  Kenji Miyazawa/farmer's arts, 106, 107
  Taisho democracy, 105, 106

K
Kabuki (traditional Japanese drama), 105
Kaleidoscope view, 212
Kaleidoscopic approach
  biomedical dimension, 208
  Chagas problem, 205
  Ecology of Knowledge, 203
  epidemiological dimension, 208, 209
  kaleidoscopic puzzle, 198, 200
  political dimension, 209
  socio-cultural dimension, 209
kalimba instrument (*mbira*), 93
Kenji Miyazawa/farmer's arts, 106, 107
Knowledge translation
  academic tradition, 159
  arts-based methods, 160
  component, 144
  definition, 142
  intervention phase, 142
  post-intervention, 145
  traditional research, 153

L
la brega (the daily struggle), 95
"Language & Media" workshop, 59, 60
LBGTQ+ community, 131
Lesbian, gay, bisexual, trans, and queer
    (LGBTQ), 123

Lesbian, gay, bisexual, transgender, queer, or
    gender non-conforming (LGBTQ+),
    124, 128
Live drama performances, 104
Local and bilingual facilitators, 169
Logotherapy approach, 44
LOMA-local food
  art-based approach, 54
  art teacher, 55
  creative collaboration, 57
  creative imaginations, 55, 57, 64
  deep learning, 57, 63, 64
  Denmark, 54
  digital creative learning activities,
      iPads, 60, 61
  dimensions
    didactic and socio-cultural, 59
    organizational, 59
    physical, 59
  evaluation, 63
  implications, 63
  integrated approach, 54, 64
  limitations, 63
  logo, 55
  Nottingham Apprenticeship Model, 57
  nurturing creativity, children, 57
  Ottawa Charter, 56
  primary level, 62
  professional learning systems, 63
  social constructivist theory, 56
  teachers, 63
  teacher-training courses, 56, 58
  universe, 55, 56, 63
  vegetable-art, 60
  whole school approach, 58, 60, 64

M
Maasai pastoralists, 157
Manageability, 20, 23, 36, 37
Mapping mechanism, 226
Meaningfulness, 20, 23, 37
Meaning-making, 44–46, 48
Mental disorders, 295–299, 304–306, 308, 309
Mental health, 20
  challenges, 307, 308
  democracy, 296
  human rights violations, 296
  Movimiento Ventana (*see* Movimiento
      Ventana)
  Nicaragua, 295
  successes, 306
  volunteers experience, 305, 306

Migration-related traumas, 176
Monochromatic kaleidoscope, 198
Month of Chagas, 203
Movimiento Ventana
  activities
    art therapy, 303–305
    Biodanza, 303–305
    coordination, 301
    execution, 301, 302
    social volunteer, 300
  art therapy, 296, 299, 300
  Biodanza, 300
  gender, 298
  human rights, 298
  logo, 297
  mental health, 298, 299
  personal recovery model, 299
  public health services user, 299
  social movement, 298
Multidimensional matrix, 212
Mural, 142, 143, 145–147, 154, 156, 318, 332,
    333, 335, 337, 338
Music, 7, 9, 68, 93, 142, 147, 183, 201, 218,
    220, 239, 252, 259, 281, 300, 303,
    308, 318, 320, 335, 336

N
Nagano prefecture, 105, 108
NAM's Culture of Health Program,
    318, 319
The National Aboriginal Health Strategy,
    269
National Academy of Medicine (NAM)
  arts, 314
  clinician resilience, 320
  clinician well-being, 320, 322–325
  community engagement, 314
  health, 313
  health equity (*see* Health equity)
  private, non-profit institutions, 313
  stakeholders, 313, 314
  vision, 313
National Organization of Arts in Health
    (NOAH), 103
Natural disasters, 85
  Hurricane Maria, 7, 85–100, 347
  tsunami-related disaster, 89
Ngorongoro Conservation Area (NCA), 143
Ningyou-jyoruri (puppet plays), 105
Non-communicable diseases (NCDs),
    279
Nottingham Apprenticeship Model, 57
Nutrition and hygiene problems, 170

O
Online-based educational opportunities, 116
Open defecation mapping, 144
Ottawa Charter, 87, 88, 181, 194

P
Painting, 10, 68, 89, 142, 145, 287, 288, 316,
    318, 320, 333
Participatory action research, 166, 175
Participatory video, 137
Passive characters analysis, 211
Peer educators, 246
Peer-reviewed qualitative research, 225
Peers, 31
Personal recovery model, 299
Photo discussion sessions (PDS), 149,
    151–153, 157, 159
Photo exhibition, 173
Photovoice exhibitions, 352
Photovoice facilitator (PI), 150
Photovoice photograph exhibition, 153
Photovoice process
  advocacy through dissemination, 173
  CBPAR approach, 174
  community involvement, 174
  data analysis, 170, 172, 173
  exhibition, 153
  experiences, 174
  formative research and adaptation, 149
  goals, 166, 169
  gold standard approach, 184
  group discussions, 176
  health promotion, 167, 176
  inductive mneumonic questioning
      technique, 151
  information meeting, 150, 151
  methodology, 193
  mixed-methods, 167
  participants, 166, 167
  participatory research, 175, 184
  partnerships, 174
  PDS, 149, 151, 152
  photographs, 151
  purposive sampling strategy, 149
  qualitative interviews, 175
  qualitative study, 176
  setting, 167
  SHINE India adaptation, 153
  SHINE school curriculum, 152
  SHOWeD guide, 169
  social cohesion/ties improvement, 175
  students training, 151
  timeline and steps, 168–170

Place-based narrative, 181
Poetic inquiry
    aboriginal recovery, 190
    colonization, 193
    demonstration, 192
    idea transformation, 188
    research methodology, 188
    types, 188
Poetry, 44–46
Policy makers, 173
Political dimension, 201, 209
Popular agents, 261
"Popular Agents of Health Promotion and
        Vigilance", 261, 262
Post-disaster trauma, 89
Poverty, 20, 30, 33
Practice
    art, 5
    commentaries, 219
    health promotion, 5, 10
    and research, 5
    social justice, 4
    transformative, 11
Primary/secondary traumatic experiences, 95
Primary/secondary traumatic stress, 100
Professional learning systems, 63
Project SHINE
    arts-based methods, 160
    assets-based approach, 142
    empowerment, 157
    goals, 156
    India (see SHINE India)
    interventions, 153
    school-based intervention, 142
    Tanzania (see SHINE Tanzania)
Proletarianism, 106
Proliferation, 225
Pseudonyms, 23
Public and fiscal policies, 100
Public health, 279
Public Health Advocacy Institute of Western
        Australia (PHAIWA), 269–271
Public health services user, 299
Purple Caravan, 90, 91

Q
Qualitative construction, 212
Qualitative-critical investigation, 202
Qualitative research methods, 166, 180
Quality of care, 320
Quantitative needs assessment study, 167
Quantitative review, 212
Queer-centered programming, 132

R
Recovery model, 299
Reductionism, 227
Refugees
    barriers, 170
    data analysis, 170
    data collection, 169
    definition, 165
    and local youth, 168, 175
    origins, 168
    participation. refugee-related research, 177
    registered, 166, 170
    social cohesion, 176
    UNHCR, 165
    vulnerable/disadvantaged groups, 167
    young, 174
Registered refugees, 170
Relatives, 32
Research
    arts-based, 8
    community arts, 6
    health promotion, 11
    interdisciplinary team, 10
    and practice, 5
Residential care
    local-authority-funded, 69
Resources and strategies
    community leaders, 33
    community members, 34
    peers, 31
    relatives, 32
    social workers, 32
    spirituality, 34
Roebourne Art Group, 272

S
Salutogenic therapy of drawing
    Balekane EARTH, 22–23
    comprehensibility, 35, 36
    framework, 35
    HIV/AIDS, 20
    manageability, 36, 37
    meaningfulness, 37
    narrative sessions, 35
    resources and strategies (see Resources and
        strategies)
    SOC, 20, 21, 23, 36
    stressors, 24–30
    verbal narrations, 34
    written and verbal narratives, 34
Sanitation and Hygiene INnovation in
        Education (SHINE), 142
Sanitation mural, 145

Sanitation science fair, 144
Scaling up, 224, 225
Schools, 53, 54, 64
Science, technology, engineering, and
        mathematics (STEM), 254
Science, technology, engineering, arts and
        mathematics (STEAM), 254
Scientific conferences
    art-based presentations, 331
    forum, 330
    group poses questions, 329
    health promotion field, 330
    parallel panel sessions, 330
    poster presentations, 330
    scientific events, 331
    scientific fields, 329
    structure, 330
    ways of knowing, 330, 331
Scientific grounds, 227
Scottish Sculpture Workshop (SSW), 72
Secondary traumatic stress, 88
Self-care, 98
Sense of Coherence (SOC), 20, 21, 23, 36, 349
Sensitization, 92
Sensory motor skills, 19
Setotwane, 28
Seva activities, 155
Sexual and gender minority (SGM), 124
Sexual and Reproductive Health Policy, 280
Sexually transmitted infections (STIs), 280
Shared meaning making, 229
SHINE arts-based school/community event
    digital stories, 147
    knowledge translation, 145
    sanitation mural, 145
    stations, 145
    time capsule, 147
SHINE India
    adaptation, 149
    arts-based research methods, 148
    community members, 155
    curriculum, 153, 159
    knowledge translation, 157
    mutual interests, 148
    participants, 150
    photovoice (see Photovoice sub-study)
    sanitation-related challenges, 148
SHINE interventions
    arts-based methods, 158–160
    health promotions, 157, 158
    meaningful participant
            engagement, 154–155
    research and implementation phases, 154
    youth encouragement, 156, 157

SHINE PDS, 157
SHINE Tanzania
    arts-based school/community event, 145
    curriculum, 152
    implementation, 159
    intervention, 143, 158
    NCA, 143
    open defecation mapping, 144
    purpose, 143
    sanitation science fair, 144
SHOWeD guide, 169
SIDAJoc, 240, 241, 248
Silent silhouettes
    approach, 286, 287
    challenges, 290, 291
    civil society actors, 283
    domestic violence, 282, 284
    gender-based violence, 282, 283
    impact, 288, 290
    interpersonal violence, 282
    preparation, 285
    process, 287, 288
    psycho-social support, 283
    SIDs, 283
    Silent Witness, 285
    Trinbagonian, 282
    victims' ages, 285
    WOMANTRA, 284
Singing, 183, 184, 221, 300, 303, 333
Small Island Developing States (SIDS),
        283
Social constructivist theory, 56
Social determinants, 67, 218
Social determinants of health (SDOH),
        314, 319
Social impact, 218, 228
Social interaction, 300
Social isolation and loneliness, 69
Social justice, 4–6, 11
    art amplifies voices, 351, 352
    health promotion, 351
    power, 352, 353
    ways of knowing, 353
Social media, 255
Social movement, 298
Social networks, 246
Social policy, 227
Social representations, 209
Social stigma, 297, 305
Social subjectivities and collectivities, 226
Social workers, 32
Societal changes, 69
Socio-cultural dimension, 209
Socio-natural disaster, 86, 88

Spiritual health
    art, 44
    existentialism, 44
    human health, 44
    initiative, 46
    life satisfaction, 44
    Logotherapy approach, 44
    poetry, 44, 45
    Rumi, 45
Spirituality, 34
Stakeholders, 155, 173
Stigma, 20
Storyboarding
    definition, 186
    highlights, 192
    implications, 187
    inclusion, 193
    visual method, 186
Storybooks
    Aboriginal Australians, 268, 269, 275
    Aboriginal Steering Committee, 268
    advocacy tool, 276
    creative tool, 275
    evaluation, 273, 274
    forum and opportunity, 275
    literature, 267
    patience, 276
    PHAIWA, 275
    storytellers, 276
    traditional storytelling, 268
    West Australian Indigenous Storybook
        project, 267, 269, 271, 276
    yarning/storytelling, 268
Storytellers, 271, 273, 274, 276
Stressors
    caregiver suicide, 28–32
    ghosts and dead, 27–29
    poverty, 30, 33
    sudden death, 25–28
    witchcraft, 24, 25
Sudden death, 25–28
"Supermarketization", 53
Sustainable Development Goals (SDGs), 295
Synergy, 346–348, 350, 351, 354
Systematization of experiences, 202
Systematization process, 202
Systemic networks, 206, 208
Systemization of experiences, 202

T
Taisho democracy, 105, 106
Taxonomy, 254
The "Tbactiva't" (TB activation) program, 239
TGNC resilience, 133
TGNC youth of color

discourse, 124, 132
experiences, 125, 131
knowledges, 136
network, 130
research team, 128
stories, 129
Theater-based health promotion
    audience-centered, 104
    drama script, 111
    health promoters, 117
    impacts, 111, 112, 116
    intervention, 116, 117
    medical professionals involvement, 113
    planning medical drama, 110, 111
    Saku Hospital, 113
Theater production, 181, 182
Theater techniques, 182
Thematic content analysis, 23
Theory-based evaluation, 226, 228
Theory of Change approaches, 226, 228
Therapeutic approaches, 34
Therapy, Salutogenic, *see* Salutogenic therapy
        of drawing
Thinking tools, 256, 259
Time capsule, 147
Traditional storytelling, 268
Training health professionals, 245
Trans and gender non-conforming (TGNC) youth
    complexity, 126
    health promotion, 126
    LGBTQ, 123
    LGBTQ+ youth, 124
    mainstream media coverage, 124
    mental health outcomes, 125
    participatory video, 137
    research, 124, 125
    research team, 137
    resilience and health disparities, 125
    students, 125
    traditional research methods, 136
    youth report, 125
    YPAR (*see* Youth participatory action
        research (YPAR))
The Trans List (Film), 126
Trauma
    collective, 91
    disaster-related, 90
    effects, 91
    healing, 99
    hurricanes, 86, 98
    neurobiology, 89
    personal, 100
    primary, 88
    recovery, 99
    symptoms, 98
    vicarious, 88

Trauma-related symptoms, 95
Traumatic impact, 86
Traumatic responses, 87
"Tree of Many Colours" project
    activities, 79
    aim and objectives, 71
    captured qualitative data, 77
    care home setting, 71
    challenges and considerations, 79
    evaluation, 73, 74
    filming, 79
    funding, 72
    information sign, 80
    intergenerational aspect, 78
    observations and reflections, 77, 78
    planning, 72, 73
    practical and creative considerations, 73
    questionnaires themes
        being creative and artistic, 76
        excitement, 76
        having fun doing something new, 76
        health and well-being impacts, 77
        memory, 77
    team, 72
Tsunami-related disaster, 89

U
UK All-Party Parliamentary Group (APPG), 67
UK Office of National Statistics (ONS), 69
Unhealthy living conditions, 170
United Nations High Commission for
            Refugees (UNHCR), 165
Universal health coverage, 108
Upstream health determinants, 223
U.S. Federal Government and support groups, 90
Usuda village, 108

V
Vector (vinchuca), 208
Verbal narrations, 34
Vertical models of communication, 251
Vicarious trauma, 88–90, 100
Victimization, 124
Video-based observational research (VOR), 73
Visual and symbolic expression, 91
Visual art pieces, 335
Volunteering, 298

W
Wakatsuki's strategy, see Theater-based health
            promotion
WASH interventions, 142

Water, sanitation, and hygiene (WASH),
            142–144, 148, 153, 160
Ways of knowing, 5, 11, 180, 203, 228, 330,
            331, 346, 351, 353–355
Welfare-like approach, 228
Well-being, 68, 70, 103
West Australian Indigenous Storybook project
    Aboriginal Australians, 270
    Aboriginal Steering Committee, 270
    art-based activity, 352
    artwork, 267
    autobiographical stories, 267
    negative media, Aboriginal
            Australians, 269
    PHAIWA, 269, 271
    public health practice gaps, 276
    regional launch, 271
    Roebourne Art Group, 272
    stories, 270 (see also Storybooks)
    storytellers, 271
    yarning/storytelling, 270, 271
Whole school approach, 58, 60, 64
Witchcraft, 24, 25
WOMANTRA, 281, 282, 284, 286–288,
            290, 291
Word cloud, 206
World Health Organization (WHO), 89, 251

X
The XarChagas (ChagasNet) program, 239

Y
Yarning/storytelling, 268, 270, 271, 275, 276
Young refugees, 166, 167, 169
Youth participatory action research (YPAR)
    adult advisors, 127
    challenges, 134, 135
    drawings, 135, 136
    formal procedures, 127
    funding, 128
    in-progress film, 131–132
    marginalized youth's experiences, 127
    mission, 127
    participants, 128
    partnerships, 128
    possibilities, 132, 133
    TGNC youth of color, 132
    throughputs, 129–131
Youth Trans List (Film), 127

Z
Zika virus, 251, 252, 257

Printed in the United States
by Baker & Taylor Publisher Services